# New Procedures in Spinal Interventional Neuroradiology

**Series Editor**
Luigi Manfrè
Catania, Italy

In recent years, the dramatically increasing demand for new minimally invasive procedures for the treatment of spinal diseases has led to the development of a wide variety of new devices designed to foster a new "covert" surgical approach that is based on only a small incision, without major muscle involvement and with excellent maintenance of normal anatomy. The use of a CT guided technique (with performance of surgery in a CT unit rather than in a conventional operating room) offers a wide range of new possibilities and many advantages in comparison to conventional open surgical procedures. These include in particular the reduction of side effects and complications, shortening of the operative time, lowering of the risks of anesthesia (especially in severely ill or elderly patients), and decreased total cost. This series provides up-to-date information on these important advances and their application in different scenarios. It will consist of 5 handy volumes designed for ease of consultation. Each volume will include a concise but comprehensive introduction on biomechanics, relevant clinical syndromes, and diagnostic imaging. The principal emphasis of the series, however, will be description of the various procedures using either an X-ray or a CT guided approach. Owing to its practical orientation, the series will fill a gap in the literature and meet the need, identified by numerous specialists (including interventional neuroradiologists and radiologists, neurosurgeons, and orthopedists), for topical and handy guides that specifically illustrate the materials and methods presently available within spinal interventional neuroradiology.

More information about this series at http://www.springer.com/series/13394

Luigi Manfrè • Johan Van Goethem
Editors

# The Disc and Degenerative Disc Disease

## Remove or Regenerate?

Springer

*Editors*
Luigi Manfrè
Minimal Invasive Spine Therapy Department
Mediterranean Institute of Oncology
Catania
Italy

Johan Van Goethem
Department of Medical of
Molecular Imaging
AZ Nikolaas
Sint-Niklaas
Belgium

Department of Neuroradiology
University of Antwerp
Antwerpen
Belgium

ISSN 2570-2203 ISSN 2570-2211 (electronic)
New Procedures in Spinal Interventional Neuroradiology
ISBN 978-3-030-03714-7 ISBN 978-3-030-03715-4 (eBook)
https://doi.org/10.1007/978-3-030-03715-4



This Springer imprint is published by the registered company Springer Nature Switzerland AG
The registered company address is: Gewerbestrasse 11, 6330 Cham, Switzerland

# Foreword

It was with singular delight that I accepted the honor of preparing this foreword for *The Disc and Degenerative Disc Disease. Remove or Regenerate?* knowing that Drs. Luigi Manfrè and Johan Van Goethem are the editors.

As if it were a scientific novel, chapters build on each other to tell a complete story. The foundation of disc treatments necessarily starts with anatomy and biomechanics (Chap. 1). Our understanding of discal pathology emanates from the imaging findings of disc disease and physical examination (Chaps. 2 and 3). As neuroradiologists, we are simultaneously focused on conventional as well as latest and greatest in advanced imaging (Chaps. 4–6). As treating physicians, we must be familiar with the role and evidentiary basis of current interventions (Chaps. 7–10). The percutaneous approach is becoming ever more powerful in terms of both devices to navigate and treatments employed as do traditional surgical approaches which continue to evolve (Chaps. 11–14).

In preparation for writing this foreword, I had the unique opportunity to read all 14 chapters. These pages contain numerous clinical pearls ranging from spectroscopic findings to the futuristic materials that may be widely utilized to treat abnormal discs. In this context, the future is bright for patients suffering from disc disease.

The reader is thus treated to fourteen outstanding chapters conceived from the outset to exist in harmony with each other. The editors did not limit themselves to just thinking through a broad array of topics, but they complemented the topical diversity with a tapestry of subject matter experts drawn from no fewer than three continents.

While the chapter authors hail from many points in distant lands, I am writing this foreword in Boston, Massachusetts, USA. In my hometown, it would be fair to say that Drs. Manfrè and Van Goethem have "hit a home run" with this book. The honor of writing this foreword will only be exceeded by the enjoyment of those reading the material contained herein.

Joshua A. Hirsch
Massachusetts General Hospital
Boston, MA, USA

# Foreword 2

The human spine is an unmatched masterpiece of biomechanical engineering. In vertebrates, the spinal column has evolved as a protective conduit for the spinal cord and nerve roots, which are contained within the spinal canal and intervertebral foramina. The complex anatomy of the human spinal column provides the upright individual with strength and structural balance to support the weight of the body, while at the same time allowing great flexibility and freedom of movement. The human spine can accommodate an astounding range of motions: standing upright, sitting, lying down, bending, twisting, rotating, and all possible combinations and permutations thereof. These functions are made possible by a combination of osteo-articular components (bones and joints) and soft tissue elements (spinal cord and nerve roots, cerebrospinal fluid, blood vessels, ligaments, tendons, muscles, etc.). And in the centre of it all, there is the mysterious intervertebral disc, a gelatinous nucleus enclosed by a fibrous capsule, held in place by ligaments and vertebral body endplates. The intervertebral disc is the linchpin, the keystone of the spine, hidden in the deep inner recesses of the vertebral column, and it constitutes the topic of this book.

While the 3-dimensional spinal complexity provides strength and flexibility, it also means that the vertebral column, and especially the intervertebral disc, represents a formidable diagnostic and therapeutic challenge. For most medical professionals, patients with spine-related problems constitute *a riddle wrapped in a mystery inside an enigma*, to paraphrase a statement by Winston Churchill. With the discovery of X-ray imaging, 125 years ago, there was great hope that standard radiographs of the spine would deliver a key to unravel the secrets of back pain and neck pain. Throughout the greater part of the twentieth century, diagnostic evaluation of the spine was predominantly based on radiographs in different patient positions and projections. However, the intervertebral disc could not be directly visualised on plain radiographs. Invasive X-ray-based techniques evolved which required the injection of iodine-based contrast agents into the thecal sac (myelography), the facet joints (arthrography), the epidural veins (spinal phlebography), and directly into the intervertebral disc (discography) to detect abnormalities. The arrival of computed tomography (CT), in the 1970s, and magnetic resonance imaging (MRI), in the 1980s, heralded a new era in spinal imaging, because these techniques allowed direct visualisation of the intervertebral disc. These cross-sectional imaging modalities brought spectacular diagnostic improvements and, so it was thought, largely obviated the need for invasive spinal imaging. In recent decades, multi-detector CT (MDCT) and MRI have become the standard of practice for patients with spine-related problems and provide exquisite anatomical detail in axial, coronal, and sagittal imaging planes.

Yet, despite all these wonderful medical innovations, the spine, and especially the intervertebral disc, continues to challenge our diagnostic and therapeutic abilities. In any human being, the spine bears the marks of age-related wear and tear, acquired during a lifetime of active living, walking, running, sitting, dancing, playing sports, getting injured, or, simply, becoming older and frailer. Cross-sectional imaging techniques are prone to detect a panoply of incidental findings that are commonly found in asymptomatic individuals (such as intervertebral disc degeneration). Overuse of diagnostic imaging modalities, and overinterpretation of imaging findings, has led to a significant amount of overdiagnosis, which can interfere with adequate provision of care. Stigma associated with diagnostic labels, based on erroneous interpretation of imaging findings, has led many patients to undergo invasive, potentially harmful, and unnecessary surgical procedures. Imaging of the spine, and especially the intervertebral disc, should focus on finding the particular abnormality that is causing pain or loss of function, or any combination thereof. Unfortunately, the complex spinal anatomy constitutes a challenge for our imaging techniques; it remains exceptionally difficult to precisely identify the anatomical substrate that is the root cause of the patient's symptoms.

Many excellent books have been written about the spine, so is there really a need for another book about the "The disc and degenerative disc disease"? The answer to that question is a resounding YES. There are two very good reasons why this book fills a need.

- **The first reason** is that ongoing advances in medical imaging technology are rapidly changing the way we think about disc-related problems. In the past, imaging methods have mainly focused on providing comprehensive morphological information about the spinal anatomy. Today, advanced imaging techniques provide a better insight into the functional aspects of the spine. Diffusion-weighted imaging (DWI), diffusion tensor imaging (DTI), perfusion-weighted imaging (PWI), and MR-spectroscopy (MRS) are unravelling the secrets of the normal and degenerative intervertebral disc. Imaging helps to understand the post-operative spine. Recent research has focused on merging CT with SPECT (CT-SPECT) scans, thus enabling accurate identification of areas with increased osteoblastic activity, which may reflect pain generators. Imaging should not only provide an accurate interpretation of morphology, but should lead to a better understanding of the cause of a patient's complaints, against a backdrop of degenerative changes due to wear and tear of the spine.
- **The second reason** is that recent years have seen nothing short of spectacular advancements in percutaneous and minimally invasive ways to treat spinal disorders related to the intervertebral disc. The chapters in the second part of this book offer a comprehensive overview of how to treat painful discs with epidural injections, percutaneous discectomy, how to remove herniated disc material with physical and chemical tools, and how to support and potentially replace the degenerated intervertebral disc with biomaterials.

The editors of this book have brought together an outstanding team of experienced and internationally renowned experts, to cover both advanced diagnostic methods and state-of-the-art treatment options. This book really helps medical practitioners understand the diagnostic issues and guide clinical management of degenerative intervertebral discs. Readers will become familiar with the advantages and disadvantages of the various diagnostic and therapeutic methods. The chapters in the first part of the book give the reader a deeper understanding of anatomy, physiology, and diagnostic imaging procedures, whereas the chapters in the second part of the book provide advice and guidance pertaining to a broad range of minimally invasive treatment options, which, today, constitute a very valuable alternative to open surgery. The editors, Luigi Manfrè and Johan Van Goethem, have done an excellent job to integrate the various contributions and to provide a comprehensive update of current knowledge and future developments. This book will inspire readers to update their knowledge about advanced imaging diagnosis and state-of-the-art minimally invasive treatment options for patients with degenerative disc disease. Let us hope that this will lead to the delivery of better health care to our patients.

Paul M. Parizel
Royal Perth Hospital (RPH)
and University of Western Australia (UWA)
Perth, WA, Australia

National Imaging Facility (NIF)
St Lucia, QLD, Australia

Royal Australian and New Zealand
College of Radiology (RANZCR)
Sydney, NSW, Australia

# Preface

The intervertebral disc is considered as a simple anatomic structure by many doctors, which holds no secrets, but probably one of the least well-understood components of the spine and of the human body in general. It is a deceivingly simple structure, yet intrinsically much more complex than what meets the eye. Central to the core of the body, the human spine is a mechanically and physiologically complex, fine-tuned, and ingenious piece of equipment. It is central to what we are and how we are as a living creature. Our spine gave us the ability to walk upright about 6 million years ago, which in turn was crucial for our species to survive in diverse habitats all over the world. But some argue that bipedalism is also one of the reasons our species more easily develops intervertebral disc herniations.

In the first six chapters, world-renowned specialists will give you an in-depth look into the anatomy, function, imaging, and pathology of the disc.

Dr. Sumeet Kumar presents a unique look into the anatomy and biomechanics of the intervertebral disc. You will learn about hydrostatic and osmotic pressure, permeability, viscoelasticity, and much more. How does a disc respond to loading, bending, and torsion, and what is mechanotransduction? A complex structure is clearly explained in Chap. 1.

Disc degeneration is a complex process and is explained by Dr. Bosmans and Prof. Vanhoenacker in Chap. 2. Spondylosis deformans and intervertebral osteochondrosis together with inflammatory and infectious disease are well illustrated, as are secondary changes including calcification and ossification.

What should you know about clinical examination and history taking in patients with suspected disc disease? Drs. Gorrepati, Boylan, and Johnson describe this in Chap. 3. They also address appropriate imaging for further management and treatment decisions.

In Chap. 4, Prof. Thurnher and Prof. Van Goethem dive deeper in imaging the degenerative intervertebral disc. Conventional radiography, computed tomography (CT), and magnetic resonance imaging (MRI) form the cornerstones of neuroradiology of the disc. How should you grade disc degeneration on imaging, what is the appropriate nomenclature to use, and what can you expect to find in the vertebra aligning a degenerative disc?

In Chap. 5, the reader will learn about advanced imaging of the intervertebral disc. Prof. Van Goethem, researcher Caro De Weerdt, Dr. Becker, and Prof. Lotz explore diffusion-weighted imaging (DWI), diffusion tensor imaging (DTI), diffusion kurtosis imaging (DKI), perfusion-weighted imaging (PWI), and MR spectroscopy (MRS) of the disc. Although sometimes technically challenging, these advanced imaging procedures are very promising and are able to probe deeper into the ultrastructure and metabolism of the intervertebral disc.

The final chapter on diagnostic imaging is on the postoperative spine. Chapter 6 by Dr. and Prof. Georgy tackles the challenging task to image the postoperative and/or postprocedural spine. Normal or expected postoperative findings should be well known to everyone that reads spines. Also recurrent disc herniation versus epidural fibrosis or fusion versus pseudarthrosis should be the basic knowledge. Read this chapter if you need to refresh.

And after the diagnosis, the treatment comes!

> *Ecco qual debba essere il vostro studio, la vostra applicazione, la vostra industria; non istancarvi mai di vederla, di conoscerla, d'ascoltarla. Le sue voci son mute, ma efficaci. Chi si familiarizza seco lei, diviene sacerdote suo vero. Domenico Cotugno (1736–1822)*
> This is what your studio, your application, your industry should be; never get tired of seeing it, of knowing it, of listening to it. His voices are silent but effective. Whoever becomes familiar with her becomes her true priest. Domenico Cotugno (1736–1822)

The idea of treating the intervertebral disc herniation comes from the mists of time. Despite the sciatica being considered the results of evil goddess punishing poor people in ancient time, Egyptians and Greeks postulated a connection between discal hernia and leg pain [1]. Then, nothing happened from Greek time up to the eighteen century when, in 1764, the Italian researcher in Naples [2] Dr. Cotugno (Fig. 1) in his

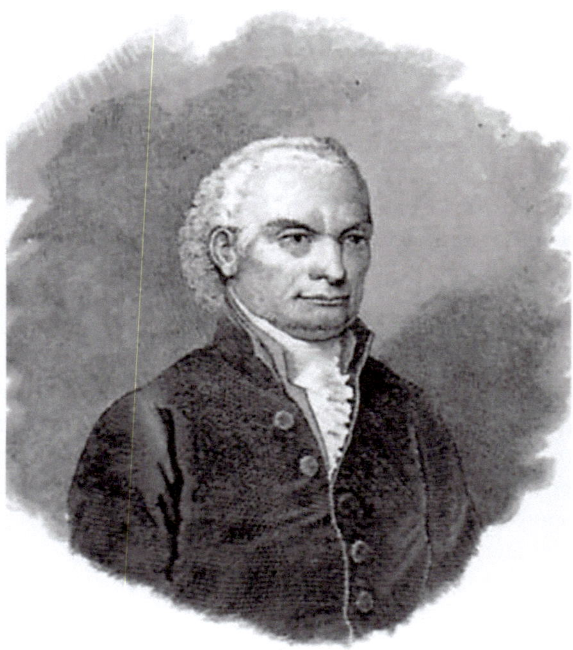

**Fig. 1** Paint of Dr. Domenico Cotugno, physician, anatomist, and surgeon, 1736–1822. (Source: public domain image)

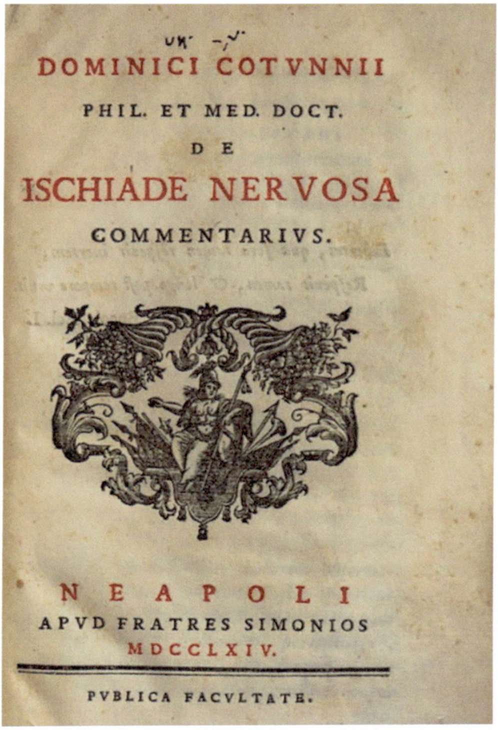


**Fig. 2** Book cover of the *De ischiade nervosa commentarius*, the first book describing sciatica scientifically. (Source: public domain image)

book *De ischiade nervosa commentarius* (Fig. 2) wrote about the "nervous" origin of sciatic pain (the term "Sciatica" or "Ischiatica" comes from Ischia, the famous isle in the gulf of Naples). The first surgical discectomy was performed by Mixter and Barr in 1932 [3]: we need almost 5000 years, from Egyptian empire to Cotugno's study, to correlate the disc to the sciatic pain, and only 80 years, from Mixter and Barr's first surgical approach, to discover an incredible variety of treatments for discal hernia.

As for the other volumes published in the Springer series on spine interventional treatments *New Procedures in Spinal Interventional Neuroradiology*, all the treatments, percutaneous, or "open surgery" have been illustrated by the Top Gun of this field.

In Chap. 7, Dr. Brook and coworkers evaluate the effects of non-surgical treatments of sciatica, talking about epidural injection, analyzing the efficacy of several anesthetics and glucocorticoids, and comparing different percutaneous approaches to the nerve (interlaminar or transforaminal) and different guidance to get the nerve, from US to fluoroscopy and CT.

It is difficult to find a disease with more controversies about the treatments to perform as for the disc herniation. In Chap. 8, Dr. Hirsch handles the extreme with skill, talking about the evidentiary basis of percutaneous discectomy, comparing most up-to-date percutaneous techniques with the "gold-standard" surgical discectomy, and looking through a tremendous amount of published papers on the topic. All the pros and cons are severely evaluated, as well as the incidence of complications and side effects, the effect of sedation, and risks of all the procedures. Talking about percutaneous treatment, we have nowadays two different approaches to get the result: we can destroy the disc using chemistry, injecting something into the disc, or we can adopt mechanics. Dr. Muto and Dr. Bonetti, two worldwide well-known pioneers in the use of intradiscal ozone, show you the effect of ozone therapy, alcohol gel, and other treatments in Chap. 9. On the other side of the moon, mechanical decompression of the disc has become more and more popular, offering an incredible variety of devices. In Chap. 10, Dr. Bonaldi and Dr. Cianfoni illustrate all the up-to-date modalities we can use, from automated lumbar discectomy to disc aspiration probes, radiofrequency ablation of the disc, coblation, PLDD, laser, and more. Nevertheless, percutaneous treatments are not the only alternative to "open surgery": during the last 3 years, endoscopic treatment of the disc has become a revolutionary method to avoid conventional surgery, demonstrating an incredible efficacy even in removing extruded disc herniation, considered the "bête noire" for all the percutaneous treatment, something that could only be removed by conventional surgery in the past. Dr. Yorukoglu and Dr. Sencer, two of the most experienced surgeons in the field of endoscopic treatments, show the powerful of endoscopic discectomy in Chap. 11. Whenever we use chemical or physical treatments, we are able to destroy the disc only. The contemporary philosopher Yuval Noah Harari stated that the cultural revolution of medicine consists of a 360° change of perspective: while the twentieth-century medicine aimed to cure sick people, the goal of the twenty-first-century medicine is to ameliorate healthy people [4]. Hence, two of the main chapters are fully dedicated to "how-to-repair" and not to "how-to-destroy" the disc. Regenerative options to restore the disc are shown by Dr. Becker in Chap. 12, and all the new biomaterials available even in the incoming future are illustrated by Dr. Beall in Chap. 13.

Finally, last but not least, comes the surgery. Because there is no one way to get Rome, and surgical treatment of the disc remains one of the most popular, important, and till now indispensable weapons, we have in case of severe disc herniation responsible for extreme pain or paresis. Dr. El-Hawary, as a skilled spine surgeon, shows in Chap. 14 all the most actual surgical treatments of the disc when everything else fails.

We hope you will enjoy reading this book, as we did.

Catania, Italy — Luigi Manfrè
Antwerpen, Belgium — Johan Van Goethem

## References

1. Truumees E. A history of lumbar disc herniation from Hippocrates to the 1990s. Clin Orthop Relat Res. 2015;473(6):1885–95.
2. Cotunii D. De Ischiade nervosa commentarius. Neapoli. Apud Fratres Simonius. MDCCLXIV.
3. Mixter W, Barr J. Rupture of the intervertebral disc with involvement of the spinal canal. N Engl J Med. 1934;211:210–5.
4. Harari YN. Homo Deus: a brief history of tomorrow. Random House Ed; 2017.

# Contents

# Anatomy and Biomechanics of the Intervertebral Disc

1

Sumeet Kumar and Vivek Pai

Walking. Running. Jumping. Bending. Climbing. The human spine has evolved beyond supporting an upright posture to permit a wide range of motions. The unique upright position along with the flexibility of the human spine is due to the presence of the paired facet joints and the intervertebral discs, which work together as a three-joint complex. The facet or zygapophyseal joints are synovial joints between the superior and inferior articular processes of adjacent vertebrae [1]. The zygapophyseal joints share the transmission of the mechanical load on the spine, limit excessive axial rotation of the vertebrae and provide passive stability [2]. The bony posterior elements of the vertebrae allow attachment of muscles which provide active stability during motion.

The intervertebral disc is sandwiched between the superior and inferior vertebral body endplates and together they constitute a spinal motion segment [3]. The spine can be viewed as consisting of 23 individual spinal motion segments, across the cervical, thoracic and lumbar regions. The sacral and coccygeal vertebrae being fused, lack intervening discs and thus spinal motion segments. The vertebral endplates are thin cartilaginous layers in the central portion of the superior and inferior surfaces of the vertebrae that allow the exchange of nutrients and metabolites between the disc and the capillaries in the vertebrae. The intervertebral discs are held in place between the vertebrae by the longitudinal ligaments continuous with the outer fibres of the disc. A schematic drawing of the spine is shown in Fig. 1.1. The function of the spinal motion segment is to provide axial stability, absorb shock and allow mobility of the segment in three dimensions. Each segment is subject to static and dynamic mechanical forces of varying kinds—compression, shear, bending and torsional forces.

S. Kumar (✉)
Neuroradiology, National Neuroscience Institute, Singapore, Singapore

Duke-NUS Medical School, Singapore, Singapore
e-mail: sumeet.kumar@singhealth.com.sg

V. Pai
Neuroradiology, National Neuroscience Institute, Singapore, Singapore



L. Manfrè, J. Van Goethem (eds.), *The Disc and Degenerative Disc Disease*, New Procedures in Spinal Interventional Neuroradiology,
https://doi.org/10.1007/978-3-030-03715-4_1

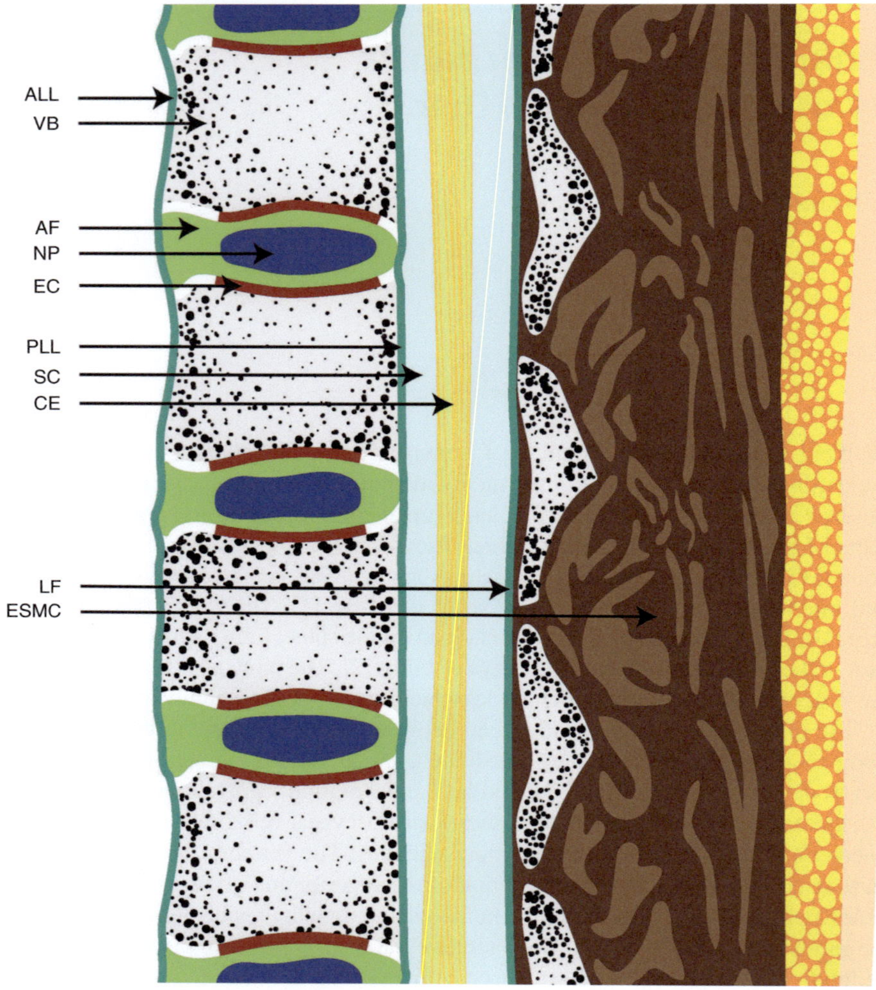


**Fig. 1.1** Sagittal illustration of the spine showing the relationship of the vertebrae, the cartilaginous endplates and the intervertebral discs

In this chapter, the focus is on the intervertebral disc; we will discuss the structure and anatomy of the disc and elaborate on the biomechanical responses of the intervertebral disc when subjected to various forces.

## 1.1 Anatomy of the Intervertebral Disc

Intervertebral discs are present in the cervical, thoracic and lumbar regions, varying in shape and volume at different anatomical levels. On gross morphology, the height of the discs in the lumbar region is the largest, measuring about 9–17 mm in adults. The height in the thoracic region is lesser, about 5 mm and it is the least, about 3 mm in the cervical region [4]. In the cervical region, the discs are thicker anteriorly than posteriorly to form the normal cervical lordotic curvature [5]. Similarly, they are thicker in the anterior portions in the lumbar region to form the lumbar lordosis. In the thoracic region, the discs are of uniform thickness from front to back [6].

On an axial cross section, the disc comprises three zones; the inner most nucleus pulposus surrounded by the inner fibres of the annulus fibrosus and the outer most zone being the outer fibres of the annulus fibrosus [7]. The inner fibres of annulus fibrosus are also sometimes referred to as the transitional zone. The nucleus pulposus is the soft and gelatinous core of the intervertebral disc, occupying about 40% of the cross sectional area in a young healthy adult. The nucleus pulposus has a high water content (about 70–90%), which varies through the time of the day and with activity [8, 9]. The remainder of the matrix of the nucleus pulposus consists of proteoglycans and collagen—primarily type II collagen [4]. The water is held within the domains of the proteoglycans, most abundant of which is aggrecan. The aggrecans attract water molecules and maintain the hydrostatic pressure of the disc [10]. This bound water is responsible for the dynamic viscoelastic properties of the disc that allow it to deform under pressure, sustain and transmit the load in all directions. The type II collagen fibres are fine interconnected fibres that form a meshwork in the matrix and connect with the inner annulus fibres and with the vertebral endplates. Histologically, the nucleus pulposus contains few chondrocyte-like cells which secrete and maintain the abundant extracellular matrix, the predominant component of which is the proteoglycans [11].

Surrounding the nucleus pulposus circumferentially is the ring-shaped annulus fibrosus, which limits the nucleus pulposus forming its outer boundary [12]. The annulus fibrosus is a fibrous structure, consisting of concentric series of collagenous lamellae [13]. Collagen forms about 70% of the dry weight of the annulus fibrosus. Interspersed between the collagen fibrils are proteoglycans, glycoproteins, elastic fibres and fibroblast-like connective tissue cells that secrete these products [14]. The peripheral or outer annulus fibrosus is a more collagenous region than the inner annulus, which forms a transitional layer and lies in contact with the nucleus pulposus. Type I collagen predominates the structure of the outer annulus fibrosus, while type II collagen is abundant in the inner annulus fibrosus [15]. The architecture and composition of the annulus fibrosus change gradually from the outer to the inner layers, being more organised in the outer layers.

The outer annulus is a highly organised lamellated structure made of about 15–25 concentric, densely packed, lamellae of collagen. The number of lamellae is highest in the lumbar discs, up to 25 lamellae [16]. Each lamella varies in thickness from 200 to 400 μm, being thicker towards the periphery [17]. The collagen fibres within each lamella are uniformly oriented in a plane but differ in orientation to the adjacent lamella by about 60° [12]. This alignment leads to the parallel orientation of alternate lamella, referred to as "radial-ply" formation, which provides exceptional strength to the annulus. This arrangement is illustrated in the schematic drawing, Fig. 1.2. The deformation characteristics of the annulus fibrosus are believed to be related to the difference in the angles between adjacent lamella [18, 19]. The lamellae are interconnected through translamellar bridges. The number of translamellar bridges per unit area determines the balance between strength and flexibility. A greater number of bridges provide greater resistance to compressive forces but limit flexibility [12]. In the lumbar discs, the annulus is thicker anteriorly than posteriorly, the lamellae being more numerous anteriorly and spreading out in the peripheral aspects of the disc [20]. The peripheral lamellae connect with the fibres of the longitudinal ligaments, more intimately with the anterior longitudinal ligament than with the posterior longitudinal ligament [21]. The lamellae in the peripheral annulus also attach to the bony edges of the vertebrae by Sharpey's fibres, and the lamellae in the inner annulus are continuous with the cartilaginous endplates [21, 22].

In adults, the intervertebral disc is an avascular structure. It receives its nutrition through diffusion of nutrients through the endplates from the bone vasculature. The vertebral endplates are thin cartilaginous plates composed of hyaline cartilage, about 1 mm thick, at the interface of the vertebral bone and the intervertebral disc. The collagen fibres in the endplates are continuous with the collagen fibres in the disc [23].

Embryologically, the disc originates from two distinct entities. The central nucleus pulposus arises from remnants of the notochord which eventually disappear by the age of 10 years and are replaced by cells which closely resemble chondrocytes [12, 24]. The annulus fibrosus arises from the sclerotome as "annular" condensation of mesenchymal cells between the primordial vertebral bodies [12, 24]. The cells of outer annulus have an oblong, fibroblast-like appearance.

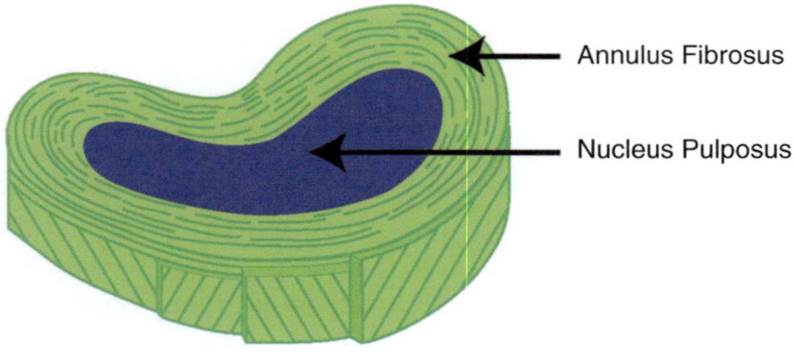


**Fig. 1.2** Diagrammatic representation of the intervertebral disc showing the central nucleus pulposus (blue) surrounded circumferentially by the multilayered annulus pulposus (green)

In adulthood, there is a sharp fall in the number of viable cells within the intervertebral disc and with it, the onset of disc degeneration [25]. The nucleus hardens, loses its gel-like consistency and translucent appearance due to a reduction of its proteoglycan and water content and an increase in the density and size of the collagen fibrils within it [26]. Consequent to these structural alterations within the nucleus, there is an overall reduction of the size of the nucleus pulposus and expansion of the inner layer of the annulus. The outer layer of the annulus remains stable in size [26]. The composition of the annulus remains unchanged in adulthood, but areas of myxomatous degeneration occur which eventually progress to fissuring [26, 27]. With degeneration, the collagen fibrils are thinned and their arrangement loses its regularity [28]. With advancing degeneration, the intervertebral disc is no more than a hard fibrocartilage. The volume of the disc reduces markedly with multiple fissures extending to the centre of the disc. The nucleus may be imperceptible from the rest of the annulus.

## 1.2 Biomechanical Properties of the Intervertebral Disc

The extracellular matrix of the intervertebral disc, consisting predominantly of three macromolecules—collagen, proteoglycans and glycoproteins, is responsible for many of the biomechanical properties of the disc. The relative proportion of water and the macromolecules varies in different regions of the disc, imparting distinct mechanical properties to the nucleus pulposus, inner and outer annulus fibrosus. For instance, the proteoglycans are most abundant in the nucleus pulposus. This gives the nucleus pulposus higher hydrostatic and osmotic pressures and thus more compressive properties. Highly organised collagen fibres are more abundant in the annulus, giving the annulus a higher tensile loading capacity. During axial loading (axial force is a force applied along the long axis of the spine) compression is experienced by both the nucleus pulposus and the annulus fibrosus. However, their responses vary due to the relative differences in their composition. The relative composition and architectural arrangement not only vary in different regions, but they also vary with the anatomical level (i.e. cervical versus thoracic versus lumbar level) and with age [29–32]. For example the lumbar intervertebral discs have the highest proteoglycan content in the nucleus pulposus, whereas the nucleus pulposus in the cervical discs show the highest collagen content [30]. Some of the important properties of the disc that influence biomechanical behaviour are discussed below.

### 1.2.1 Hydrostatic Pressure

The proteoglycans, being hydrophilic, attract water molecules and this maintains the hydrostatic pressure of the nucleus pulposus. The hydrostatic pressure is responsible for maintaining the height of the disc which separates the adjacent vertebrae and expands the annulus fibrosus outwards. The magnitude of hydrostatic pressure varies diurnally depending on the spinal alignment and physical activity, being in the magnitude range of 0.1 MPa at sleep to 0.5 MPa in quiet standing to more than 3 MPa, with increased loading [31–34]. With advancing age, lower proteoglycan and thus lower water content of the disc result in reduced hydrostatic pressure. This is accompanied by a decrease in the height of the disc along with altered mechanical properties of the disc.

### 1.2.2 Osmotic Pressure

Osmotic pressure in the disc is due to the differences in the concentration of macromolecules and ions in the extracellular matrix [35]. The presence of charged ions in the disc creates an osmotic pressure, which pulls water into the tissue and keeps the disc hydrated. The proteoglycans in the disc are composed of long chains of glycosamine attached to protein and are responsible for the negative charge. Within the nucleus pulposus, the most abundant proteoglycan is aggrecan, which is composed of negatively charged side chains of chondroitin sulphate and keratan attached to filaments of hyaluronic acid. These large molecules are trapped inside the collagen fibres and cannot diffuse out [36–38]. The negative charge attracts the positively charged Na+ ions creating an imbalance of cations. This draws in water that maintains the osmotic turgor of the nucleus pulposus, causes swelling of the disc and increases the stiffness of the tissue. The osmotic pressure within the disc shows diurnal variation, with changes in standing and supine positions and variations due to posture and activity with about 20–25% water exchange in every diurnal cycle [39].

### 1.2.3 Permeability

Permeability refers to the ability of fluid to flow in and out of the disc and is a key mechanical property of the nucleus pulposus. During axial loading, fluid flows out of the disc into the plasma. Inward movement of water into the disc is through passive diffusion on removal of the applied forces, for example on lying down. The movement of water into the disc and efflux of water out of the disc is thought to occur through two routes, predominantly through the vertebral endplate. The vertebral endplate is a hyaline cartilage similar to that found in the joints. It is perforated by vascular buds from the bone marrow at the bone endplate interfaces [40]. The other, probably less important route is through the annulus into the blood vessels adjacent to the annulus [40]. The permeability of the disc has been tested using confined compression techniques in which harvested nucleus pulposus tissue is compressed axially with methods to prevent lateral expansion. It has been observed that when subjected to small deformations, the nucleus pulposus demonstrates a constant permeability with a linear relationship between stress and strain. (Stress is a measure of force intensity, that is, force or load per unit area. Strain is a measure of deformation, that is, change in length divided by the original length.) This relation however is non-linear for moderate and large strain.

The hydrostatic and osmotic pressures are related to the permeability of the disc and are mediated by the binding and releasing of water molecules by the aggrecans in the nucleus pulposus [41]. This diurnal and load responsive alteration in the water content of the disc is also referred to as the poroelastic behaviour of the disc [41].

### 1.2.4 Viscoelasticity

The nucleus pulposus is highly hydrated and has a gelatinous consistency. This makes it a classic example of a biological viscoelastic material, i.e. it demonstrates the properties of both fluid and solid. A fluid is defined as a substance that constantly deforms when subjected to a shear stress (shear stress is a force applied tangential to a surface), irrespective of magnitude of the applied force. Solids, on the other hand, resist shear stress (though minimal initial deformation is possible) and do not continue to deform like fluids, reaching a state of equilibrium with the applied stress. In experimental conditions, it has been found that nucleus pulposus shows a fluid-like behaviour under slow deformation rates and solid-like behaviour under dynamic conditions; its behaviour varying as a function of the rate of loading [42]. The viscoelasticity of the nucleus pulposus is attributed to ionic or osmotic effects and non-ionic or solid effects related to the proteoglycans [43].

### 1.2.5 Nonlinearity

Non-linear response of the annulus fibrosus to stress refers to a response that is not proportional to the applied loading force. In other words, the stiffness of annulus fibrosus varies with the magnitude of the applied load and is a property imparted by the collagen fibres. The annulus shows low stiffness for smaller deformations and higher stiffness for larger deformations [44–46]. This is related to the zigzag shape or "crimp" of the collagen fibres in the annulus and the gradual "uncrimping" with increasing stretch [47, 48]. On application of a stretching force "crimp" of the collagen fibres is straightened, and the stiffness and load-bearing capacity of the annulus increase with increasing stretch. Progressively further stretching after all the fibres are straightened can disrupt and break the collagen fibres. This important feature allows the annulus to restrain the swelling pressure in the nucleus pulposus.

### 1.2.6 Elasticity

The elastic properties of the annulus are related to its extra-fibrillary matrix, that is, the material excluding the collagen fibres. The elastic properties have been described in ex vivo studies using shear and compression tests (which may be uniaxial or biaxial), obtaining the Young's modulus (from the slope of stress and strain response) and using mechanical models.

### 1.2.7 Anisotropy

Anisotropic behaviour of the disc is a property of the annulus. It means that the stress in the annulus fibrosus varies in different axes. This is a function of the collagen fibre orientation with respect to the applied stress [20, 49].

## 1.3 Biomechanics of the Intervertebral Disc

### 1.3.1 Unloaded Disc

There are baseline forces at work within the intervertebral disc even in the absence of external loading. These forces arise mainly due to the internal tissue inhomogeneities within the disc. The higher proteoglycan concentration in the nucleus causes a higher hydrostatic and osmotic pressure within it. This is resisted in the axial plane by the vertebral endplates and in the radial plane by the tensile stress of the annulus, also referred to as the "hoop stress" (tensile stress tends to pull and elongate the material in the direction of applied force). These multidirectional "residual" stresses are present in the unloaded state within the disc and have been studied by measuring the opening angle after an incision on the annulus fibrosus of an animal disc and by needle pressure gauge studies [50–52]. When an external load is applied, it creates additional stresses on top of the baseline "residual" stress.

### 1.3.2 Response to Compression

Compression is a force that has the action of shortening the material in the direction of the applied force. The direction of axial compression on the disc is depicted schematically in Fig. 1.3. The key function of the intervertebral disc is transmission of compression load in the spinal column, together with facet joints. The discs and facet joints work synergistically, the disc supports the compressive forces anteriorly and the facet joints posteriorly. To maintain spinal stability, the net load vector passes through the centre of rotation of each adjacent spinal motion segment in the sagittal axis, also described as follower load path [53]. Using this strategy, the spine can support static loading for physical tasks more than physiological demands while maintaining flexibility [54–56]. Muscle activation occurs in vivo so that during static conditions, the primary loading of the disc is axial compression.

The amount of compression loading force on the disc depends on the weight of the upper body, action of the muscles and posture of the spine. For example in erect standing position and erect sitting position, the intervertebral disc transmits 84% and 100% of the compression load, respectively. The response of the disc depends on the duration of the loading, the frequency of change of loading and on the spinal level (cervical vs. lumbar).

The water content of the disc and movement of water inside and out of the disc are major determinants to the biodynamic mechanical behaviour of the disc to

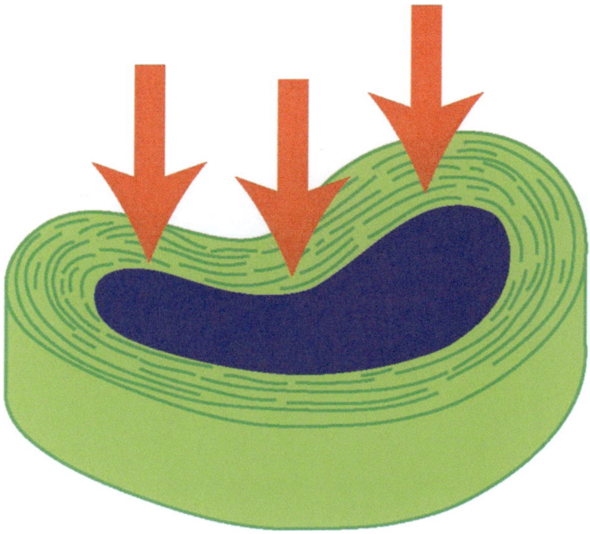

**Fig. 1.3** Illustration of the direction of axial compressive force on the disc

compression loading [57–60]. The disc tends to maintain an equilibrium with respect to the external loading and internal disc swelling [61]. Upon application of a compressive load, the initial changes in the disc are different from the later changes. Initially, the hydrostatic pressure rapidly rises within the disc, more specifically, within its core, the nucleus pulposus. The nucleus pulposus behaves as an incompressible material and dissipates the pressure radially outwards to the annulus fibrosus and axially to the vertebral endplates—both of which restrain the nucleus pulposus. The hydrostatic pressure transferred to the outer fibres of the annulus causes them to experience a radial stretch or tensile stress and bulge outwards [62, 63]. This outward tensile force on the annulus is schematically represented in Fig. 1.4. The lamellae of the annulus fibrosus also experience axial compressive stress, which causes the inner lamellae to buckle inwards. The inward buckling of these lamellae is counteracted by the circumferentially outwardly directed hydrostatic pressure from the nucleus pulposus, thus stabilising these lamellae. This mechanism fails in the degenerating disc, which allows the inner lamellae of annulus to buckle inwards. The axial compression experienced by the inner fibres of annulus fibrosus is eventually transferred to adjacent vertebrae [63]. During prolonged external compressive loading, interstitial fluid is forced out of the nucleus pulposus towards the annulus and the endplates [64]. This causes a decrease in the disc height and increased outward bulging of the annulus. During this state, the nucleus pulposus bears less of the axial compression, and the contribution of the annulus fibrosus towards bearing the compression load increases [65].

As the fluid is expressed out from the nucleus pulposus, the concentration of the proteoglycans and fixed charge density within it increases. This causes a build-up of

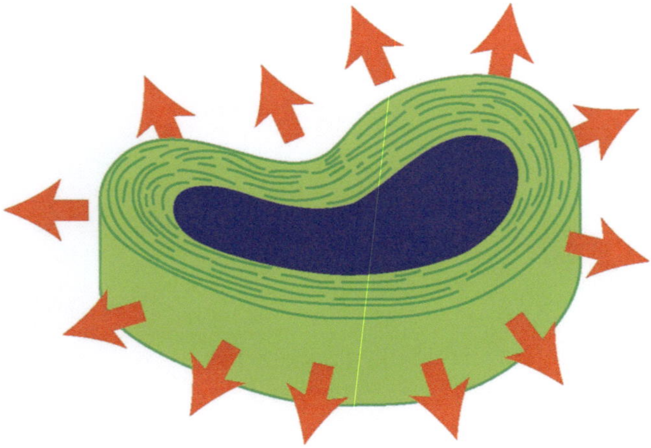

**Fig. 1.4** Illustration of the outwardly directed tensile stress on the annulus fibrosus

osmotic pressure within the disc which tries to recover equilibrium [61]. The direction of water movement is reversed during rest, restoring the mechanical properties of the disc [66]. The water content is re-imbibed into the disc when the loading pressure is released, for example in supine position [67–70]. Sleeping or supine position is a low loading state that facilitates re-entry of fluid into the disc and decrease in disc osmolality. Correspondingly, the height of the disc (or its axial stiffness) changes, showing reduction in height during the loading cycle (during the day) and increase in height in the recovery (sleeping) phase. In vivo MRI studies have shown an increase in the water content of the discs and increase in height of the discs after a night of rest [66, 71, 72].

The response of the disc to loading depends on the type of compression loading, whether it is static or dynamic, duration of the loading and the frequency of the loading. The responses to various loading and recovery protocols have been studied extensively in many animal models [64, 66, 73–75]. Since most of these properties have been studied by application of loads in cadaveric animal intervertebral disc experiments, it is worth keeping in mind that the biological properties of the discs studied in vitro may not precisely simulate the in vivo behaviour of discs in humans.

The healthy disc remains soft under low compression loads but stiffens under high compression loads, to increase the stability [76]. A degenerated disc is less hydrated than a disc in health and is unable to generate enough hydrostatic pressure, and the pressure transfer mechanisms fail [76]. As a consequence, the load is transferred predominantly to the annulus rather than the vertebrae. In other words, in a degenerating disc, the annulus is subjected to a larger tensile stress [63].

While the compressive load is absorbed by the healthy nucleus pulposus, tensile force is resisted by the healthy annulus fibrosus. As mentioned previously, due to its unique structure, the annulus fibrosus is able to resist the tensile stress transmitted to it by the nucleus pulposus [77]. The alignment of the fibres within the annulus is responsible for absorbing a high magnitude of the tensile stress [63].

### 1.3.3 Response to Bending and Torsion

Much of the stress exerted on the spine is due to changes in posture. Bending and torsional movements are common movements of the spine associated with activity. These result in a combination of shear, compression and tensile forces on the spine [59, 63, 78]. Bending forward (spinal flexion), backward (spinal extension) or lateral bending are movements that result in rotation of the segments perpendicular to the axis of the spine. This causes a tensile stress on the annulus on the convex aspect of the spine and a compressive stress on the annulus on the concave aspect of the spine. For example on forward bending of the torso, the anterior annulus fibrosus experiences most of the compression. The outer fibres of the anterior annulus bulge outwards and the inner fibres of the anterior annulus buckle inwards. The posterior annulus on the other hand does not contribute to compression loading. It is subjected instead to a tensile or stretching stress in the axial direction. The nucleus pulposus pressurises and shifts backwards (opposite to the direction of bending) [43]. Effectively, there is asymmetric distribution of forces in different aspects of the annulus, the one side under the tensile stress stretching and the other side bulging under the weight of the body [59, 63, 78].

Torsion of the spine along its long axis is resisted by the zygapophyseal joints and is limited to 1–3° during physical activities [79]. It causes a combination of tensile and shear stresses in the annulus. Shear stress occurs in the horizontal plane in relation to the axis of rotation and perpendicular to the annulus fibres. Shear stress on the disc is schematically shown in Fig. 1.5. The oblique orientation of the lamellae of annulus results in tensile stress being generated within the fibres resisting the rotation [63] but not in the other fibres. When subjected to torsion, the peripheral or outer portion of the annulus is subjected to the largest stresses, thus developing the greatest strains. The strain on the annulus being directly proportional to the distance between the axis of rotation and the peripheral fibres [80, 81]. In the lumbar disc, this stress is maximum at the posterolateral portions of the annulus.

Therefore, bending and twisting movements of the spine when performed individually or in combination, especially when superimposed with a compressive load, result in increased stress and strain on the intervertebral disc. The effects of these

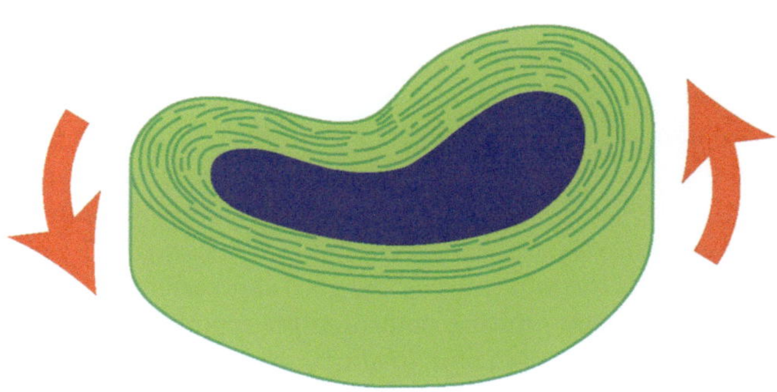

**Fig. 1.5** Illustration of the shear stress acting on the disc in torsion

movements are magnified when applied to an already degenerating disc and account for disc injury.

The physical forces acting on the disc are translated into chemical signals which induce a cellular response. The cellular responses influence the biomechanical properties of the disc. This is dealt within the subsequent section of mechanotransduction.

## 1.4 Mechanotransduction in Intervertebral Disc

Three-dimensional mechanical forces acting on the disc cause biological responses at a cellular level within the disc through the phenomenon of mechanotransduction. For example on application of a compressive load, there is a physical deformation or a decrease in height of the nucleus pulposus. This results in a series of important intracellular changes, such as gene expression, protein synthesis and proliferation in response to this mechanical stress.

The mechanical stimuli are received by receptors, the mechanoreceptors, located in the nerve endings that begin the biological response by firing an action potential. In the spine, mechanoreceptors have been found in the peripheral lamellae of the annulus fibrosus and the longitudinal ligaments, most populous of which are the Golgi tendon organs [77]. The others are Pacinian corpuscles and Ruffini endings [77]. The Golgi tendon organs are primarily related to pain stimuli while the others are related to posture [77, 82]. On stimulation by mechanical stress, the mechanoreceptors activate various pathways which depend on the type and magnitude of the load, the duration, frequency and the anatomical zone where it is applied. These pathways induce biological effects by altering the gene expression that affects intracellular processes such as enzyme synthesis and apoptosis via signalling pathways [77]. The cellular pathways are different in a healthy disc versus a degenerated intervertebral disc, for example mechanosensing in healthy disc cells is via the arginine-glycine-aspartic acid (RGD) integrin protein whereas in the degenerated discs it is shown to trigger a different pathway that involves calcium [83, 84] and nitric oxide [84, 85].

On application of compressive stress, different responses are seen in distinct parts of the intervertebral disc. Most responses of the inner annulus fibrosus and the nucleus pulposus are similar, while the outer annulus fibrosus is not equally responsive to low-to-moderate magnitudes of load [34]. The compressive stress also regulates transport of nutrients and cell receptor signalling. Dynamic compression stress increases the oxygen concentration and consumption in the disc and reduces the accumulation of lactate [86]. On the other hand, static compression inhibits transport and metabolism of oxygen and lactate [86]. When exposed to in vivo static compression, changes in the biosynthesis and gene expression for molecules such as collagen, proteoglycans and protease activation are reported in some studies [34]. Most studies have found that dynamic loading largely leads to an anabolic effect, while static loading leads to catabolism [34, 87]. Short periods of loading elevate gene expression of collagens I and II as well as proteoglycans (e.g. aggrecan, decorin and biglycan) in isolated annulus fibrosus cells and long duration of loading disrupt the transport of oxygen and nutrients [34, 88]. The age of the cells also plays a role in the response to dynamic compression, the younger cells maintaining the homeostasis better than the mature cells [89].

These studies give a glimpse of how the mechanical forces of the three-dimensional environments of the cells regulate the cells and their most fundamental cellular processes through complex pathways.

## 1.5 Summary

To summarise, the structure of the intervertebral disc is closely coupled with its biomechanical properties, allowing the spine to sustain load and maintain flexibility. The biomechanics vary at different levels of the spine, there being more rotation, less compression in the cervical segments and more compression, less rotation in the lumbar segments. The constitution of the intervertebral discs and the morphology of the facet joints are adapted for these mechanically different forces.

The composition of the central core of the intervertebral disc—the nucleus pulposus is geared towards retaining hydration through its proteoglycan rich matrix, which bequeaths it with hydrostatic properties. The annulus fibrosus or the outer restraining ring of the intervertebral disc, on the other hand, is rich in type I collagen and has a unique cross-ply design so that it can withstand high tensile forces.

Mechanical and cellular responses to loads through alterations in gene expression, enzyme synthesis and signalling pathways maintain a complex homeostasis to preserve disc structure and execute repair pathways. Failure of these mechanisms to cope with the applied loads leads to injury and initiates degeneration of the disc. The understanding of the anatomy and the biomechanics of load transfer in the intervertebral disc is important in understanding how we perform our day-to-day activities in health.

## References

1. Singh V. General anatomy. 2nd ed. Gurgaon: Elsevier; 2015. p. 108.
2. Jaumard N, Welch W, Winkelstein B. Spinal facet joint biomechanics and mechanotransduction in Normal, injury and degenerative conditions. J Biomech Eng. 2011;133(7):071010. https://doi.org/10.1115/1.4004493.
3. Dennison C, Wild P, Wilson D, Cripton P. A minimally invasive in-fiber Bragg grating sensor for intervertebral disc pressure measurements. Meas Sci Technol. 2008;19(8):085201.
4. White T, Malone T. Effects of running on intervertebral disc height. J Orthop Sports Phys Ther. 1990;12(4):139–46.
5. Cifu D. Braddom's physical medicine & rehabilitation. 5th ed. Amsterdam: Elsevier; 2015. p. 688.
6. Mirab SMH, Barbarestani M, Tabatabaei SM, et al. Measuring dimensions of lumbar intervertebral discs in normal subjects. Anat Sci. 2017;14(1):3–8.
7. McCann M, Séguin C. Notochord cells in intervertebral disc development and degeneration. J Dev Biol. 2016;4(1):3.

8. DePalma AF, Rothman RH. The intervertebral disc. Philadelphia, PA: W.B. Saunders Company; 1970.
9. Bogduk N. Clinical anatomy of the lumbar spine and sacrum. 3rd ed. Churchull Livingstone: New York, NY; 1997.
10. Gawri R, Moir J, Ouellet J, et al. Physiological loading can restore the proteoglycan content in a model of early IVD degeneration. PLoS One. 2014;9(7):e101233.
11. Yoon S, Patel N. Molecular therapy of the intervertebral disc. Eur Spine J. 2006;15(S3):379–88.
12. Waxenbaum J, Reddy V, Futterman B. Anatomy, back, intervertebral discs. Ncbi.nlm.nih.gov. https://www.ncbi.nlm.nih.gov/books/NBK470583/.
13. Beadle OA. The intervertebral discs: observations on their normal and morbid anatomy in relation to certain spinal deformities. Issued by the Medical Research Council. Royal 8vo. Pp. 79, with 47 illustrations. 1931. London: His Majesty's stationery office. 2s. Net. Br J Surg. 1932;19(76):667.
14. Adams M. Intervertebral disc tissues. Eng Mater Process. 2014;2014:7–35.
15. Hayes A, Isaacs M, Hughes C, et al. Collagen fibrillogenesis in the development of the annulus fibrosus of the intervertebral disc. Eur Cells Mater. 2011;22:226–41.
16. Roberts S. Disc morphology in health and disease. Biochem Soc Trans. 2002;30(Pt 6):864–9.
17. Inoue H. Three-dimensional observation of collagen framework of intervertebral discs in rats, dogs and humans. Arch Histol Jpn. 1973;36:39–56.
18. Horton W. Further observations on the elastic mechanism of the intervertebral disc. J Bone Joint Surg Br. 1958;40-B(3):552–7.
19. Naylor A. The biophysical and biochemical aspects of intervertebral disc herniation and degeneration. Ann R Coll Surg Engl. 1962;31(2):91–114.
20. Galante J. Tensile properties of the human lumbar annulus fibrosus. Acta Orthop Scand. 1967;38(Sup100):1–91.
21. Hirsch C, Schajowicz F. Studies on structural changes in the lumbar annulus fibrosus. Acta Orthop Scand. 1952;22(1–4):184–231.
22. Tandon P, Ramamurthi R. Ramamurthi and Tandon's textbook of neurosurgery. New Delhi: Jaypee Brothers Medical Publishers; 2012.
23. Scott JE, Bosworth TR, Cribb AM, Taylor JR. The chemical morphology of age-related changes in human intervertebral disc glycosaminoglycans from cervical, thoracic and lumbar nucleus pulposus and annulus fibrosus. J Anat. 1994 Feb;184(Pt 1):73–82.
24. Subhadra DV. Inderbir Singh's human embryology. New Delhi: Jaypee Brothers Medical Publishers; 2016.
25. Buckwalter JA, Pedrini-Mille A, Pedrini V, Tudisco C. Proteoglycans of human infant intervertebral disc. Electron microscopic and biochemical studies. J Bone Jt Surg. 1985;67(2):284–94.
26. Buckwalter JA. Aging and degeneration of the human intervertebral disc. Spine (Phila Pa 1976). 1995;20(11):1307–14.
27. Buckwalter JA, Smith K, Kazarien L, et al. Articular cartilage and intervertebral disc proteoglycans differ in structure: an electron microscopic study. J Orthop Res. 1989;7(1):146–51.
28. Coventry MB, Ghormley RK, Kernohan JW. The intervertebral disc: its microscopic anatomy and pathology. Part III Pathological changes in the intervertebral disc. J Bone Jt Surg. 1945;27:460.
29. Antoniou J, Steffen T, Nelson F, et al. The human lumbar intervertebral disc: evidence for changes in the biosynthesis and denaturation of the extracellular matrix with growth, maturation, ageing, and degeneration. J Clin Invest. 1996;98:996–1003.
30. Scott JE, Bosworth TR, Cribb AM, Taylor JR. The chemical morphology of age-related changes in human intervertebral disc glycosaminoglycans from cervical, thoracic and lumbar nucleus pulposus and annulus fibrosus. J Anat. 1994;184(Pt 1):73–82.
31. Demers CN, Antoniou J, Mwale F. Value and limitations of using the bovine tail as a model for the human lumbar spine. Spine (Phila Pa 1976). 2004;29(24):2793–9.
32. Wilke HJ, Neef P, Caimi M, et al. New in vivo measurements of pressures in the intervertebral disc in daily life. Spine (Phila Pa 1976). 1999;24(8):755–62.

33. Vergroesen P, Kingma I, Emanuel K, et al. Mechanics and biology in intervertebral disc degeneration: a vicious circle. Osteoarthr Cartil. 2015;23(7):1057–70.
34. Fearing B, Hernandez P, Setton L, Chahine N. Mechanotransduction and cell biomechanics of the intervertebral disc. JOR Spine. 2018;1(3):e1026.
35. Urban J. The role of the physicochemical environment in determining disc cell behaviour. Biochem Soc Trans. 2002;30(6):858–63.
36. Urban JP, Maroudas A. Swelling of the intervertebral disc in vitro. Connect Tissue Res. 1981;9(1):1–10.
37. Melrose J, Ghosh P, Taylor TK. A comparative analysis of the differential spatial and temporal distributions of the large (aggrecan, versican) and small (decorin, biglycan, fibromodulin) proteoglycans of the intervertebral disc. J Anat. 2001;198(Pt 1):3–15.
38. Kiani C, Chen L, Wu YJ, et al. Structure and function of aggrecan. Cell Res. 2002 Mar;12(1):19–32.
39. Chan S, Ferguson S, Gantenbein-Ritter B. The effects of dynamic loading on the intervertebral disc. Eur Spine J. 2011;20(11):1796–812.
40. Ogata K, Whiteside LA. Volvo award winner in basic science. Nutritional pathways of the intervertebral disc. An experimental study using hydrogen washout technique. Spine (Phila Pa 1976). 1981;6(3):211–6.
41. Vergroesen P, van der Veen A, Emanuel K, et al. The poro-elastic behaviour of the intervertebral disc: a new perspective on diurnal fluid flow. J Biomech. 2016;49(6):857–63.
42. Iatridis J, Setton L, Weidenbaum M, Mow V. The viscoelastic behavior of the non-degenerate human lumbar nucleus pulposus in shear. J Biomech. 1997;30(10):1005–13.
43. Cortes D, Elliott D. The intervertebral disc: overview of disc mechanics. New York, NY: Springer; 2013. p. 17–31.
44. McGraw-Hill PS. McGraw-Hill dictionary of scientific and technical terms. New York, NY: McGraw-Hill; 2003.
45. Guerin HL, Elliott DM. Quantifying the contributions of structure to annulus fibrosus mechanical function using a nonlinear, anisotropic, hyperelastic model. J Orthop Res. 2007;25(4):508–16.
46. Wu HC, Yao RF. Mechanical behavior of the human annulus fibrosus. J Biomech. 1976;9(1):1–7.
47. Diamant J, Keller A, Baer E, et al. Collagen; ultrastructure and its relation to mechanical properties as a function of ageing. Proc R Soc Lond B Biol Sci. 1972;180(60):293–315.
48. Kastelic J, Baer E. Deformation in tendon collagen. Symp Soc Exp Biol. 1980;34:397–435.
49. Setton L, Chen J. Cell mechanics and mechanobiology in the intervertebral disc. Spine. 2004;29(23):2710–23.
50. Michalek AJ, Gardner-Mose MG, Iatridis JC. Large residual strains are present in the intervertebral disc annulus fibrosus in the unloaded state. J Biomech. 2012;45(7):1227–31.
51. Nachemson AL. Disc pressure measurements. Spine (Phila Pa 1976). 1981;6(1):93–7.
52. Panjabi M, Brown M, Lindahl S, et al. Intrinsic disc pressure as a measure of integrity of the lumbar spine. Spine (Phila Pa 1976). 1988;13(8):913–7.
53. Patwardhan AG, Havey RM, Meade KP, et al. A follower load increases the load-carrying capacity of the lumbar spine in compression. Spine (Phila Pa 1976). 1999;24(10):1003–9.
54. Rohlmann A, Neller S, Cleas L, et al. Influence of a follower load on intradiscal pressure and intersegmental rotation of the lumbar spine. Spine (Phila Pa 1976). 2001;26(24):E557–61.
55. Patwardhan AG, Havey RM, Ghanayem AJ, et al. Load-carrying capacity of the human cervical spine in compression is increased under a follower load. Spine (Phila Pa 1976). 2000;25(12):1548–54.
56. Patwardhan AG, Havey RM, Carandang G, et al. Effect of compressive follower preload on the flexion-extension response of the human lumbar spine. J Orthop Res. 2003;21(3):540–6.
57. Lanir Y. Mechanisms of residual stress in soft tissues. J Biomech Eng. 2009;131(4):044506.
58. Iatridis JC, Setton LA, Weidenbaum M, Mow VC. Alterations in the mechanical behavior of the human lumbar nucleus pulposus with degeneration and aging. J Orthop Res. 1997;15:318–22.
59. White A, Panjabi M. Clinical biomechanics of the spine. Philadelphia, PA: J.B. Lippincott; 1990. p. 14–5.

60. van Dieen JH, Kingma I, Meijer R, et al. Stress distribution changes in bovine vertebrae just below the endplate after sustained loading. Clin Biomech (Bristol, Avon). 2001;16(Suppl 1):S135–42.
61. Urban JP, McMullin JF. Swelling pressure of the lumbar intervertebral discs: influence of age, spinal level, composition, and degeneration. Spine (Phila Pa 1976). 1988;13(2):179–87.
62. Inoue N, Espinoza OA. Biomechanics of intervertebral disk degeneration. Orthop Clin N Am. 2011;42(4):487–99.
63. Jensen G. Biomechanics of the lumbar intervertebral disk: a review. Phys Ther. 1980;60(6):765–73.
64. van der Veen AJ, van Dieen JH, Nadort AETAL. Intervertebral disc recovery after dynamic or static loading in vitro: is there a role for the endplate? J Biomech. 2007;40(10):2230–5.
65. O'Connell GD, Johannessen W, Vresilovic EJ, Elliott DM. Human internal disc strains in axial compression measured noninvasively using magnetic resonance imaging. Spine (Phila Pa 1976). 2007;32(25):2860–8.
66. Malko JA, Hutton WC, Fajman WA. An in vivo MRI study of the changes in volume (and fluid content) of the lumbar intervertebral disc after overnight bed rest and during an 8-hour walking protocol. J Spinal Disord Tech. 2002;15:157–63.
67. Adams MA, Dolan P, Hutton WC, Porter RW. Diurnal changes in spinal mechanics and their clinical significance. J Bone Joint Surg Br. 1990;72(2):266–70.
68. Kraemer J. Dynamic characteristics of the vertebral column, effects of prolonged loading. Ergonomics. 1985;28(1):95–7.
69. MacLean JJ, Lee CR, Grad S, Ito K, Alini M, Iatridis JC. Effects of immobilization and dynamic compression on intervertebral disc cell gene expression in vivo. Spine (Phila Pa 1976). 2003;28(10):973–81.
70. McMillan DW, Garbutt G, Adams MA. Effect of sustained loading on the water content of intervertebral discs: implications for disc metabolism. Ann Rheum Dis. 1996;55(12):880–7.
71. McGill SM, Axler CT. Changes in spine height throughout 32 hours of bedrest. Arch Phys Med Rehabil. 1996;77:1071–3.
72. Reilly T, Tyrrell A, Troup JD. Circadian variation in human stature. Chronobiol Int. 1984;1:121–6.
73. Ayotte DC, Ito K, Perren SM, Tepic S. Direction-dependent constriction flow in a poroelastic solid: the intervertebral disc valve. J Biomech Eng. 2000;122:587–93.
74. Tyrrell AR, Reilly T, Troup JD. Circadian variation in stature and the effects of spinal loading. Spine (Phila Pa 1976). 1985;10:161–4.
75. Johannessen W, Vresilovic E, Wright A, Elliott D. Intervertebral disc mechanics are restored following cyclic loading and unloaded recovery. Ann Biomed Eng. 2004;32(1):70–6.
76. Oktenoglu T, ECE K. Biomechanics of the lumbar spine and lumbar disc. 2019. https://www.turknorosirurji.org.tr/TNDData/Books/426/biomechanics-of-lumbar-spine-and-lumbar-disc.pdf.
77. Tsai T, Cheng C, Chen C, Lai P. Mechanotransduction in intervertebral discs. J Cell Mol Med. 2014;18(12):2351–60.
78. Farfan HF, Farfan H. Mechanical disorders of the low back. Philadelphia, PA: Lea & Febiger; 1973. p. 13–24, 63, 90, 201.
79. Pearcy M, Portek I, Shepherd J. Three-dimensional x-ray analysis of normal movement in the lumbar spine. Spine (Phila Pa 1976). 1984;9(3):294–7.
80. Frankel VH, Burstein AH. Orthopaedic biomechanics. Philadelphia, PA: Lea & Febiger; 1971. p. 40–76.
81. Frost HM. Orthopaedic biomechanics. Springfield, IL: Charles C Thomas; 1973. p. 49–56, 146–163.
82. Roberts S, Eisenstein SM, Menage J, et al. Mechanoreceptors in intervertebral discs. Morphology, distribution, and neuropeptides. Spine (Phila Pa 1976). 1995;20(24):2645–51.
83. Pritchard S, Erickson GR, Guilak F. Hyperosmotically induced volume change and calcium signaling in intervertebral disk cells: the role of the actin cytoskeleton. Biophys J. 2002;83:2502–10.

84. Le Maitre C, Frain J, Millward-Sadler J, Fotheringham A, Freemont A, Hoyland J. Altered integrin mechanotransduction in human nucleus pulposus cells derived from degenerated discs. Arthritis Rheum. 2009;60(2):460–9.
85. Benallaoua M, Richette P, Francois M, Tsagris L, Revel M, Corvol M, et al. Modulation of proteoglycan production by cyclic tensile stretch in intervertebral disc cells through a post-translational mechanism. Biorheology. 2006;43:303–10.
86. Huang C, Gu W. Effects of mechanical compression on metabolism and distribution of oxygen and lactate in intervertebral disc. J Biomech. 2008;41(6):1184–96.
87. Wuertz K, Godburn K, MacLean J, Barbir A, Stinnett Donnelly J, Roughley P, et al. In vivo remodeling of intervertebral discs in response to short- and long-term dynamic compression. J Orthop Res. 2009;27(9):1235–42.
88. Chen J. Static compression induces zonal-specific changes in gene expression for extra-cellular matrix and cytoskeletal proteins in intervertebral disc cells in vitro. Matrix Biol. 2004;22(7):573–83.
89. Korecki C, Kuo C, Tuan R, Iatridis J. Intervertebral disc cell response to dynamic compression is age and frequency dependent. J Orthop Res. 2009;27(6):800–6.

# Imaging of Degeneration, Inflammation, Infection, Ossification, and Calcification of the Intervertebral Disk

2

Frederik Bosmans, Johan Van Goethem, and Filip M. Vanhoenacker

## 2.1 Introduction

The intervertebral disk is a complex structure located between two adjacent vertebrae in the spine. Its main functions are to act as a load distributing shock absorber and to allow for flexibility with multiaxial spinal motion. The intervertebral disks are vulnerable to a wide array of pathological processes which may cause significant morbidity. From the radiologist's perspective, familiarity with the structure of the disk and the pathophysiology of disk disease is pivotal in order to understand the natural history of disk-related disease, which in turn helps in developing an appropriate diagnostic strategy. The purpose of this chapter is to discuss and illustrate the semiology of the different intervertebral disk pathologies on conventional radiography, computed tomography (CT), and magnetic resonance imaging (MRI).

F. Bosmans
Department of Radiology and Antwerp University Faculty of Medicine and Health Sciences, Antwerp University Hospital, Edegem, Belgium

General Hospital Sint-Maarten Mechelen, Mechelen, Belgium
e-mail: Frederik.bosmans@emmaus.be

J. Van Goethem
Department of Radiology and Antwerp University Faculty of Medicine and Health Sciences, Antwerp University Hospital, Edegem, Belgium

AZ Nikolaas, Sint-Niklaas, Belgium
e-mail: johan.vangoethem@uantwerpen.be

F. M. Vanhoenacker (✉)
Department of Radiology and Antwerp University Faculty of Medicine and Health Sciences, Antwerp University Hospital, Edegem, Belgium

General Hospital Sint-Maarten Mechelen, Mechelen, Belgium

Faculty of Medicine and Health Sciences, University of Ghent, Ghent, Belgium
e-mail:filip.vanhoenacker@telenet.be



L. Manfrè, J. Van Goethem (eds.), *The Disc and Degenerative Disc Disease*, New Procedures in Spinal Interventional Neuroradiology,
https://doi.org/10.1007/978-3-030-03715-4_2

## 2.2 Imaging of the Disk: Normal and Variants with Imaging Correlation

### 2.2.1 The Normal Intervertebral Disk

Intervertebral disks are located between the vertebral bodies of C2–C3 to L5–S1. The normal anatomy of the intervertebral disk is discussed in detail in Chap. 1 and summarized schematically in (Fig. 2.1). This paragraph will focus on imaging of the normal disk and its variations.

### 2.2.2 Plain Radiographs

The intervertebral disk is indirectly evaluated by the disk height on lateral plain films. In the normal cervical (C) spine (Fig. 2.2a), disk spaces are roughly equal in height at both the anterior and posterior margins across the different spinal segments [1]. In the thoracic (T) spine, the height of the intervertebral disk decreases from C7–T1 toward T4–T5, increases caudally to T10–T11, to finally decrease again at the T11–T12 level. In general, the disk height at the posterior margins is slightly smaller than at the anterior margin (Fig. 2.2b) [2]. At the lumbar spine, the height of the disks increases from cephalad to caudad up to the L4–L5 level. At the L5–S1 segment, the disk height is slightly less most noticeable at the posterior

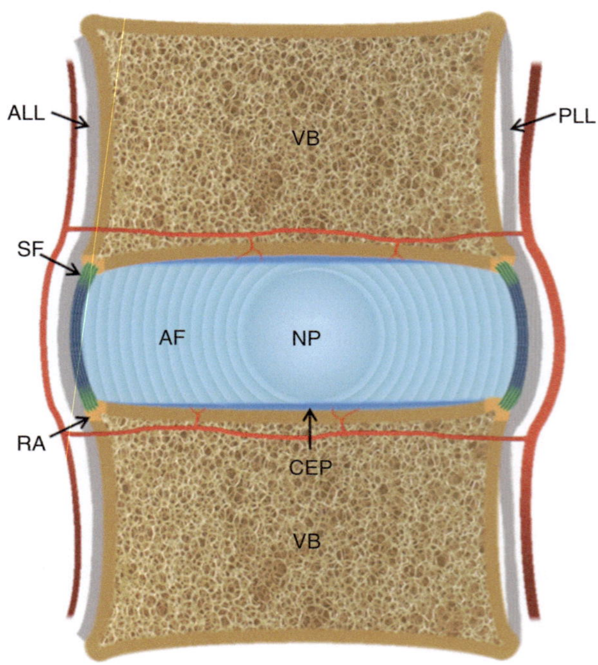


**Fig. 2.1** Schematic representation of the normal lumbar discovertebral complex. Vertebral bodies (VB), nucleus pulposus (NP), annulus fibrosus (AF), Sharpey's fibers (SF), anterior longitudinal ligament (ALL), posterior longitudinal ligament (PLL), and cartilaginous endplates (CEP)

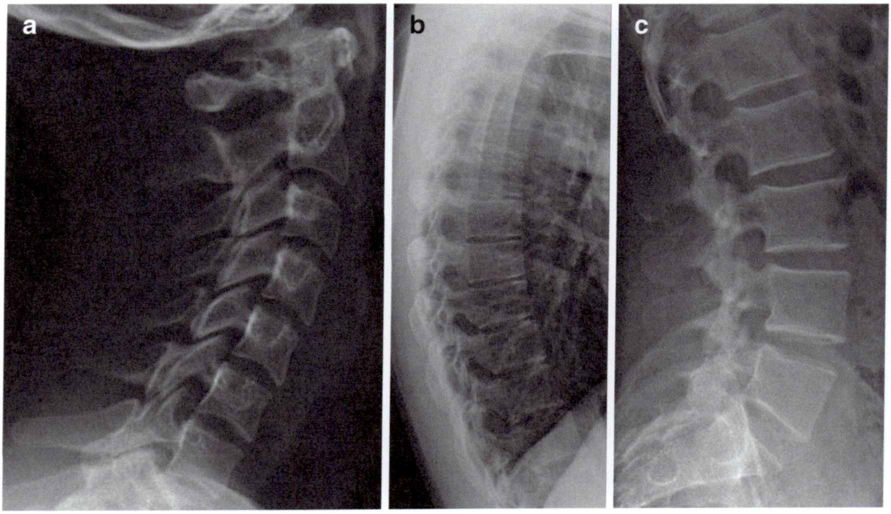


**Fig. 2.2** Lateral plain films of the normal cervical (**a**), thoracic (**b**), and lumbar (**c**) intervertebral disk s. (**a**) At the cervical spine, the disk spaces are roughly equal in height across the different spinal segments. (**b**) The normal height of the intervertebral disks decreases from C7–T1 toward T4–T5, increases caudally to T10–T11, and finally decreases again at the T11–T12 level. (**c**) At the lumbar spine, the height of the disks increases from T12–L1 until the L4–L5 level. At the L5–S1 segment, the disk height declines slightly and this is most pronounced posteriorly

margin (5) (Fig. 2.2c). Morphometric studies have shown that the height, width, and diameter of the intervertebral disk can vary significantly depending on age and sex of the patient. Detection of decreased disk heights should therefore rather be based on abrupt changes in the height of disk spaces than on small changes from the normal craniocaudal pattern [3].

### 2.2.3 CT Scan

Due to the limited contrast between various soft tissues, the internal architecture can only be grossly evaluated, and its sensitivity for the early stages of disk degeneration is weak. In young adults, the normal intervertebral disk does not extend beyond the interspace on axial CT scans [4] (Fig. 2.3).

### 2.2.4 MRI Scan

MRI is the imaging modality of choice to evaluate the intervertebral disk and to provide excellent anatomic detail of the disk. On MRI, the normal adult disk is of intermediate to low signal intensity on T1-weighted images and of high signal intensity on T2-weighted images, compared to the bone marrow in the adjacent

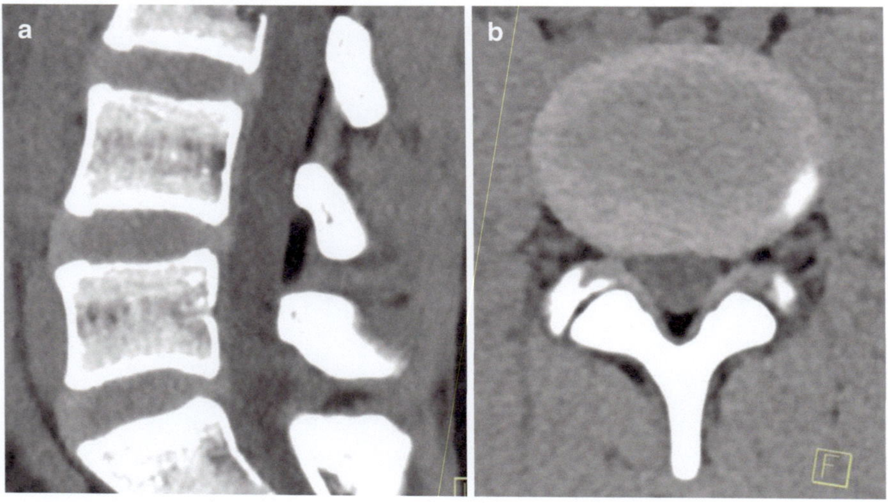


**Fig. 2.3** Sagittal reformatted (**a**) and axial (**b**) CT images in soft-tissue window of normal lumbar intervertebral disks. In young adults, the normal intervertebral disk does not extend beyond the interspace on axial CT images

vertebral bodies. On T2-weighted images, the normal bright nucleus pulposus and the inner annulus are indistinguishable. The outer annulus, which contains densely packed fibers, is hypointense on all pulse sequences (Fig. 2.4). As early as in the third decade, a horizontal band of decreased signal intensity on T2-weighted images appears in the nucleus pulposus. This is known as the intranuclear cleft and represents a fibrous transformation of the nucleus pulposus. The bright signal intensity of the intervertebral disks on T2-weighted images gradually decreases, until the disks eventually become hypointense. The loss of signal intensity is due to a decrease in water and proteoglycan content [4, 5]. There is a high interindividual variability in this sequence of normal aging (see Sect. 2.3).

### 2.2.5 Anatomical Variants

Block vertebrae are developmental anomalies due to failure of segmentation of the vertebral column during fetal development. There is fusion of the adjacent vertebrae at the intervertebral disk, but the posterior elements are usually involved as well. While block vertebrae can be completely fused, there often is a disk remnant that may be calcified. A "wasp-waist" sign can be seen at the level of the intervertebral disk between the fused segments. This finding is often absent in acquired vertebral fusions (Fig. 2.5). Another important diagnostic clue with acquired fusion is that the height of the individual vertebral bodies is preserved. Congenital block vertebrae most commonly occur at the cervical spine [6]. Block vertebrae may predispose to accelerated degeneration at the adjacent disk levels similar to what has been reported after surgical spinal fusion [7, 8]. Unilateral failure of segmentation is characterized by a bony bar between adjacent vertebra (Fig. 2.7e) [9]

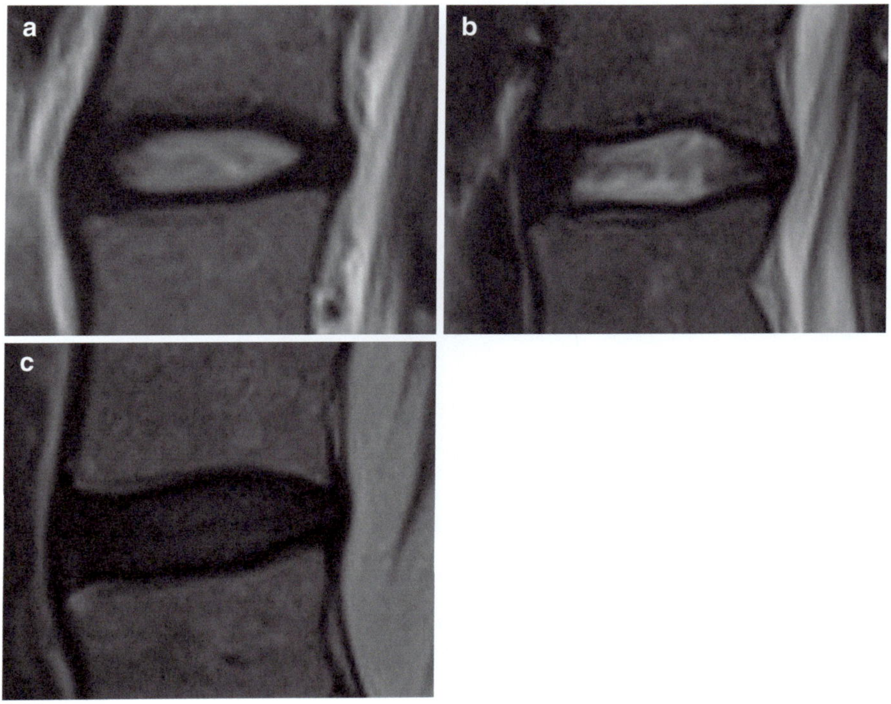


**Fig. 2.4** Normal aging process of the intervertebral disk on sagittal T2-weighted images. (**a**) Normal intervertebral disk in a 25-year-old adult. (**b**) The intranuclear cleft presenting as a thin hypointense band in the center of the nucleus pulposus in a 35 year old. (**c**). Normal intervertebral disk in a 65-year-old patient. The intervertebral disk has become hypointense. There is preservation of the disk height in all three patients

Lumbosacral transitional vertebrae are congenital spinal variants ranging between complete sacralization of the L5 vertebra to complete lumbarization of S1. When sacralization of L5 is present, there is a decrease in disk height between the lumbar transitional segment and the sacrum. Similarly, when a lumbarized S1 is present, the disk space between S1 and S2 is larger than the rudimentary disk that is most often seen. Castellvi et al. described a radiographic classification system identifying four types on the basis of morphologic characteristics (Fig. 2.6) [5, 10].

Hemivertebrae are incompletely formed vertebral column segments and can be classified into three types: fully segmented, semi-segmented, and non-segmented. A fully segmented hemivertebra has a normal disk space above and below (Fig. 2.7a). When a fully segmented vertebra is encapsulated by the adjacent vertebrae, it is also called incarcerated (Fig. 2.7b). Semi-segmented hemivertebrae are fused to one of the adjacent vertebral bodies and have a normal intervertebral disk on the opposite side (Fig. 2.7c). Finally, non-segmented hemivertebrae are in direct contact with surrounding vertebra without interposition of a disk (Fig. 2.7d) [6]. Simultaneous occurrence of hemivertebrae and unsegmented bars can occur, creating a mixed type (Fig. 2.7f) [9]. Unilateral failure of segmentation failures and hemivertebrae may cause secondary scoliosis [11].

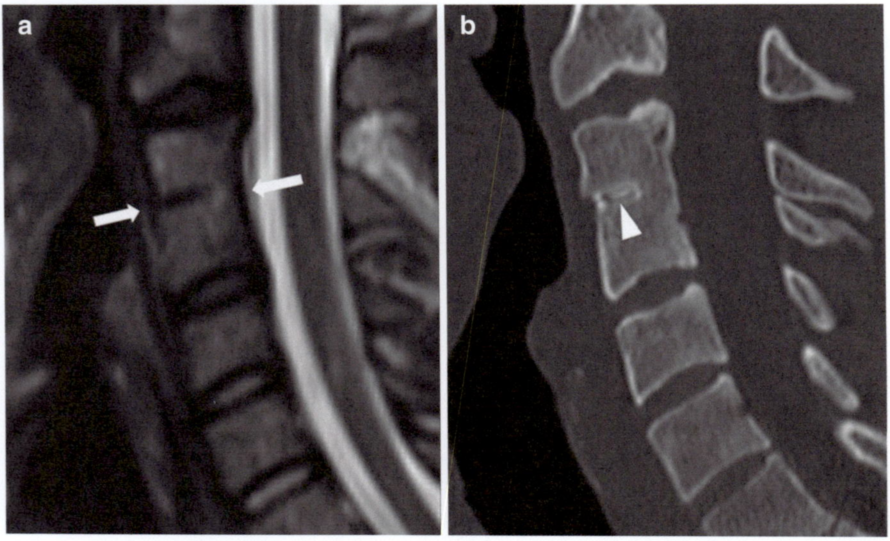


**Fig. 2.5** Sagittal T1-weighted image (**a**) and sagittal reformatted CT image (**b**)with bone window settings in a 53-year-old female demonstrates a block vertebra at the C3–C4 level. There is a calcified disk remnant between the fused vertebrae (arrowhead). Note the wasp-waist sign (arrows) as the diameter at the level of the disk remnant is smaller than the diameter at the superior and inferior limits of the vertebrae adjacent to uninvolved disks

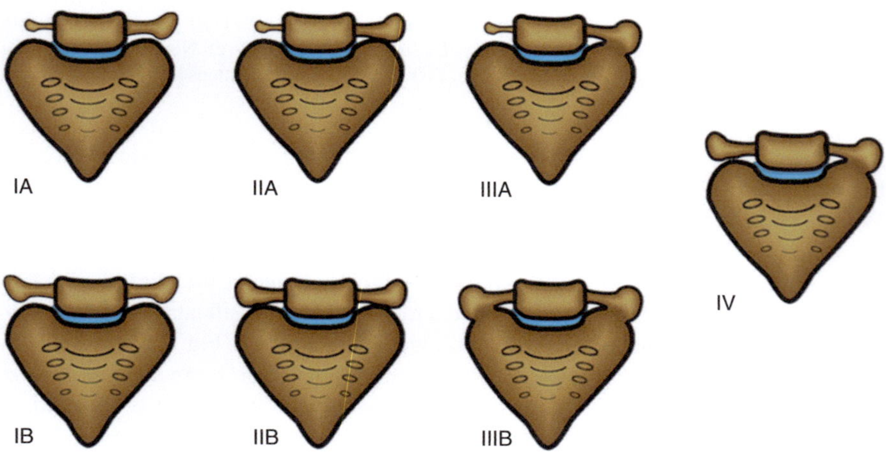


**Fig. 2.6** Schematic representation of the Castellvi classification. Type I consists of unilateral (IA) or bilateral (IB) dysplastic transverse processes, measuring at least 19 mm (superoinferior). Type II consists of incomplete unilateral (IIA) or bilateral (IIB) sacralization with an enlarged transverse process that has a diarthrodial joint between itself and the sacrum. Type III describes unilateral (IIIA) or bilateral (IIIB) lumbarization (or sacralization) with complete osseous fusion of the transverse process(es) to the sacrum. Type IV involves a unilateral type II transition with a type III on the contralateral side

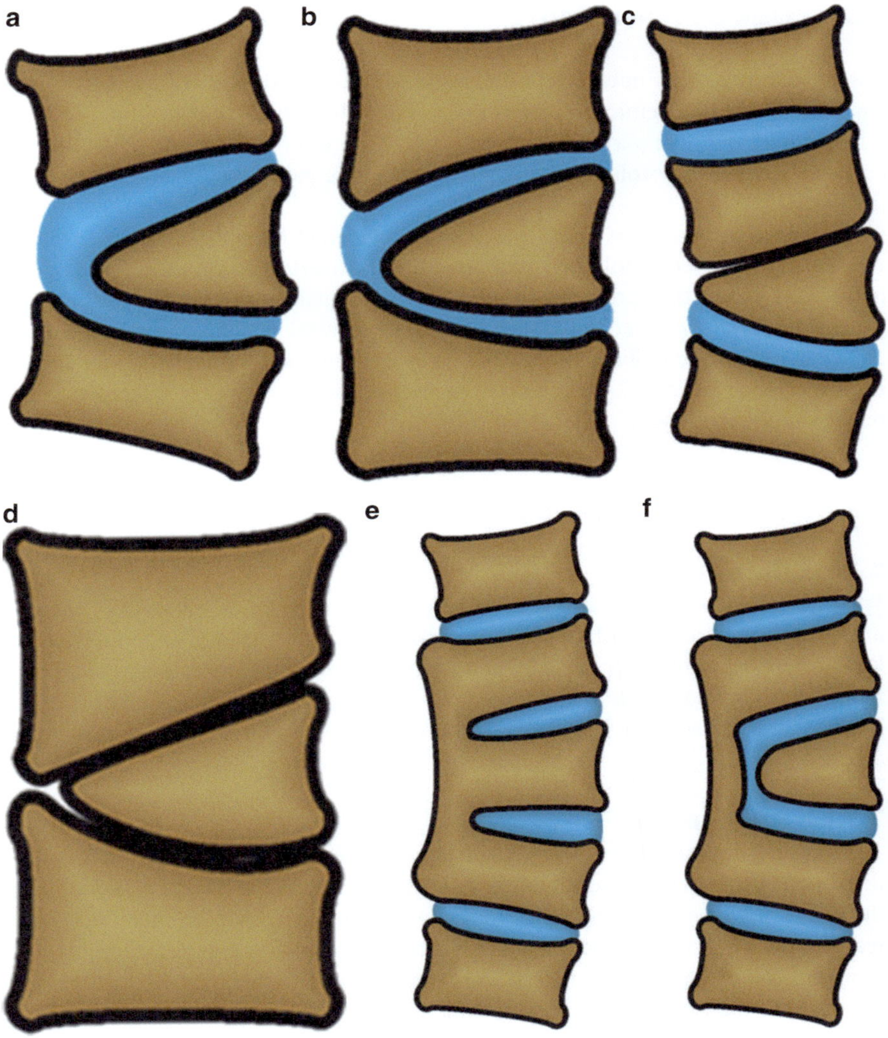


**Fig. 2.7** Defects of segmentation and formation: schematic representation. Fully segmented vertebra (**a**) with disk spaces on either side. Fully segmented incarcerated vertebra (**b**), demonstrating a hemivertebra encapsulated within the adjacent vertebrae. Compared to (**a**), there is absence of scoliosis. Semi-segmented vertebra (**c**) with a normal disk on the one side and an absent disk on the opposing side. A non-segmented vertebra (**d**) lies in direct contact with the adjacent vertebrae without interposing disks. Unsegmented bar vertebra (**e**) due to unilateral failure of segmentation. Finally, mixed type (**f**), which may be a combination of the above

## 2.3 Disk Degeneration

The appearance of an intervertebral disk on MRI is age-dependent because of the anatomical and biochemical changes that occur within the disk over time. There is a high interindividual variability of the normal aging process of the disk, and the borders between physiological disk aging and disk pathology is not always distinct [12].

Degenerative processes in the spine can be divided into three categories based on the primary involved histologic structure of the discovertebral complex. *Spondylosis deformans* affects the peripheral annulus fibrosus together with the adjacent apophyses. *Intervertebral osteochondrosis* affects the central nucleus pulposus and the adjacent vertebral endplates. It consists of a combination of peripheral and central disk disease [13]. In reality, however, these processes are closely linked and may occur simultaneously.

### 2.3.1 Spondylosis Deformans

#### 2.3.1.1 Definition

*Spondylosis deformans* is a degenerative process of the spine involving the outer annulus fibrosus and vertebral body apophysis, characterized by osteophytes (also known as spondylophytes at the level of the spine) arising from the vertebral body, most commonly at the anterolateral edges. The intervertebral disk height remains normal or decreases only slightly. Spondylosis deformans is usually not symptomatic [14].

#### 2.3.1.2 Pathogenesis

Tears of the annulus fibrosus may result in microinstability and cause anterolateral displacement of the intervertebral disk. Posterior displacement is uncommon due the firm attachment of the posterior longitudinal ligament. Displacement of the disk leads to traction on the attachments of Sharpey's fibers at the anterior longitudinal ligament and triggers the formation and growth of spondylophytes. Marginal osteophytes have their osseous site of attachment at the Sharpey's fibers enthesis, while nonmarginal phytes originate 2 to 3 mm away from the vertebral apophysis at the attachment of the anterior longitudinal ligament. Both follow an initial horizontal course before curving upward or downward, partially or completely bridging the intervertebral disk. Osteophytes are continuous with the spongiosa and cortical bone of the vertebral body (Fig. 2.8) [15]. In case of larger fissures at the outer annulus fibrosus, gas can occasionally accumulate and produce a linear radiolucency at the periphery of the intervertebral disk. Distraction of the vertebral surfaces or extension of the spine creates an environment with negative pressure. This "vacuum phenomenon" attracts nitrogen gas from the surrounding tissue into the clefts or disk [16, 17].

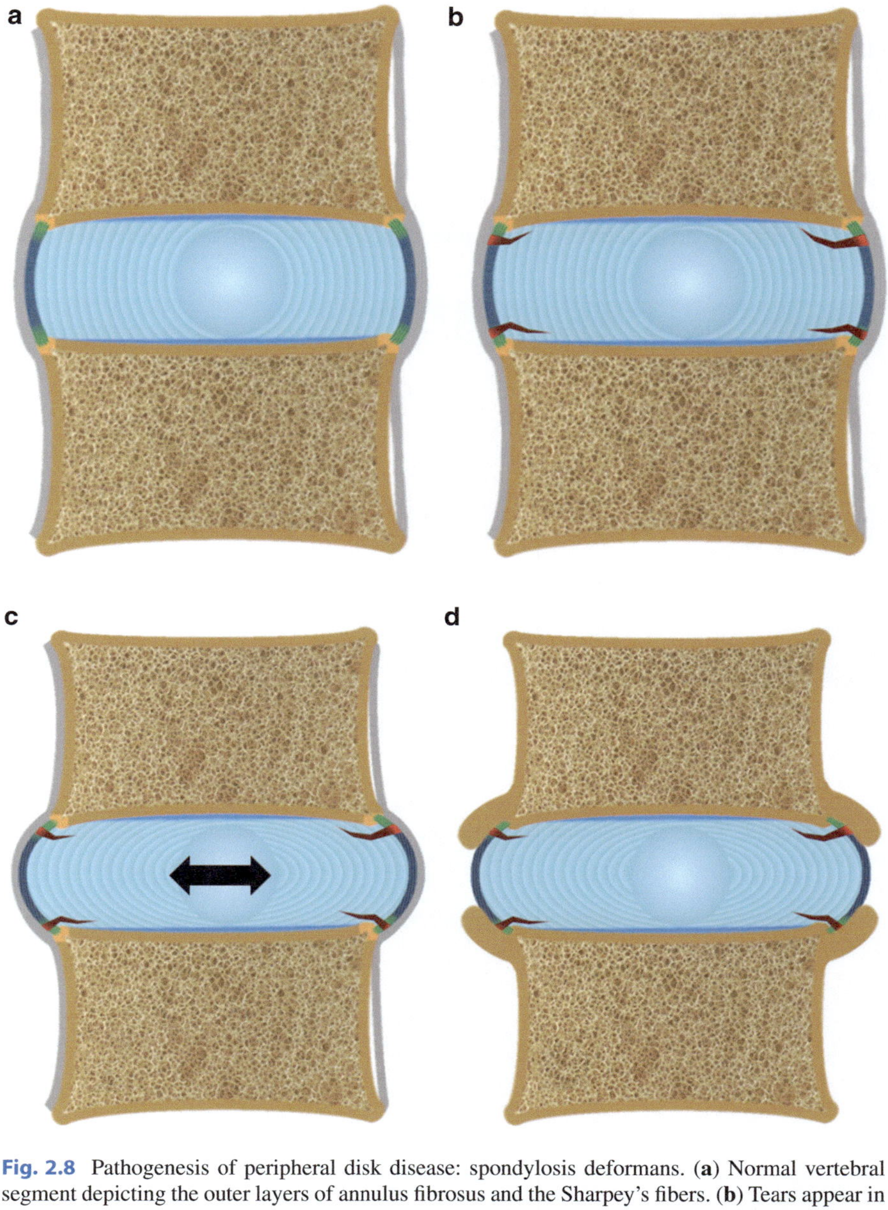


**Fig. 2.8** Pathogenesis of peripheral disk disease: spondylosis deformans. (**a**) Normal vertebral segment depicting the outer layers of annulus fibrosus and the Sharpey's fibers. (**b**) Tears appear in the outer annulus fibrosus due to degenerative processes. (**c**) These tears lead to microinstability of the discovertebral complex with resulting disk displacement (double arrow) with traction on the anterior longitudinal ligament and Sharpey's fibers. (**d**) Ultimately, there is formation of traction osteophytes

### 2.3.1.3 Imaging

Plain films (Fig. 2.9) and CT depict spondylophytes while the height of the intervertebral disks is preserved. Small amounts of gas are often seen at the periphery, located in annular tears [16]. Similar findings are found on MRI imaging together with "age-related" changes of the central intervertebral disks [17] (Fig. 2.10). Small spondylophytes can be difficult to detect on MRI. Spondylophytes are hypointense on both T1- and T2-weighted images and may blend in with the surrounding tissue. Annular fissures can be seen in asymptomatic patients and can be considered as part

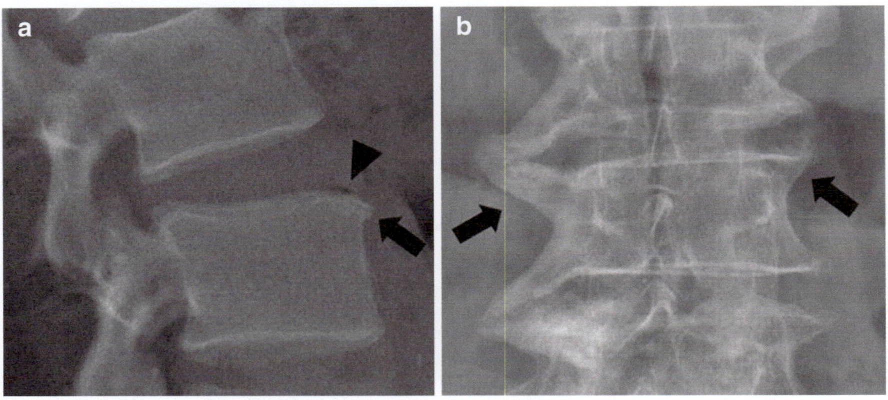


**Fig. 2.9** Radiography of spondylosis deformans. Lateral (**a**) plain films of the lumbar vertebra showing marginal osteophytes (arrows) and peripheral vacuum phenomenon (arrowheads). Anteroposterior (**b**) in another patient shows prominent lateral osteophytes also called claw spondylophytes (arrows). Fusion of spondylophytes of adjacent levels may result in so-called bridging spondylophytes. The spongiosa and cortex of the osteophytes are contiguous with the vertebral body

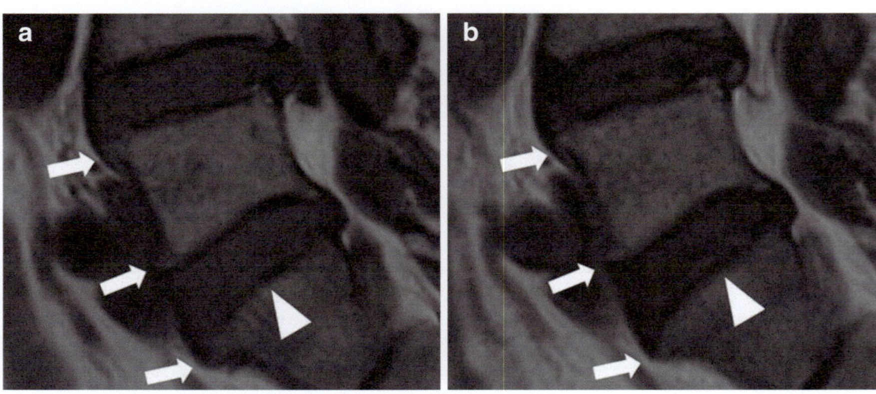


**Fig. 2.10** MRI of spondylosis deformans. Sagittal T1- (**a**) and T2-weighted (**b**) images of spondylosis deformans in a 67-year-old patient. There are anterolateral osteophytes at the L4–L5–S1 levels (arrows). There is preservation of the intervertebral disk height with an age appropriate-signal intensity of the disk (arrowhead)

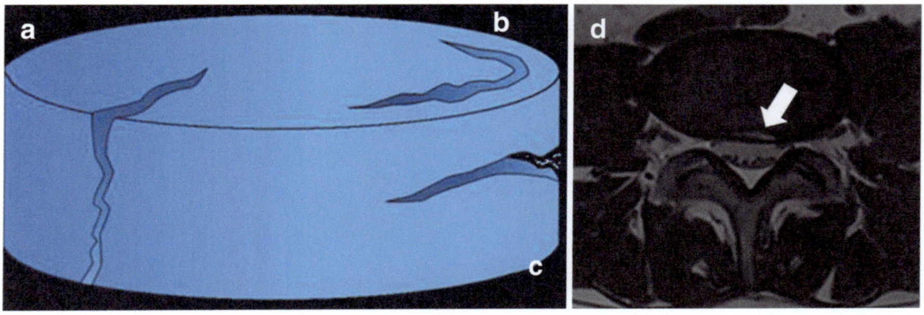


**Fig. 2.11** Schematic representation of the different annulus fibrosus fissures subtypes. (**a**) Radial, (**b**) concentric, and (**c**) transverse. Axial T2-weighted image of the L3–L4 segment depicts an abnormal linear hyperintensity in the posterior margin of the annulus fibrosus, indicating annular fissure (arrow)

of the aging normal process. These fissures can be concentric, radial, or transverse (Fig. 2.11). After administration of Gadolinium there is contrast enhancement is observed due to the presence of vascular granulation tissue [12]. On T2-weighted images, these tears present as hyperintense foci within the low signal annulus fibrosus as these fissures contain fluid.

## 2.3.2 Intervertebral (Osteo)Chondrosis

### 2.3.2.1 Definition

*Intervertebral (Osteo)chondrosis* is a degenerative process of the nucleus pulposus and the vertebral endplates. The term osteochondrosis is used if there are accompanying spondylophytes. It is not necessarily symptomatic [18].

### 2.3.2.2 Pathogenesis

With disk degeneration, there is dehydration and tissue loss of the nucleus pulposus leading to a decrease in disk height and the formation of fissures (Fig. 2.12). With further progression, the crevices extend more peripherally to the inner and subsequently to the outer fibers of the annulus fibrosus [19]. Due to negative pressure, gas from neighboring tissues is attracted into these fissures. Large amounts of gas in the central disk space are highly indicative of degeneration of the nucleus pulposus. Rarely, gas may occur with infection due to gas-forming organisms [16]. Similar to spondylosis deformans, tears in the annulus fibrosus may lead to displacement of the disk with subsequent reactive formation of osteophytes. With degeneration, microscopic calcifications occur in the cartilaginous endplate. These calcifications may occlude the vascular openings, decreasing nutrient supply to the disk, initiating or aggravating intervertebral chondrosis. This process of calcification and resorption together with microfractures is also responsible for the destruction of the endplates [13]. Disk material may protrude cranially or caudally through the weakened endplates into the vertebral body. These herniations are called

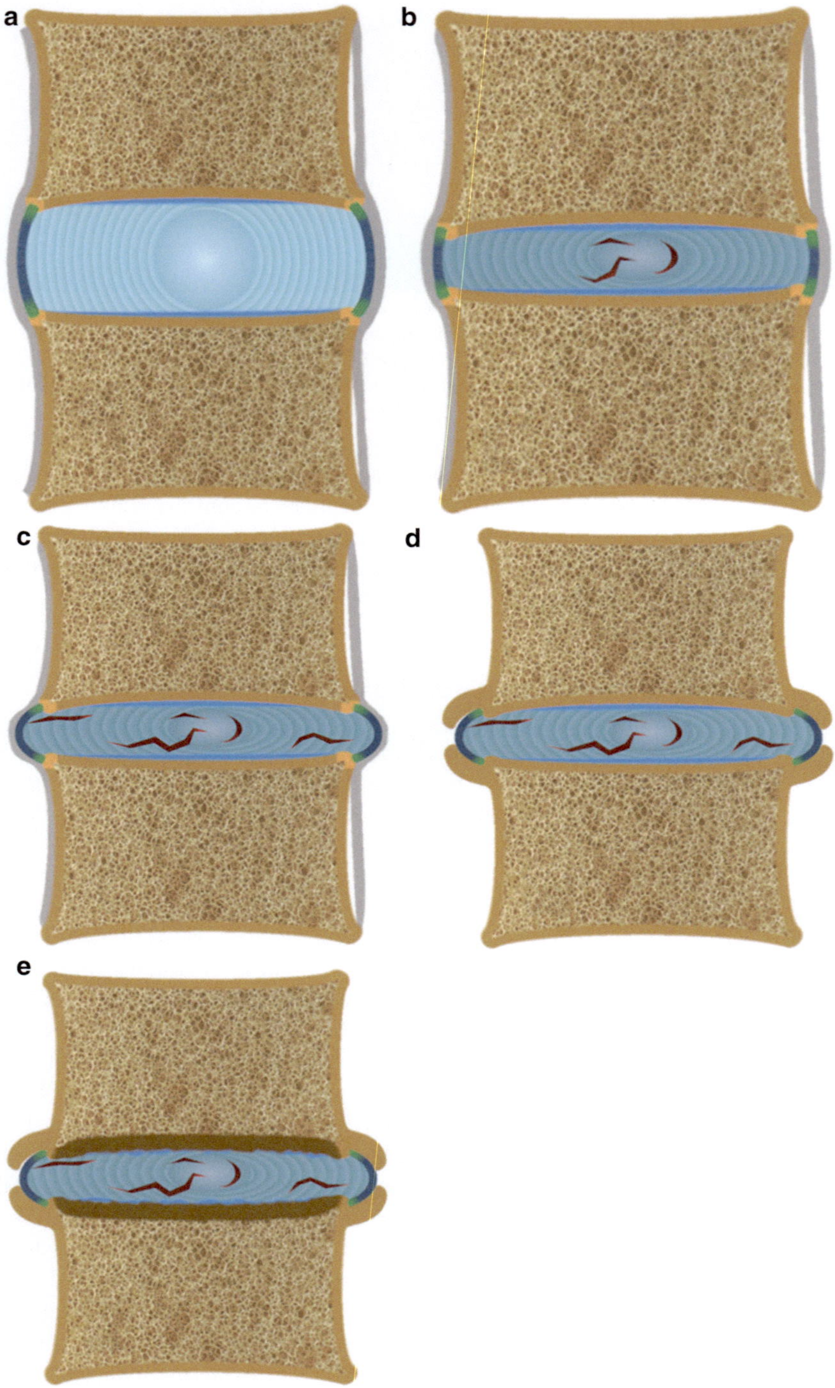
a
b
c
d
e

Schmorl's nodes [20]. Schmorl's nodes will be discussed in more detail in Sect. 2.3.4.

#### 2.3.2.3 Imaging

Standard radiography (Fig. 2.13a) and CT (Fig. 2.13b) show subchondral sclerosis of the vertebral endplates, loss of disk space height, spondylophytes, and a vacuum phenomenon located centrally in the disk space, manifesting as radiolucent stripes or rounded areas [21].

MRI is the imaging modality of choice to depict (early) changes of intervertebral (osteo)chondrosis (Fig. 2.13c, d). Degeneration of the disk was classified by Pfirrmann et al. based on a combination of T2-weighted characteristics: structure (I) and signal intensity (II) of the disk, distinction between the nucleus pulposus and the annulus fibrosus (III), and the intervertebral disk height (IV) (Fig. 2.14) [4]. A modified grading system by Griffith et al. adds three more stages and includes a quantitative measurement of the disk height reduction in severely dehydrated disks to allow better discrimination when assessing disks in the elderly spine (Table 2.1) [18].

Changes in the vertebral body endplates and bone marrow observed with degenerative disk disease were first described by Modic et al. [22]. These changes are classified into three categories depending on the T1- and T2-weighted characteristics (Fig. 2.15) (Table 2.2). Type I represents bone marrow edema and inflammation. On MRI, a low signal intensity on T1-weighted and a high signal intensity on T2-weighted images are seen. In type II, red bone marrow is replaced by fatty yellow bone marrow due to ischemic changes. These changes are of high signal intensity on both T1- and T2-weighted images. Type III changes are due to subchondral fibrosis and sclerosis and are of low signal intensity on both T1- and T2-weighted images [12]. Type II changes are the most common, with type III changes being the least common [23]. Previous studies have shown that Modic type I changes have the strongest association with low back pain [24]. A recent systematic review by Herlin et al. suggests rather an association between pain and type II changes. This discrepancy could be attributed to the fact that Modic type I and II changes can coexist at the same vertebral level or at different levels within the same individual [25].

**Fig. 2.12** Schematic pathogenesis of intervertebral (osteo)chondrosis. (**a**) Normal vertebral segment depicting the annulus fibrosus and the Sharpey's fibers. (**b**) Dehydration of the nucleus pulposus results in loss of disk height and the formation of fissures or tears centrally within the disk. (**c**) With further progression, the fissures extend more peripherally to the inner and subsequently to the outer fibers of the annulus fibrosus. (**d**) Similar to spondylosis deformans, peripheral tears in the annulus fibrosus may lead to displacement of the disk with subsequent reactive formation of osteophytes. (**e**) Simultaneously with disk degeneration, reactive endplate changes may occur

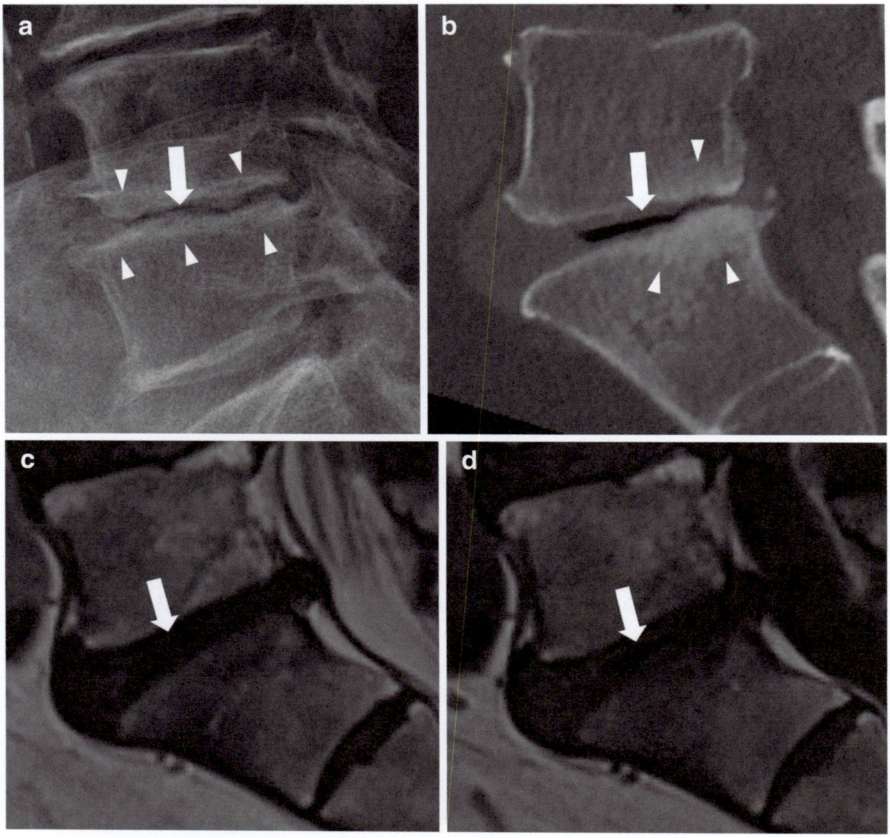


**Fig. 2.13** Imaging abnormalities of intervertebral osteochondrosis. Lateral plain film (**a**) vacuum phenomenon at the level of L4–L5 presenting as a linear radiolucency in the disk space (arrow). There is loss of the disk space with reactive sclerosis of the vertebral body endplates (arrowheads). Osteophytes are seen on the anterolateral aspect of the vertebral body. Sagittal reformatted CT with bone window settings (**b**). There is loss of the disk space height with reactive sclerosis of the vertebral body endplates at the L5–S1 level (arrowheads) and a centrally located vacuum phenomenon (arrows). Posterior osteophytes are seen at the L5–S1 level. On T2-Weighted image (**c**) and T1-Weighted image (**d**) in the same patient as (**b**) the hypointense vacuum phenomenon (arrows) is visible as a hypointense band on all pulse sequences. Endplate sclerosis (Modic type III) is hypointense as well on both pulse sequences

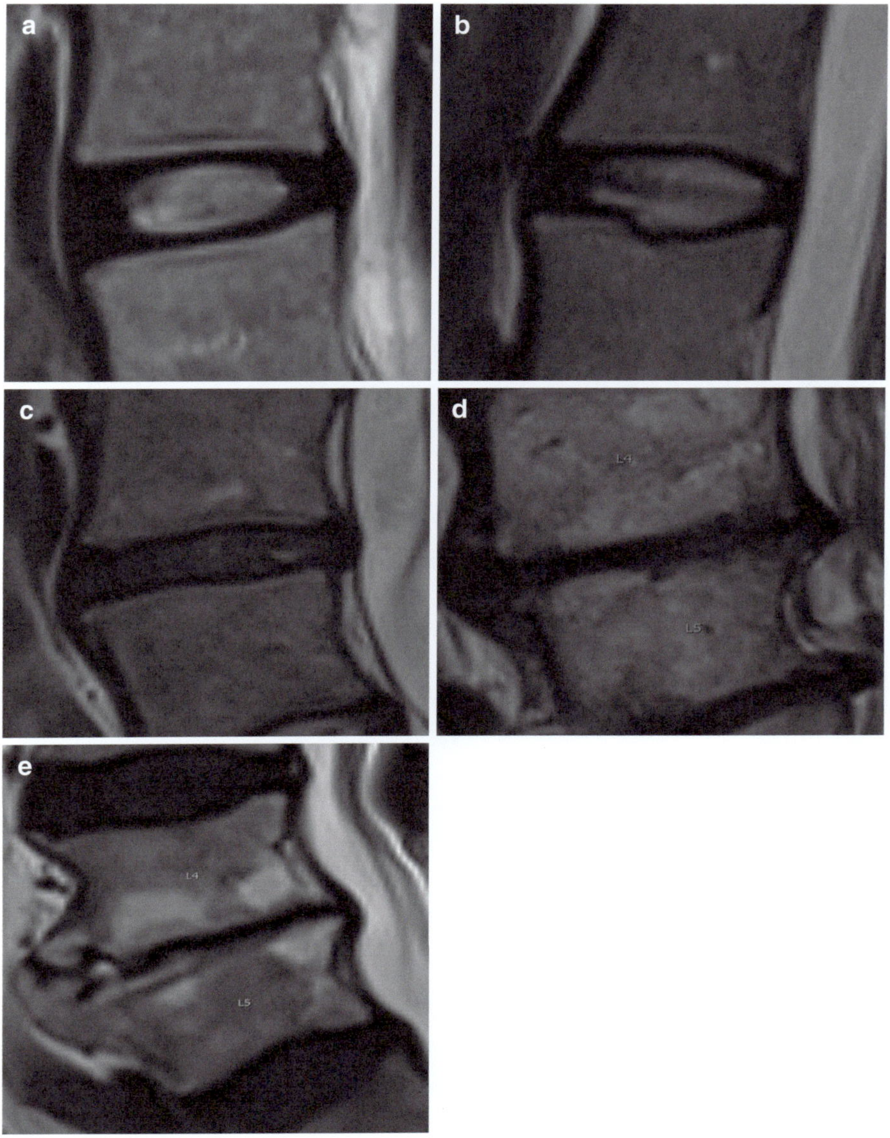


**Fig. 2.14** Pfirrmann grading system for lumbar disk degeneration on sagittal T2-weighted MRI images. Grade I (**a**), homogeneous disk with a hyperintense signal intensity, and a normal disk height. Grade II (**b**), the internal structure of the disk is inhomogeneous. A hyperintense signal surrounds the intranuclear cleft and the latter representing as a central hypointense band. There is a clear distinction between nucleus and annulus, and the disk height is normal. Grade III (**c**), the disk is inhomogeneous, with an intermediate signal intensity. The distinction between nucleus and annulus is unclear, and the disk height is normal or slightly decreased. Grade IV (**d**), the structure of the disk is inhomogeneous, with a hypointense signal. The distinction between nucleus and annulus is lost, and the disk height is markedly decreased. Finally, in Grade V (**e**), the disk space is collapsed

**Table 2.1** Comparison between the lumbar disk classification systems of Pfirrmann and Griffith on T2-weighted images with fat saturation

| Grade | | Structure | | Signal intensity | | Distinction NP and AF | | Disk height | |
|---|---|---|---|---|---|---|---|---|---|
| P | G | Pfirrmann | Griffith | Pfirrmann | Griffith | Pfirrmann | Griffith | Pfirrmann | Griffith |
| I | 1 | Homogenous | | Hyperintense | | Clear | | Normal | |
| II | 2 | Inhomogeneous ± intranuclear cleft | | Hyperintense + horizontal hypointense band | SI > CSF | Clear | | Normal | |
| | 3 | | | | SI < CSF | | | | |
| III | 4 | Inhomogeneous | | Intermediate | Intermediate | Unclear | | Normal or slightly decreased | Normal |
| | 5 | | | | Hypointense | | | | |
| | 6 | | | | | | | | <30% |
| IV | 7 | Inhomogeneous | | Hypointense | | Indistinct | | Moderately decreased | 30% < H < 60% |
| V | 8 | Inhomogeneous | | Hypointense | | Indistinct | | Collapse | >60% |

*G* Griffith, *H* height, *P* Pfirrmann

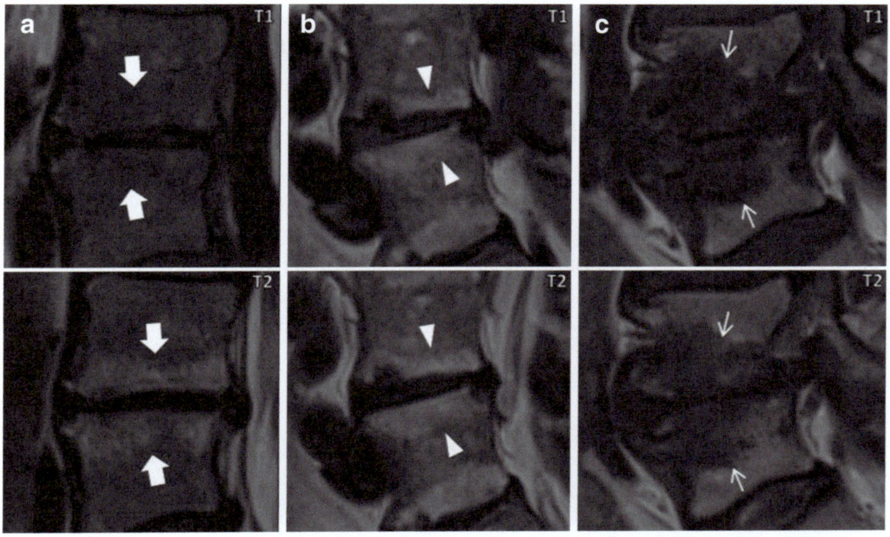


**Fig. 2.15** Modic type endplate changes. Sagittal T1- and T2-weighted images. Modic type 1 (**a**) changes at L4–L5 level. There is decreased signal intensity on T1-weighted images and increased signal intensity on T2-weighted images (thick arrows), indicating inflammation with bone marrow edema. There is a loss of the intervertebral disk height with posterior bulging. Modic type 2 (**b**) changes at L4–L5 level. There is increased signal intensity on T1-weighted images and mildly increased signal intensity on T2-weighted images (arrowheads), in keeping with conversion to fatty bone marrow. Note a Schmorl's node in the lower endplate of L4. Modic type 3 (**c**) changes at L4–L5 level. There is decreased signal intensity on T1-weighted images and decreased signal intensity on T2-weighted images (thin arrows), in keeping with reactive sclerosis

**Table 2.2** Modic type endplates changes

| | Signal intensity | | |
|---|---|---|---|
| Type | T1 | T2 | Histology |
| I | Low | High | Edema (fibrovascular tissue) |
| II | High | High | Fat |
| III | Low | Low | Sclerosis |

## 2.3.3 Kümmel Phenomenon

### 2.3.3.1 Definition

Kümmel disease is the eponymous name for avascular necrosis with delayed vertebral collapse after a vertebral fracture. Inadequate revascularization of bone marrow predisposes to ischemic necrosis of the vertebral body and may result in subsequent vertebral collapse [26].

### 2.3.3.2 Imaging

On plain radiographs, Kümmel disease typically presents as an intravertebral air-filled cleft and a linear radiolucency within the subchondral bone of the vertebral body (Fig. 2.16a). This cleft represents fractures of necrotic bone, similar to the crescent sign seen in osteonecrosis at the femoral or humeral head. Although the process is not primarily located in the intervertebral disk, it may secondarily involve the adjacent disk space. If the intravertebral gas extends into the intervertebral disk, it may mimic degenerative disk disease [27]. Pseudoarthrosis of the intervertebral body is another classic sign of Kümmel disease and can be detected on flexion or extension radiographs. CT scans depict these changes more accurately but are not always mandatory for the diagnosis. On MRI, the intravertebral vacuum cleft is seen as low signal intensity area on all pulse sequences. In early stages of Kümmel disease intravertebral fluid can be seen [28]. The combination of gas and fluid may cause an air-fluid level on T2-weighted images (Fig. 2.16c).

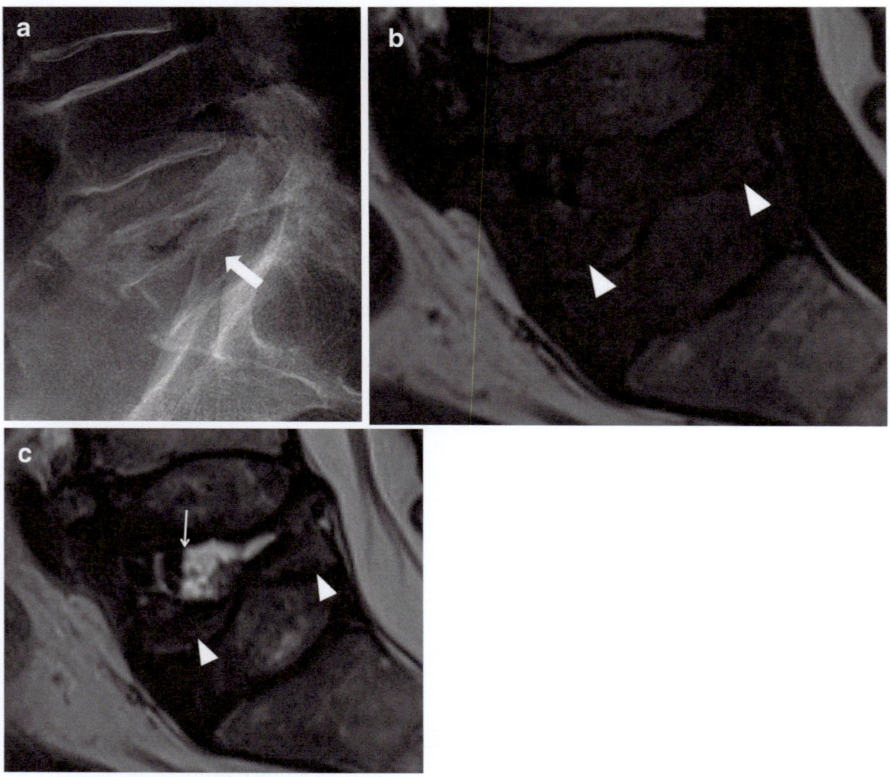


**Fig. 2.16** Imaging of Kümmel disease. Lateral (**a**) plain film of the lumbar spine demonstrates an intravertebral vacuum cleft sign at L5 as a band-like radiolucency within the collapsed vertebral body of L5 (arrow). Sagittal T1- (**b**) and T2- (**c**) weighted images show an abnormal hypointense bone marrow signal in the vertebral body of L5 due to vertebral collapse (arrowheads). The area of signal void on both sequences seen anteriorly in the disk represents a collection of gas. On the T2-weighted image in supine position, an air-fluid level is seen (thin arrow)

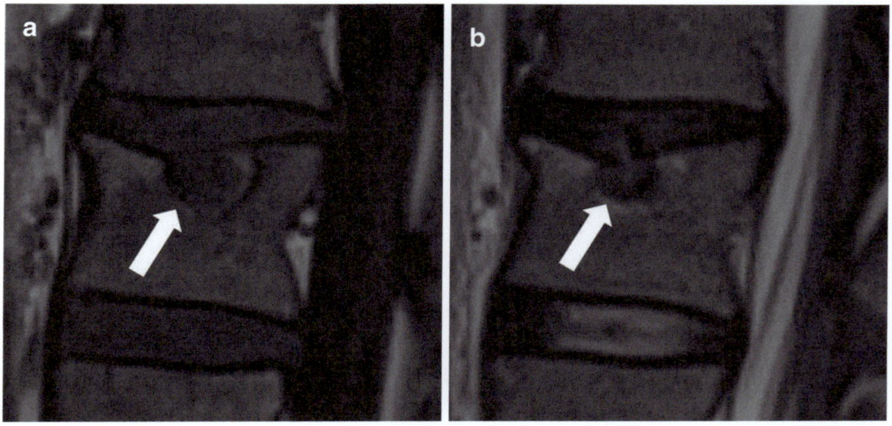


**Fig. 2.17** Sagittal T1- (**a**) and T2-weighted (**b**) images demonstrate a large Schmorl's node (arrows) at the upper endplate of Th8. The herniated disk has retained a signal intensity similar to the adjacent disk

### 2.3.4 Schmorl's Nodes

According to most authors, Schmorl's nodes is caused by herniations of the nucleus pulposus through the cartilaginous endplates into the vertebral body (Fig. 2.17). These intravertebral discal displacements may occur in a variety of disease processes such as degeneration, trauma, or Scheuermann's disease [20]. Others have attributed the occurrence of Schmorl's nodes due to subchondral necrosis. This pathogenetic mechanism may explain why the disk has a normal imaging appearance (Fig. 2.18) [29]. Whatever the etiology may be, the radiological appearance is similar. Schmorl's nodes appear as radiolucent depressions surrounded by a sclerotic rim at the vertebral endplates on plain films and CT. A branching pattern of gas within the herniations may be seen. On MRI, these lesions have the same signal characteristics as the adjacent disk [30].

In Scheuermann's disease, these protrusions are commonly found in the thoracic spine located in the anterior third of the vertebral body. There may be compensatory bone overgrowth of the opposing endplate (Edgren-Vaino sign) (Fig. 2.19). Schmorl's nodes need to be differentiated from notochord remnants. These focal depressions are typically located in the posterior third, usually in the two opposing endplates, and span several segments of the thoracic spine or the thoracolumbar junction [31].

## 2.4 Inflammation

*Spondyloarthritis* (SpA) represents a group of inflammatory disorders with interrelated clinical features and an association with HLA-B27. SpA includes ankylosing spondylitis, psoriatic arthritis, reactive arthritis, and SpA associated with

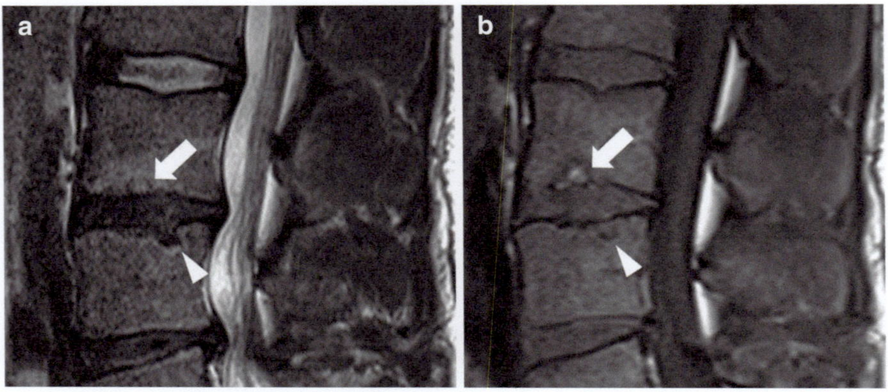


**Fig. 2.18** Sagittal T2- (**a**) and T1-weighted (**b**) images show a well-delineated early Schmorl's node (arrows) at the lower endplate of L3. These are believed to represent focal zones of osteonecrosis. There is subtle surrounding bone marrow edema. A second Schmorl's node with subtle disk herniation is seen in the upper endplate of L4 (arrowhead)

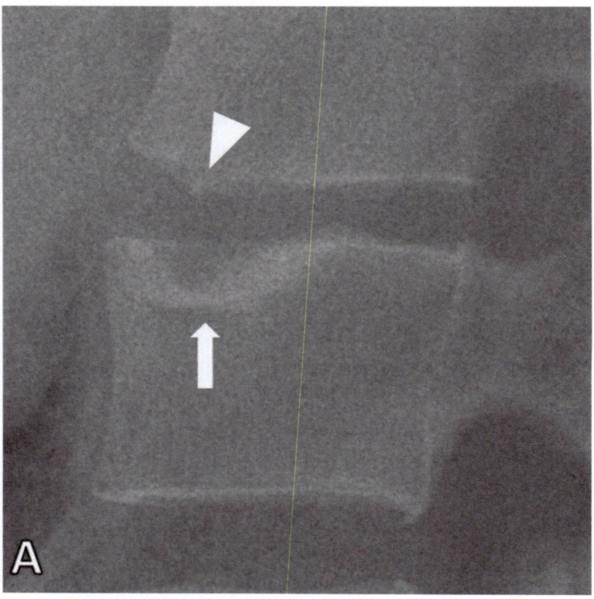


**Fig. 2.19** Lateral plain film of the thoracic spine depicting the Edgren-Vaino sign. There is a Schmorl's node in the upper vertebral endplate of Th10 (arrow). Reactive compensatory bony overgrowth (arrowhead) at the opposing endplate of Th9 is seen

inflammatory bowel disease (Table 2.3) [32]. The characteristic targets of the inflammatory process in SpA in the spine are the entheses corresponding to the site where ligaments (and tendons elsewhere in the body) attach to the bone. SpA with predominant axial involvement and sacroiliitis on plain films are labeled "axial

**Table 2.3** Overview of the subtypes of Spondylarthropathies (SpA)

| Spondylarthropathies |
|---|
| Ankylosing spondylitis |
| Psoriatic arthritis |
| Reactive arthritis |
| SpA associated with inflammatory bowel disease (Crohn, ulcerative colitis) |
| Juvenile |
| Undifferentiated |

spondyloarthritis" (axSpA). SpA without radiographic sacroiliitis is designated as "nonradiographic axial spondyloarthritis" (nr-axSpA) [33]. This section will focus on the imaging manifestations of spondylarthritis at the entheses of the discovertebral junction. The different SpA subtypes may have similar imaging characteristics. As ankylosing spondylitis (AS) is the prototype of SpA, most of the discussion will focus on AS.

### 2.4.1 Ankylosing Spondylitis

#### 2.4.1.1 Definition

The peak onset is around 15–30 years, and AS rarely manifests after the age of 50. The most typical symptom is low back pain with morning back stiffness that lasts for 30 min or more, improves with activity, and worsens after periods of inactivity [33]. Sacroiliitis is the earliest site of onset and the hallmark of the disease. Detailed discussion of sacroiliitis however is not within the scope of this book. In the spine, the thoracolumbar region is the preferred site of involvement, while the cervical spine may be affected in later stages of the disease.

#### 2.4.1.2 Pathogenesis

The exact mechanism that triggers the inflammatory response in ankylosing spondylitis is unknown. The entheses of the discovertebral junction are the primary targets of spinal ankylosing spondylitis and the anterior edges are most commonly involved (Fig. 2.20) [34]. An inflammatory reaction with accompanying bone marrow edema may lead to erosions of the bone. Healing of erosion may cause reactive bone formation. Ultimately, the fibrosis and ossification of the eroded defect between the bone and Sharpey's fibers lead to the formation of syndesmophytes. Finally, spread of this ossification process underneath the anterior longitudinal ligament may result in ankylosis of the spine (so-called bamboo spine formation). These pathogenic processes occur simultaneously rather than consecutively, leading to a mixed pattern of lysis, sclerosis, and ankylosis [35, 36].

#### 2.4.1.3 Imaging

The most early radiographic signs of AS in the spine are erosions at the insertion of the outer layers of the annulus fibrosus at the vertebral rim apophysis. On plain films, these erosions, called "Romanus lesions," can be seen at the superior and

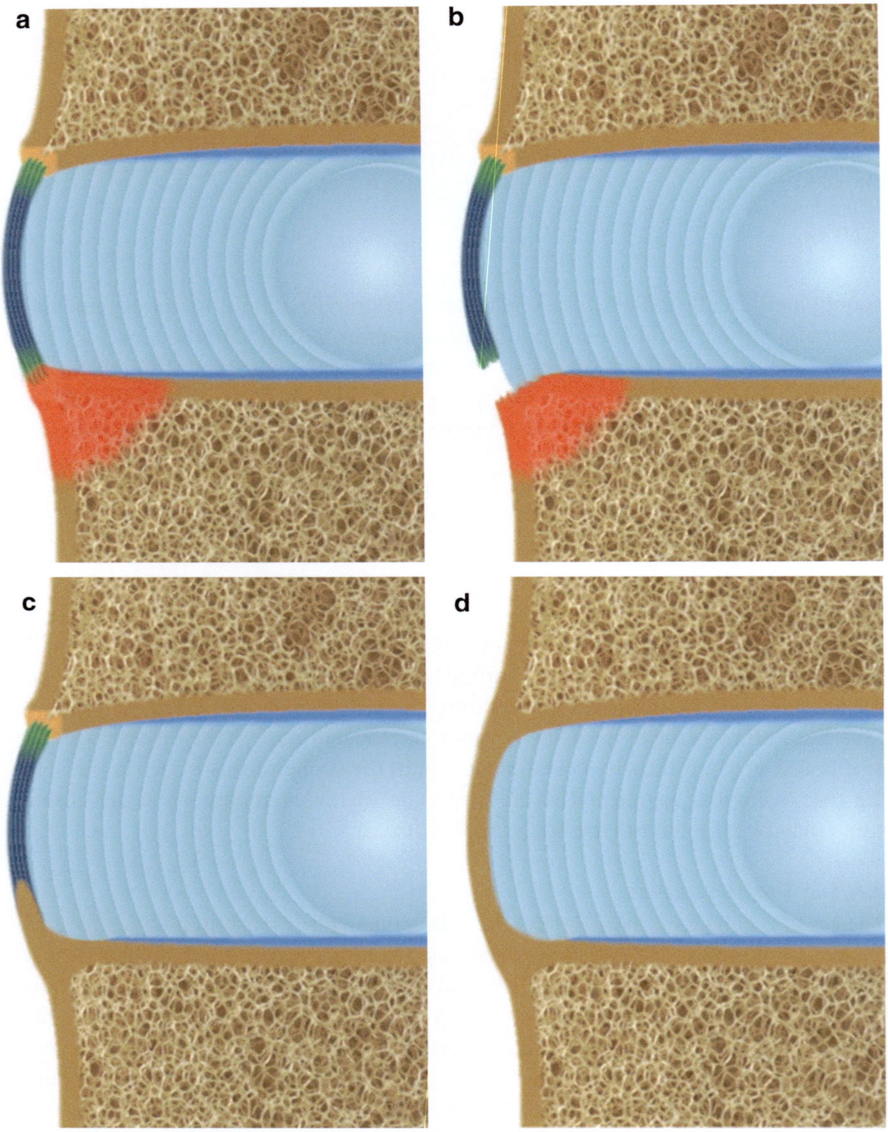


**Fig. 2.20** Schematic representation of the pathogenesis of ankylosing spondylitis in the spine. Inflammation and bone marrow edema (**a**) at the entheses. This inflammatory process leads to erosions and reactive sclerosis of bone at the enthesis (**b**). Vertically oriented reactive bone formation may result in an osseous bridge between the altered margins of the entheses and the Sharpey's fibers (**c**). Finally, spread of this ossification process may result in ankyloses of the spine with bamboo spine formation (**d**)

inferior vertebral margins [37] (Fig. 2.21a). The reactive bone formation and sclerosis at the site of these Romanus lesions lead to the appearance of "shiny corners" on radiographs [38]. When the periosteal deposition of new bone extends along the anterior edge of the vertebrae, the normal concavity is replaced by a more squared appearance of the vertebral body (Fig. 2.21b). This phenomenon is most obvious at the lumbar spine where normal vertebrae are always concave anteriorly, whereas normal thoracic and cervical vertebra have more variable contours [13]. With disease progression, the characteristic finding of spinal disease in AS is the development of syndesmophytes (Fig. 2.22a) when ossification occurs at the Sharpey's fibers and outer annulus fibrosus. These syndesmophytes are slender and bilaterally and vertically oriented the new bone formations originating from the apophyseal ring of the vertebra and growing along the periphery of the intervertebral space. Ultimately, syndesmophytes form osseous bridges across the intervertebral space resulting in a bamboo spine appearance (Fig. 2.22b) [39]. Supra- and interspinous ligaments may ossify as well and are visible on frontal radiographs as an ossified band between the spinous processes called the *dagger sign*. When this ligamentous ossification is accompanied by the fusion of the facet joints, three vertical

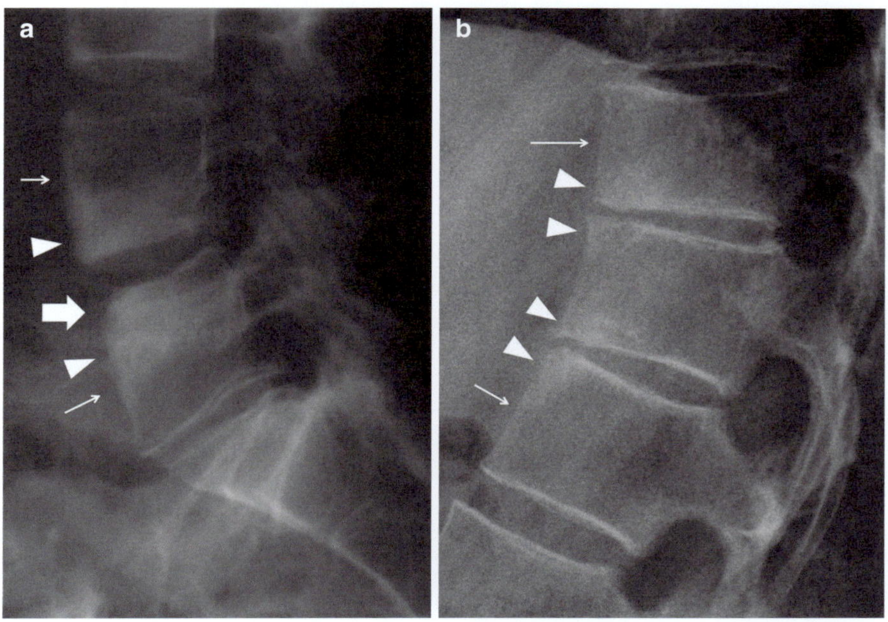


**Fig. 2.21** Lateral plain film (**a**) of the lumbar spine and thoracolumbar junction (**b**) in patients with ankylosing spondylitis. There is a Romanus lesion (arrow) at the anterosuperior margin of the L5 vertebra. Erosions are the earliest finding of AS on radiographs. Simultaneously, there is reactive bone formation with squaring of the vertebrae (thin arrows) and sclerosis of the vertebral margins in keeping with shiny corners (arrowheads)

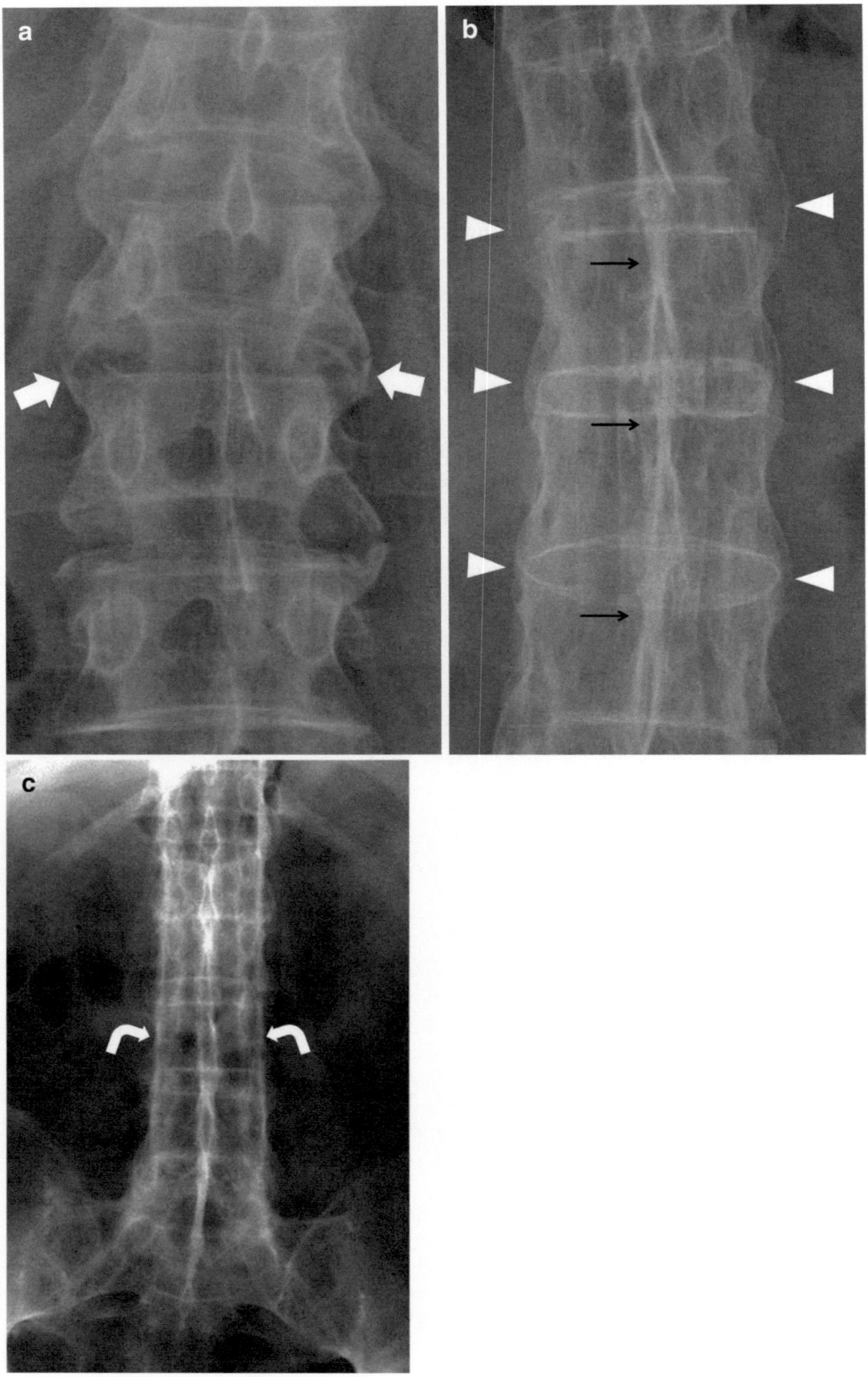
a
b
c

radiopaque lines, the *trolley-track sign*, are visible on anteroposterior radiographs (Fig. 2.22c) [38].

Andersson lesions, another late feature of AS, are characterized by extensive involvement of the intervertebral disk (Fig. 2.23a). There is destruction of the disco-vertebral complex with erosions extending into the subchondral bone of the vertebral body. The exact etiology is unknown, but traumatic events or chronic mechanical stress are thought to play an important role [40]. On plain films, this process is depicted by erosions or destruction of the vertebral endplates with surrounding areas of reactive sclerosis. Andersson lesions or occult fractures may lead to instability and movement of the ankylosed spine, creating pseudo-arthrosis-like changes and reactive osteophytes [41].

Patients with an ankylosed spine are at risk for spine fracture with minor trauma due to the accompanying disuse osteoporosis and ankylosis. Chance fractures involve the three spinal columns and often occur at the cervicothoracic and thoracolumbar junctions. Mechanical stress near these junctions is increased due to the transition from kyphosis to lordosis or vice versa [42]. As these fractures may be difficult to visualize on radiographs, additional CT of the spine may be necessary [43]. In case of a neurological deficit, MRI is mandatory for the evaluation of spinal cord lesions.

CT allows visualization of the same pathological processes as plain radiographs (erosion, sclerosis, ossification, ankylosis, and bone demineralization) with the benefit of multiplanar imaging and greater sensitivity for fractures [42].

MRI is the most sensitive imaging method to detect early inflammatory changes of the spine and to detect subchondral bone marrow edema, commonly at the anterior edges of the vertebral body, at the silent radiograph stage. Early Romanus lesions (Fig. 2.24) are hypointense on T1-weighted MR images and hyperintense on T2-weighted images. There is enhancement on T1-weighted post-gadolinium images. Romanus lesions may be easily confused with Modic type I marrow changes of degenerative disease. However, in AS (and SpA in general) three or more vertebral corners are involved with the absence of degenerative disk disease [44]. Furthermore, AS and SpA are more frequent at the thoracolumbar junction while degenerative disease has a predilection for the lower lumbar spine [45]. As the disease progresses, fatty bone marrow deposition at the apophyseal rim increases the signal intensity of T1-weighted images. These areas of fatty deposition characterize the inactive Romanus lesions and are believed to be predictive of formation of syndesmophytes [46]. However, this is still a matter of ongoing debate in the current literature [47]. According to some authors [48], the presence of more than five fatty corners is

**Fig. 2.22** Anteroposterior radiographs of the upper lumbar spine (**a**) show multiple syndesmophytes (arrows) as thin, vertical bony outgrowths. The Dagger sign (thin arrows) (**b**) is a central radiopaque band related to the ossification of the supra- and interspinous ligaments. There is ankylosis of the spine leading to the characteristic "bamboo" spine appearance (arrowheads). The trolley-track sign (curved arrows) (**c**) consists of the combination of the central band of ossification and two lateral dense bands, representing ossification of the facet joints

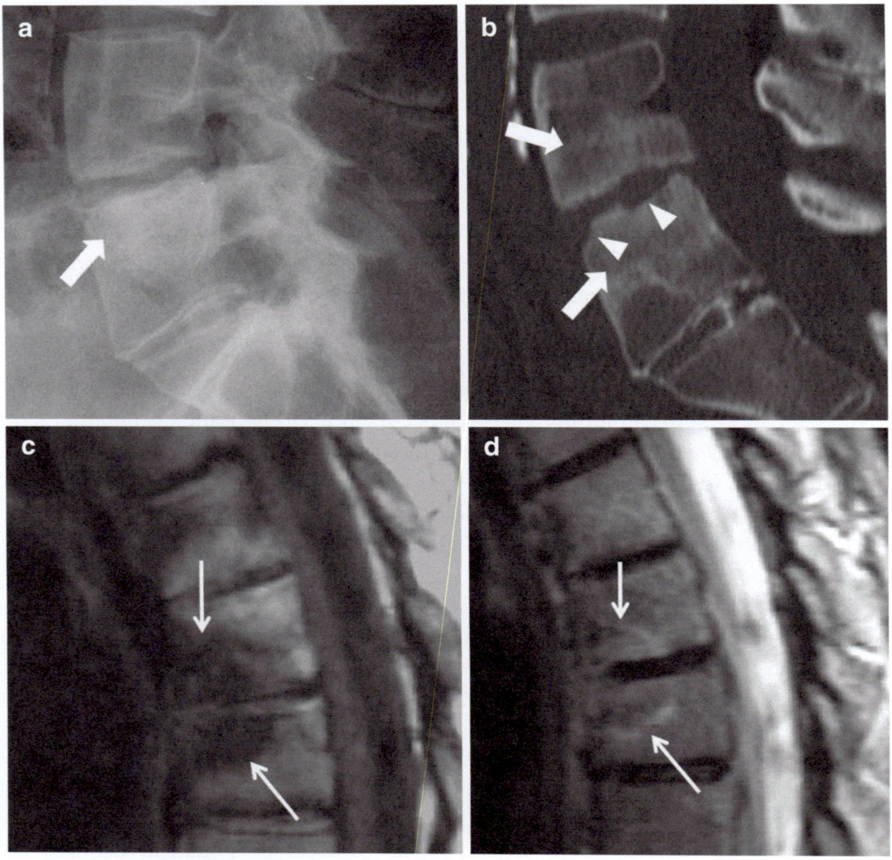


**Fig. 2.23** Andersson lesion on lateral plain film (**a**) at the L4–L5 level. There is sclerosis of the vertebral body of L5 (arrow) with irregular margins of the vertebral endplates and narrowing of the intervertebral disk space. Sagittal reformatted CT scan with bone window settings (**b**) better depicts the sclerosis (arrow) and erosions of the endplate (arrowhead) in the same patient. Note the squaring at anterior margin of L4. Sagittal T1- (**c**) and T2- (**d**) weighted images of an Andersson lesion in a different patient reveal irregular endplates and reactive sclerosis surrounded by a thin layer of bone marrow edema representing acute inflammation (thin arrows)

indicative of SpA, although this is still controversial [48]. Early syndesmophytes may be difficult to see on MRI due to their low signal intensity similar to the surrounding fibrous tissue of the anterior longitudinal ligament. Radiographs and CT are superior in detecting these lesions. Later, when syndesmophytes become larger and contain enough fatty marrow, they are more apparent on T1-weighted images (Fig. 2.25) [39].

Andersson lesions on MRI (Fig. 2.23) demonstrate a diffuse hypointense signal on T1-weighted images at the intervertebral disk and adjacent vertebral endplates. The lesions are hyperintense on T2-weighted sequences and show significant enhancement after intravenous administration of gadolinium contrast mimicking

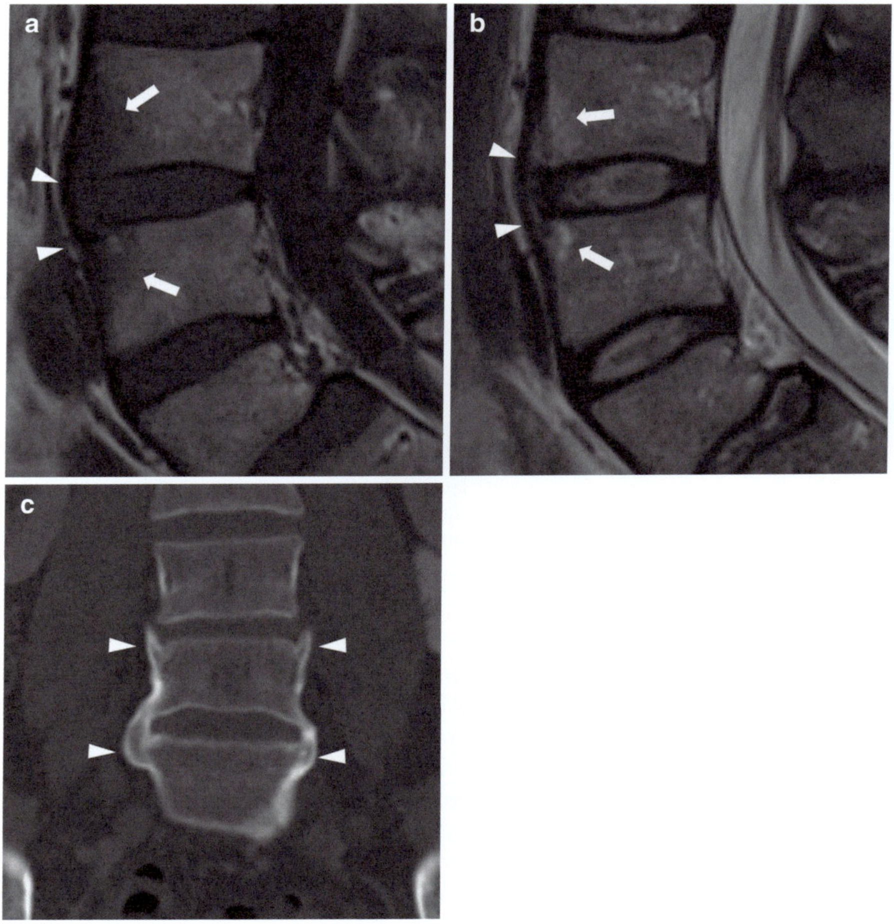


**Fig. 2.24** Sagittal T1- (**a**) and T2-weighted (**b**) images of the lumbar spine in a 39-year-old patient with ankylosing spondylitis. There are Romanus lesions (arrows) at the anterior vertebral corners of the L3 and L4 vertebrae. The low signal intensity on T1-weighted images and high signal intensity on T2-weighted images represent inflammation and edema. Note the preserved signal and contour of the intervertebral disk. Coronal reformatted CT scan with bone window settings (**c**) in the same patient depicts the syndesmophytes (arrowheads) in greater detail compared to MRI

infectious spondylodiscitis. The lack of paravertebral soft-tissue involvement of Andersson lesions is a salient finding for differentiating both entities [41].

### 2.4.2 Other Inflammatory Spondyloarthropathies

*Psoriatic arthritis* (PsA) is an inflammatory arthritis occurring with psoriasis. The peak onset of psoriatic arthritis is 30–35 years. In a minority of patients, the arthritis precedes the appearance of skin lesions. The etiopathogenesis of PsA

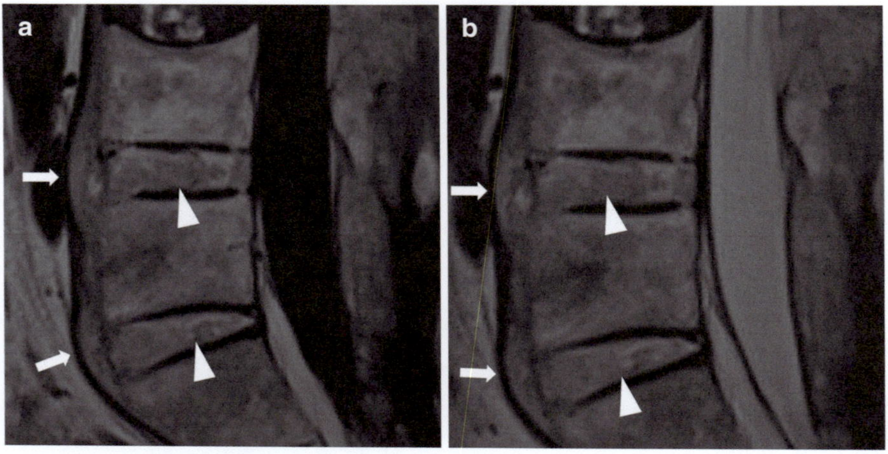


**Fig. 2.25** Sagittal MR of the lower lumbar levels in a 69-year-old patient with long-standing ankylosing spondylitis. T1- (**a**) and T2-(**b**) weighted images show ankylosis of the vertebral bodies with bridging syndesmophytes (arrows) containing fatty bone marrow. In addition there is ossification of the intervertebral disks (arrowheads)

remains unknown. Similar to SpA, the inflammatory process targets the entheses and synovial joints [49]. Axial psoriatic arthritis occurs in approximately 50% of patients with peripheral PsA [50]. Late radiographic changes in psoriatic arthritis may show parasyndesmophytes. These nonmarginal, bulky syndesmophytes-like formations occur most commonly in the thoracolumbar spine and appear as curvilinear, thick ossifications, parallel to the lateral intervertebral disk. Parasyndesmophytes tend to coalesce creating a large bony bridge. In contrast to syndesmophytes in AS, they often remain asymmetric and unilateral and therefore rarely create a bamboo spine appearance [51]. *Reactive arthritis* is a clinical entity in which arthritis develops following an infection. The peak onset is 15–35 years of age and is rarely seen in young children. The disease usually occurs within 1–3 weeks after a gastrointestinal or urogenital infection. No pathogens can be cultured from the affected joints. The proposed pathophysiologic mechanism is an autoimmune response targeting the axial skeleton or the appendicular joints, triggered by the initial infection. There is frequent involvement of the sacroiliac joints with similar radiological features of psoriatic sacroiliitis. Although rare, spinal involvement has features similar to those of psoriatic SpA with parasyndesmophytes formation [40].

*Enteropathic spondyloarthritis* (ESpA) is associated with chronic inflammatory bowel syndromes such as Crohn's disease and ulcerative colitis. The imaging features of both spondylitis and sacroiliitis are similar to those of ankylosing spondylitis [52].

## 2.5 Infection

### 2.5.1 Pyogenic Spondylodiscitis

#### 2.5.1.1 Definition

*Pyogenic spondylodiscitis* refers to infection of one or more intervertebral disks and vertebrae with frequent involvement of the paravertebral tissues. The peak age of incidence is the fifth decade. Males are affected twice as much as females [53]. The lumbar vertebral disks and adjacent vertebral bodies are frequently involved, followed by thoracic and infrequently by the cervical vertebrae. Although, the term spondylodiscitis is widely accepted, strictly spoken, it is a misnomer as the initial focus of infection is located at the subchondral bone rather than in the disk. The most prevalent cause of spondylodiscitis is *Staphylococcus aureus*, responsible for approximately 50% of cases [54]. The clinical symptoms of spondylodiscitis are nonspecific, commonly leading to a delay in diagnosis. Over 90% of patients with bacterial spondylodiscitis complain of back pain that is not relieved by rest or common analgesics. Fever is not a consistent feature of discitis and is seen in only 60–70% of cases [55].

#### 2.5.1.2 Pathogenesis

There are two main pathways in the development of a spinal infection: hematogenous and non-hematogenous. In patients without a history of surgery or a paraspinal infection, the source of infection is usually hematogenous. The most common source is the genitourinary tract; other less common sources include endocarditis, pneumonia, or infection of the oral cavity [54]. Pyogenic spondylodiscitis presents with lesions in two adjacent vertebral bodies and the corresponding intervertebral disk since supplying arteries bifurcate to supply two adjacent vertebral bodies. The anterior vertebral endplates are the physiological equivalent of the metaphysis of long bones. The endarteriole network at this location is susceptible to bacterial seeding (Fig. 2.26). In the adult, the vascular supply of the disk ends at the cartilaginous endplates, and the disk is supplied by diffusion of nutrients from the vertebral endplate. Septic emboli arrive in the vertebra via the endarterioles in the subchondral plate leading to septic bone infarction with subsequent wedging or collapse of the vertebral body [56]. Extensive vertebral destruction may result in deformity, compromise stability, and ultimately cause spinal cord compression. In essence, spinal infection in the adult consist primarily of spondylitis rather than discitis. Later, the infection spreads contiguously to the disk and the surrounding structures leading to the formation of paravertebral abscesses or may result in meningitis, epidural abscess formation [57].

The pathophysiology of spinal infections is slightly different in children. In children, the intervertebral disk is vascularized and may provide an inoculation site for bacterial infection. In addition, the extensive anastomotic arterioles in the metaphysis of children offer protection against destruction by infarction due to septic emboli [58].

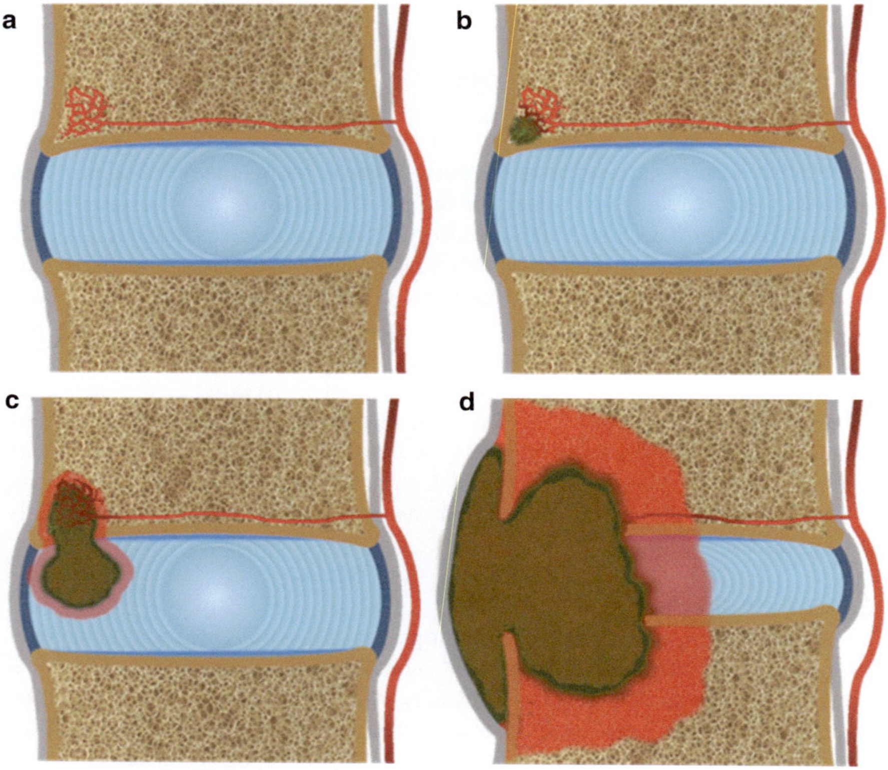


**Fig. 2.26** Pathogenesis of spondylodiscitis of the spine. (**a**) Arterial supply of the vertebral bodies in an adult. The endarterioles terminate near the anterior aspect of the vertebral endplate. (**b**) Entrapment of a septic emboli at the endarteriolar complex. (**c**) Inoculation and proliferation of the pathogen at the anterior endplate with focal destruction of cortex and extension into the disk space. (**d**) Further extension of the infectious process to adjacent vertebral levels

Contrary to tuberculosis (TB) and fungal infections, the posterior vertebral structures are rarely involved in haematogenous pyogenic infection [59]. Non-hematogenous bacterial inoculation is mainly iatrogenic after a spinal procedure. Spondylodiscitis due to contiguous spread or an adjacent infected focus is rare [54].

#### 2.5.1.3 Imaging

Findings on plain radiographs usually require 2 weeks to develop. Plain films are insensitive at detecting early changes. At least 50% of a vertebral body has to be destroyed before destruction is visible. A negative plain film does not rule out spondylodiscitis [60]. The presence of gas within the intervertebral disk is an argument against spondylodiscitis and most likely indicates degenerative disk disease, except for gas-forming pathogens [16].

The earliest findings are localized osteoporosis and progressive loss of the "white stripe" of the vertebral endplate (Fig. 2.27a, b). Later, a decrease in disk space height may occur when progression of the infection disrupts the cortical bone and extends into the adjacent disk space with disk destruction by proteolytic enzymes present in the infective agent [60]. Subsequent imaging findings consist of

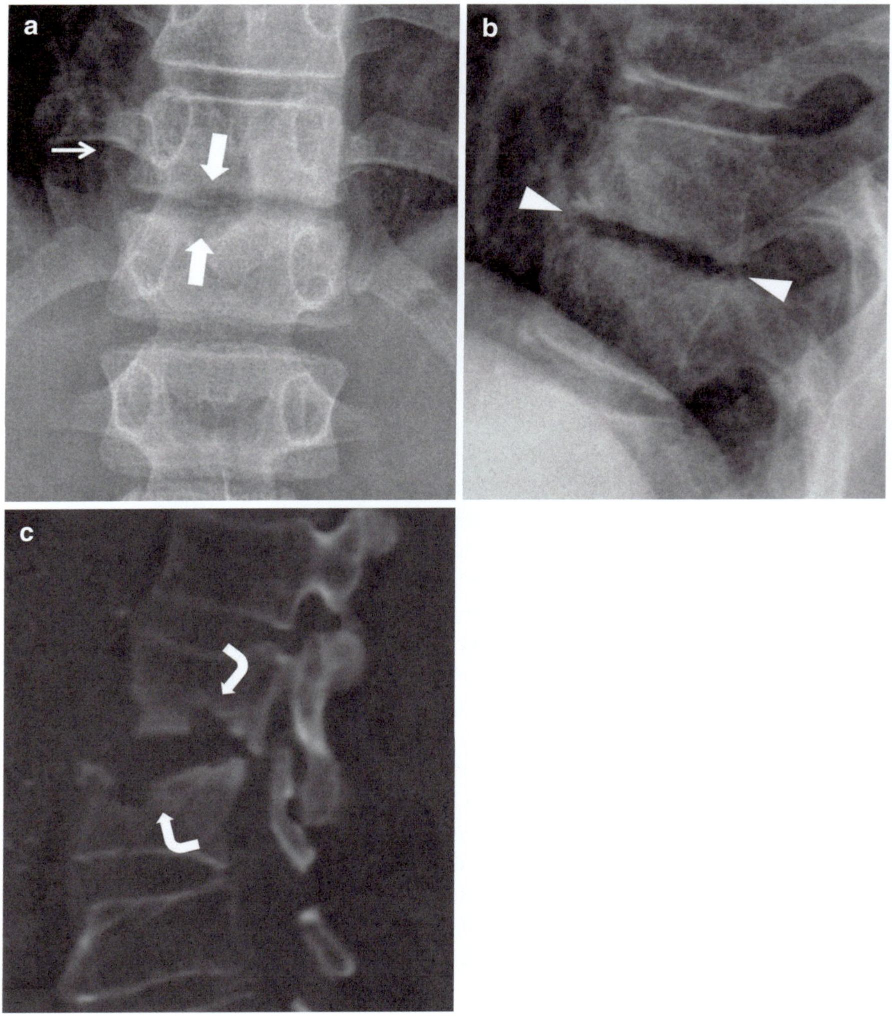


Fig. 2.27 Anteroposterior (**a**) and lateral (**b**) plain films in a 32-year-old male with acute pyogenic spondylodiscitis on standard radiography. There is narrowing of the Th11-Th12 disk space (arrowheads) with blurring of the endplates and disappearance of the "white stripe" (arrows) compared to the normal endplates. Note the subtle displacement of the right paravertebral stripe (thin arrow). Sagittal reformatted CT in another patient with long-standing spondylodiscitis (approximately 3 months) demonstrates more extensive destruction and collapse of the vertebral bodies (curved arrows)

radiolucencies of the vertebral body, loss of bone trabeculae, and ultimately marked bone destruction. Progressive kyphosis or scoliosis can develop in cases of chronic infection. In advanced stages of the disease, there is sclerosis from reparative processes and bony ankylosis [59].

CT scan allows earlier detection of endplate changes and bony destruction compared to plain films (Fig. 2.27c). Hypoattenuation of the intervertebral disk is a subtle early indicator of infection. This loss of density is related to edema and inflammatory exudate in the disk space [60]. Additionally, contrast-enhanced scans may show enhancement of the intervertebral disk and allow identification of paraspinous inflammatory changes or psoas abscesses. Multiplanar reconstructed images are helpful to define the local extent of the disease. However, compared to MRI, CT is less sensitive for early detection of spondylodiscitis [59].

MRI is the imaging modality of choice in suspected spondylodiscitis due to its capability to assess early bone marrow changes. It also allows accurate assessment of complications of spondylodiscitis, including the effect on neural structures [60].

In acute spondylodiscitis, an early sign is loss of the intranuclear cleft. However, since the intranuclear cleft cannot be identified in many unaffected disks, this sign is nonspecific [61]. A high signal intensity of the vertebral bodies and disk is seen on fluid-sensitive images representing inflammatory (bone marrow) edema and necrosis replacing the normal fatty marrow (Fig. 2.28). Accompanying hypointense signal and destruction of the endplates is seen on T1-weighted images. There is enhancement of the disk and adjacent bone marrow after administration of gadolinium contrast. Enhancement may be restricted to the periphery of the disk due to central abscess formation [59]. Post-gadolinium images are superior to assess the extent of paraspinous and epidural involvement. Uniformly, enhancing soft tissue is consistent with phlegmon, while peripheral enhancement suggests abscess formation. Epidural disease typically involves multiple vertebral levels and is located anteriorly in most cases [55]. Diffusion-weighted MRI has been advocated as an additional tool for distinguishing spondylodiscitis from degenerative endplate changes. Restricted diffusion is present in the endplates of patients with infection, but not in those with degenerative disease [60]. Another sign on DWI for the diagnosis is the claw sign, a well-delineated linear region of increased diffusion restriction situated around Modic type I changes at the interface of normal and abnormal marrow. Absence of this sign suggests infection [62].

Another confusing finding on MRI is "pseudosparing" of the endplates. When the normal fatty marrow is lost in spondylodiscitis, a decrease of the chemical shift artefact at the adjacent endplate may simulate a normal endplate, masking endplate thinning and erosion [57].

#### 2.5.1.4 Differential Diagnosis

Early in the inflammatory stage, degenerative disk disease can mimic spondylodiscitis. *Modic type 1 changes* in the vertebral endplates and bone marrow lead to a similar hyperintense signal on T2-weighted images and enhancement after the administration of gadolinium contrast. In degenerative disk disease, there is usually no hyperintensity of the disk on T2-weighted images and paraspinal inflammation

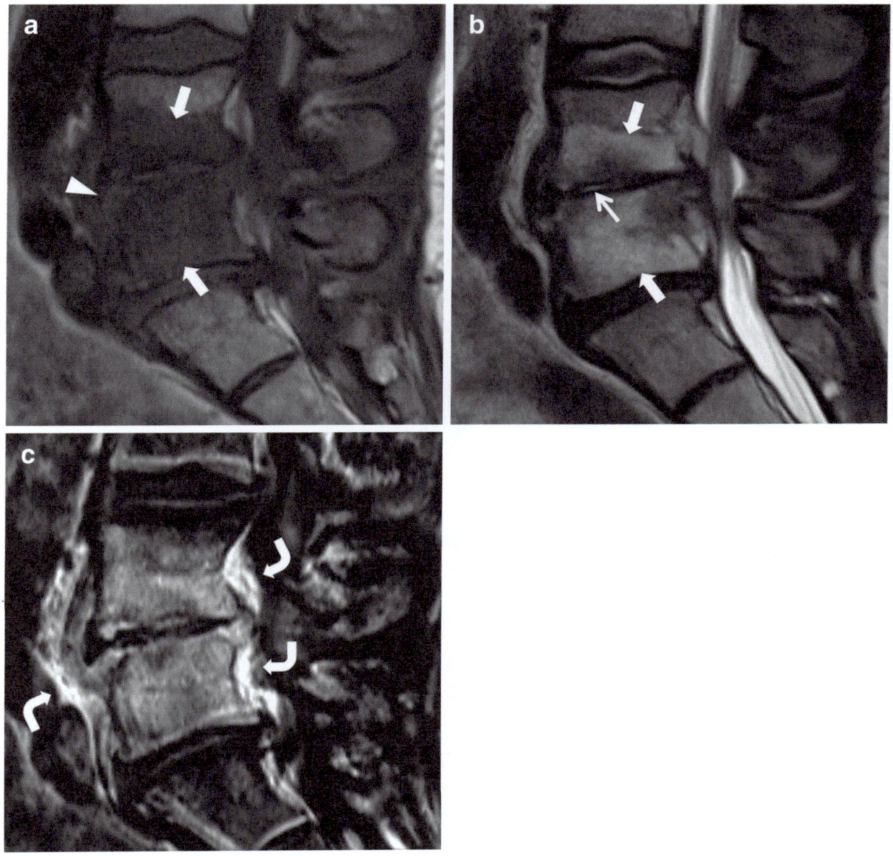


**Fig. 2.28** MRI of acute pyogenic spondylodiscitis. A 41-year-old male with history of spinal surgery, a few months prior. Sagittal T1-weighted image (**a**) demonstrates marked hypointensity of the L4–L5 disk and adjacent vertebral bodies of L4–L5 (arrows) due to inflammatory edema. There is narrowing of the intervertebral disk space with an irregularly defined endplates and focal destruction of the anterior cortex (arrowhead). Sagittal T2-weighted image (**b**) shows a hyperintense intervertebral disk with loss of the intranuclear cleft (thin arrow) and surrounding inflammatory bone marrow edema (arrows). Sagittal subtraction image (**c**) of T1-weighted images before and after intravenous gadolinium contrast administration reveal marked vertebral enhancement and uniformly enhancing soft tissue in the prevertebral and epidural space (curved arrow)

is absent. In addition, bone marrow edema in spondylodiscitis is much more extensive, and endplate destruction is usually absent in Modic type I changes [59, 63]. Finally, absence of the aforementioned claw sign is suggestive for infection [62].

*Metastases* of the spine may lead to vertebral destruction similar to spondylodiscitis. Compared to an infectious etiology, the intervertebral disk is rarely involved by metastases [64].

*Dialysis-related* disk *disease* is likely related to amyloid deposition in the disk and ligamenta flava. On conventional radiography and CT, the observed destruction of the endplates and disk space narrowing can mimic infectious discitis. On MRI, however, there is only a low-to-intermediate signal on T1- and T2-weighted images. In addition, there is often involvement of the posterior elements, and unlike spondylodiscitis, the most commonly involved area is the lower cervical spine [63].

In renal osteodystrophy, subchondral bone resorption may result in irregular destruction of the vertebral endplates. The thoracic spine is most commonly involved. The presence of chronic kidney failure and concomitant hyperparathyroidism are important clues pointing toward the correct diagnosis [65, 66].

*Neurogenic* disk *disease* can mimic spondylodiscitis on plain films and CT, but lacks a hyperintense signal on T2-weighted images [67].

*Crystal-induced inflammatory* disk *disease* may mimic spondylodiscitis on MRI. The clue to the correct diagnosis is the detection of calcification or urate deposits on (dual) energy CT, respectively [68].

Finally, the differential diagnosis of Andersson lesion in SpA has been discussed in Sect. 2.4.1.3.

## 2.5.2 Tuberculosis (Pott's Disease)

### 2.5.2.1 Definition

*Pott's disease* is the eponym for tuberculous (TB) spondylodiscitis. Spinal tuberculosis is the most common form of skeletal tuberculosis comprising approximately half of the musculoskeletal TB cases. Spinal tuberculosis most commonly involves the thoracolumbar spine and rarely the cervical spine [60]. The incidence of extrapulmonary TB is higher amongst immigrants from highly endemic areas to developed countries [69]. The most common symptom is local pain, increasing in severity over weeks to months. Fever and weight loss are observed in less than 40% of patients. A characteristic erect posture and "alderman's" gait may be present. The patient walks with short, careful steps to avoid mechanical loading of the spine [70]. Definitive diagnosis is often difficult because its clinical presentation is indistinct and nonspecific [71].

### 2.5.2.2 Pathogenesis

Spinal involvement is the result of hematogenous spread of *M. tuberculosis* to the vertebral bodies. The primary infection site is usually pulmonary or genitourinary. Spread occurs via the arterial route similar to pyogenic spondylodiscitis. Subligamentous extension underneath the anterior or posterior longitudinal ligaments spreads the infection to adjacent vertebral segments. The spread of infection within these ligamentous borders is a key finding of tuberculous spondylitis [60]. Skip lesions with sparing of vertebrae may occur. It has been proposed that the mechanism for these skip lesions is hematogenous spread via the valveless Batson's venous plexus [72]. Finally, extension into the paraspinal soft tissues leads to the formation of a paravertebral cold abscess or epidural involvement. These cold abscesses may become very large exerting a mass effect on surrounding abdominal and spinal structures. In long-standing disease, these abscesses may calcify. A rare but characteristic finding is the involvement of the posterior elements in tuberculous spondylodiscitis [60].

#### 2.5.2.3 Imaging

The disk space is relatively preserved until the late stages compared to pyogenic spondylodiscitis due lack of a proteolytic enzyme in *M. tuberculosis* [73]. Calcifications in paraspinal masses are highly suggestive of TB but will be missed on plain films unless calcifications are extensive. When the infection disseminates into adjacent spinal segments, there is multilevel involvement. In advanced stages of the disease, there is sclerosis from reparative processes and bony ankylosis. Vertebral collapse and anterior wedging lead to kyphosis and gibbus deformity. CT demonstrates abnormalities earlier than plain radiography. Other findings include soft-tissue involvement and paraspinal tissue abscesses. CT is also more sensitive for demonstration of calcifications and may depict narrowing of the spinal canal by posterior extension of infectious tissue [74].

MRI is the imaging modality of choice. Signal changes occur early in the disease. The initial infective focus can be detected as inflammatory bone marrow edema with a high signal intensity on T2-weighted images and low intensity on T1-weighted images (Fig. 2.29) [60]. Compared to pyogenic spondylitis, tuberculosis typically shows more sharply delineated destructive margins often without reactive sclerosis [75]. Inoculation of the disk space leads to similar signal changes at the intervertebral disk and blurring of the endplates, but the disk height remains relatively preserved [76]. After administration of gadolinium contrast, there is vivid enhancement of the infected vertebral body and the disk. Postcontrast T1-weighted images with fat suppression are also very useful to demonstrate paravertebral soft-tissue abscesses and epidural extension [60].

### 2.5.3 Fungal Spondylodiscitis

#### 2.5.3.1 Definition

Similar to tuberculous spondylodiscitis, fungal spondylodiscitis has a more silent clinical course compared to pyogenic spondylodiscitis. Patients at risk for developing fungal infections are immunocompromised individuals and inhabitants or visitors to endemic regions [77].

#### 2.5.3.2 Imaging

Plain radiographs and CT are similar to tuberculosis. Fungal infections tend to involve the anterior vertebral body, have a predilection for paraspinal extension, and spare the intervertebral disk due to a lack of proteolytic enzymes.

Fungal infections show more subtle signal intensity changes on MRI compared to pyogenic and tuberculous spondylodiscitis. The low T1 and high T2 signal of bone marrow edema are less pronounced compared to other causes of spondylodiscitis. It has been proposed that paramagnetic elements within the fungi contribute to the absence of signal hyperintensity in the disks [78]. Contrast enhancement is

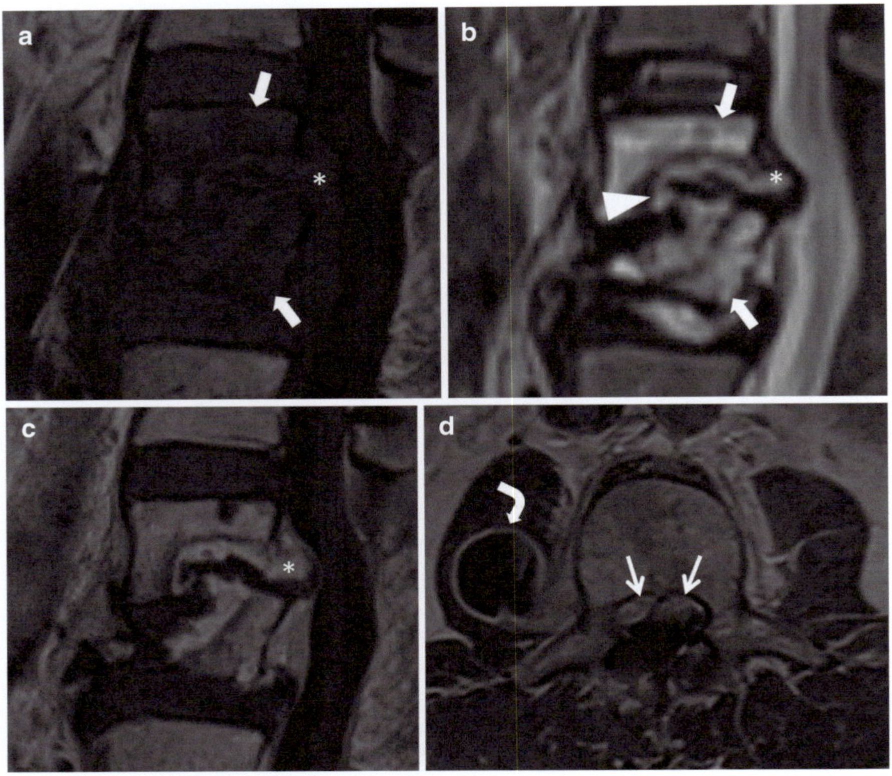


**Fig. 2.29** MRI of tuberculous spondylodiscitis. A 65-year-old male immigrant from North Africa with an indolent clinical history. Sagittal T1-weighted image (**a**) shows diffuse hypointensity of the L2–L3 vertebrae with destruction of the vertebral bodies (arrows). Sagittal STIR image (**b**) demonstrates diffuse bone marrow edema (arrows) with extension of the inflammatory process into the adjacent disk (arrowhead). There is focal displacement of the posterior vertebral wall with compression of the dural sac (asterisk). Sagittal (**c**) and axial (**d**) T1-weighted after intravenous gadolinium contrast administration reveal destruction of the endplates and extension of the infection into the anterior epidural space with the so-called "curtain sign" (thin arrows). Furthermore, there is extension into the right psoas muscle with an intramuscular rim-enhancing abscess (curved arrows)

subtle due to the milder inflammatory reaction in fungal infections. In chronic disease, particular patterns may emerge in different pathogenic fungi. Both Aspergillus and Blastomyces infections tend to involve multiple and sometimes noncontiguous vertebral bodies. In severe cases enhancement of the longitudinal ligaments and significant vertebral body destruction may occur [79, 80]. Blastomyces infection can result in vertebral body collapse and gibbus deformity like tuberculosis, but can be distinguished from tuberculosis by the presence of lesions in adjacent ribs [79].

Coccidioides infection has imaging findings similar to tuberculosis with relative sparing of the disk space [79].

### 2.5.4 Brucellosis

Brucellosis is a zoonotic organism, and its transmission occurs through fluids from infected animals. It is endemic in the Mediterranean, Middle East, and Central and South America. The infection has a broad clinical spectrum, ranging from asymptomatic disease to fatal illness [81].

Spondylitis is a serious complication of Brucellosis. It is more prevalent in older patients and patients with long-standing illness. The lumbar vertebrae are involved more frequently than the thoracic and cervical vertebrae. Spinal brucellosis has similar imaging findings as tuberculous spondylitis, however, large soft-tissue abscesses and paraspinal calcification are less common in brucellosis [82]. Serology and bacteriological examinations point toward the correct diagnosis [81].

## 2.6 Calcification and Ossification of the Intervertebral Disk and Adjacent Structures

### 2.6.1 Disk Calcification

In *hydroxyapatite deposition disease* (HADD), basic calcium phosphate crystals (BCP) may be present in the intervertebral, most often in the nucleus pulposus [83]. Concomitant evidence of degenerative changes is usually present.

*Calcium pyrophosphate dihydrate disease* (CPPD) occurs most frequently in the cervical spine, followed by the lumbar spine, and rarely the thoracic spine. The disease typically affects people older than 60 years. The incidence increases with age. Radiographic findings are disk space loss with adjacent vertebral body sclerosis. Complications depend on the size of the deposits. Spinal cord compression, myelopathy, and atlantoaxial subluxation can occur [84]. When the atlantooccipital joint is involved and the deposition is symptomatic, the term crowned dens syndrome is used. This condition results in acute neck pain with fever, stiffness, and elevated inflammatory markers, mimicking meningitis [85].

*Ochronosis or alkaptonuria (AKU)* is a rare multisystem autosomal recessive metabolic disorder. Deficiency of the homogentisate dioxygenase enzyme induces accumulation of homogentisic acid (HGA) in different tissues including the intervertebral disk. HGA irreversibly binds to collagen, and progressive deposition of HGA plaques leads to degeneration and arthropathy. Typical imaging findings are an osteoporotic appearance of the vertebrae, narrow disks with dense calcifications, and syndesmophytes (Fig. 2.30) [86, 87].

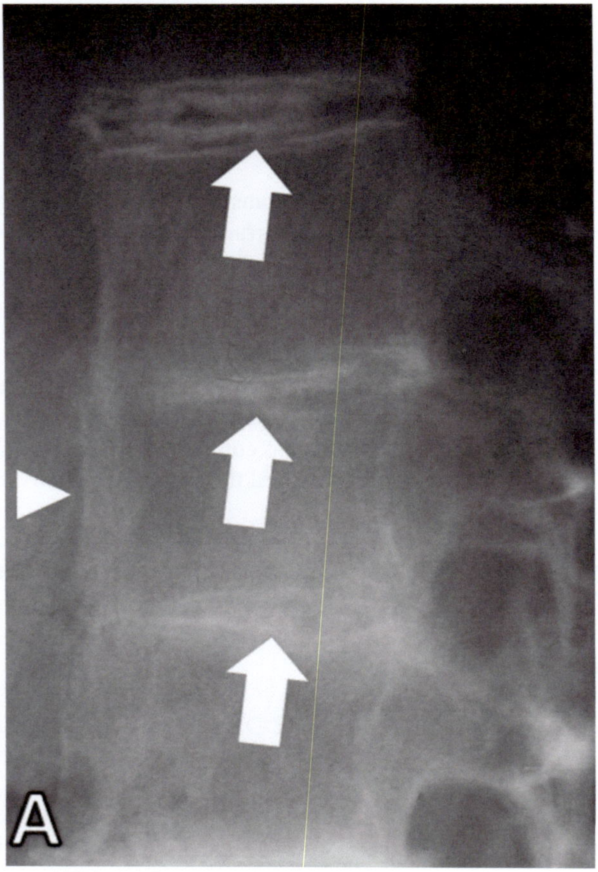


**Fig. 2.30** Lateral plain of the thoracic spine in a patient with ochronosis demonstrating calcifications of multiple intervertebral disks with associated narrowing of the intervertebral disk space (arrows). Furthermore, note the ossification of the anterior longitudinal ligament (arrowhead)

### 2.6.2 Diffuse Idiopathic Skeletal Hyperostosis

Diffuse idiopathic skeletal hyperostosis (DISH), also referred to as Forestier disease, is a flowing ossification of the anterior longitudinal ligament. DISH occurs most often in the thoracic spine, followed by cervical and lumbar spine [13]. The diagnosis of DISH in most patients is made with plain films. Flowing calcifications and ossification along the anterolateral aspect of vertebral bodies are more often on the right side than left, due to aortic pulsations [13]. These ossifications may mimic the discovertebral ankylosis of ankylosing spondylitis. There is preservation of the intervertebral disk height at the involved vertebral segments and a distinct lack of radiographic changes of degenerative disk disease. The broad anterior ossifications differ from the thin vertical syndesmophytes of SpA and sacroiliitis is absent [88].

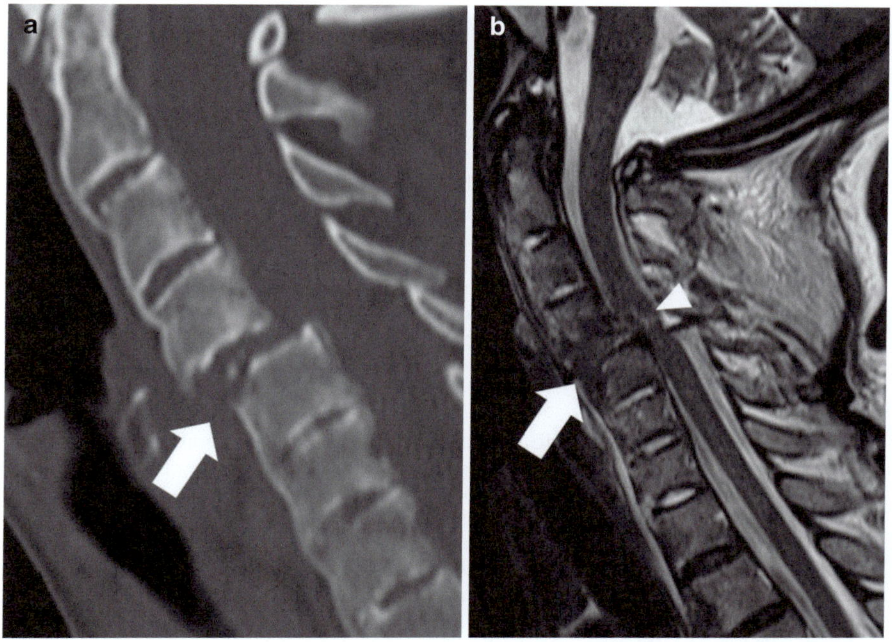


**Fig. 2.31** Chance fracture in the rigid spine. Sagittal reformatted CT with bone window settings (**a**) and sagittal T2-weighted images of the cervical spine in a patient with DISH (**b**). There is a fracture at the C4–C5 discovertebral junction (arrow). The fracture line extends posteriorly and involves all three spinal columns. There is associated traumatic myelopathy (arrowhead)

CT confirms the thick ossifications of the ALL and may show ossification anterior of the midvertebral body, an early sign of DISH. On MRI, the signal intensity depends whether the predominant process is calcification or ossification. Calcifications are hypointense on T1-and T2-weighted images while ossifications have a signal intensity similar to bone marrow fat in the vertebral body [89]. Similar to the ankylosed spine in spondyloarthritis, a rigid spine due to DISH may result in unstable chance fractures following minor trauma (Fig. 2.31).

### 2.6.3 Ossification of the Posterior Longitudinal Ligament

Ossification of the posterior longitudinal ligament (OPLL) is a rare disorder originally described in the Japanese population [90]. OPLL is observed usually in the fifth to seventh decades of life and most commonly in the midcervical region (C3–C5). Although individuals who have the disease may be entirely asymptomatic, a variety of symptoms, usually due to neurologic compression, may present. The diagnosis of OPLL in the cervical spine is established by its characteristic radiographic appearance, showing a dense ossified band of variable thickness (1–5 mm) along the posterior margins of the vertebral bodies and the intervertebral disks [91].

## References


1. Kunkel ME, Herkommer A, Reinehr M, Bockers TM, Wilke HJ. Morphometric analysis of the relationships between intervertebral disc and vertebral body heights: an anatomical and radiographic study of the human thoracic spine. J Anat. 2011;219(3):375–87. https://doi.org/10.1111/j.1469-7580.2011.01397.x.
2. Zhou SH, McCarthy ID, McGregor AH, Coombs RR, Hughes SP. Geometrical dimensions of the lower lumbar vertebrae--analysis of data from digitised CT images. Eur Spine J. 2000;9(3):242–8.
3. Biggemann M, Frobin W, Brinckmann P. The physiological pattern of lumbar intervertebral disk height. RoFo. 1997;167(1):11–5. https://doi.org/10.1055/s-2007-1015485.
4. Pfirrmann CW, Metzdorf A, Zanetti M, Hodler J, Boos N. Magnetic resonance classification of lumbar intervertebral disc degeneration. Spine (Phila Pa 1976). 2001;26(17):1873–8.
5. Konin GP, Walz DM. Lumbosacral transitional vertebrae: classification, imaging findings, and clinical relevance. AJNR Am J Neuroradiol. 2010;31(10):1778–86. https://doi.org/10.3174/ajnr.A2036.
6. Kumar R, Guinto FC, Madewell JE, Swischuk LE, David R. The vertebral body: radiographic configurations in various congenital and acquired disorders. Radiographics. 1988;8(3):455–85. https://doi.org/10.1148/radiographics.8.3.3380991.
7. Park P, Garton HJ, Gala VC, Hoff JT, McGillicuddy JE. Adjacent segment disease after lumbar or lumbosacral fusion review of the literature. Spine (Phila Pa 1976). 2004;29(17):1938–44. https://doi.org/10.1097/01.brs.0000137069.88904.03.
8. Terry YR, Rowe LJ. The essentials of skeletal radiology. Hagerstown: Williams & Wilkins; 2005.
9. Kaplan KM, Spivak JM, Bendo JA. Embryology of the spine and associated congenital abnormalities. Spine J. 2005;5(5):564–76. https://doi.org/10.1016/j.spinee.2004.10.044.
10. Castellvi AE, Goldstein LA, Chan DP. Lumbosacral transitional vertebrae and their relationship with lumbar extradural defects. Spine (Phila Pa 1976). 1984;9(5):493–5.
11. Arlet V, Odent T, Aebi M. Congenital scoliosis. Eur Spine J. 2003;12(5):456–63. https://doi.org/10.1007/s00586-003-0555-6.
12. van Goethem JWM, van den Hauwe L, Parizel PM, editors. Spinal imaging: diagnostic imaging of the spine and spinal cord. 1st ed. Berlin: Springer-Verlag; 2007. https://doi.org/10.1007/978-3-540-68483-1.
13. Resnick D, Niwayama G. Diagnosis of bone and joint disorders, vol. 3. Philadelphia, PA: Saunders; 2004.
14. Fardon DF, Williams AL, Dohring EJ, Murtagh FR, Gabriel Rothman SL, Sze GK. Lumbar disc nomenclature: version 2.0: recommendations of the combined task forces of the North American Spine Society, the American Society of Spine Radiology and the American Society of Neuroradiology. Spine J. 2014;14(11):2525–45. https://doi.org/10.1016/j.spinee.2014.04.022.
15. Pate D, Goobar J, Resnick D, Haghighi P, Sartoris DJ, Pathria MN. Traction osteophytes of the lumbar spine: radiographic-pathologic correlation. Radiology. 1988;166(3):843–6. https://doi.org/10.1148/radiology.166.3.3340781.
16. Resnick D, Niwayama G, Guerra J Jr, Vint V, Usselman J. Spinal vacuum phenomena: anatomical study and review. Radiology. 1981;139(2):341–8. https://doi.org/10.1148/radiology.139.2.7220878.
17. Yu LP, Qian WW, Yin GY, Ren YX, Hu ZY. MRI assessment of lumbar intervertebral disc degeneration with lumbar degenerative disease using the Pfirrmann grading systems. PLoS One. 2012;7(12):e48074. https://doi.org/10.1371/journal.pone.0048074.
18. Griffith JF, Wang YX, Antonio GE, Choi KC, Yu A, Ahuja AT, Leung PC. Modified Pfirrmann grading system for lumbar intervertebral disc degeneration. Spine (Phila Pa 1976). 2007;32(24):E708–12. https://doi.org/10.1097/BRS.0b013e31815a59a0.
19. Suthar P, Patel R, Mehta C, Patel N. MRI evaluation of lumbar disc degenerative disease. J Clin Diagn Res. 2015;9(4):TC04–9. https://doi.org/10.7860/JCDR/2015/11927.5761.

20. Kyere KA, Than KD, Wang AC, Rahman SU, Valdivia-Valdivia JM, La Marca F, Park P. Schmorl's nodes. Eur Spine J. 2012;21(11):2115–21. https://doi.org/10.1007/s00586-012-2325-9.
21. Modic MT, Ross JS. Lumbar degenerative disk disease. Radiology. 2007;245(1):43–61. https://doi.org/10.1148/radiol.2451051706.
22. Modic MT, Steinberg PM, Ross JS, Masaryk TJ, Carter JR. Degenerative disk disease: assessment of changes in vertebral body marrow with MR imaging. Radiology. 1988;166(1 Pt 1):193–9. https://doi.org/10.1148/radiology.166.1.3336678.
23. Kanna RM, Shanmuganathan R, Rajagopalan VR, Natesan S, Muthuraja R, Cheung KMC, Chan D, Kao PYP, Yee A, Shetty AP. Prevalence, patterns, and genetic association analysis of Modic vertebral endplate changes. Asian Spine J. 2017;11(4):594–600. https://doi.org/10.4184/asj.2017.11.4.594.
24. Kuisma M, Karppinen J, Niinimaki J, Ojala R, Haapea M, Heliovaara M, Korpelainen R, Taimela S, Natri A, Tervonen O. Modic changes in endplates of lumbar vertebral bodies: prevalence and association with low back and sciatic pain among middle-aged male workers. Spine (Phila Pa 1976). 2007;32(10):1116–22. https://doi.org/10.1097/01.brs.0000261561.12944.ff.
25. Herlin C, Kjaer P, Espeland A, Skouen JS, Leboeuf-Yde C, Karppinen J, Niinimaki J, Sorensen JS, Storheim K, Jensen TS. Modic changes-their associations with low back pain and activity limitation: a systematic literature review and meta-analysis. PLoS One. 2018;13(8):e0200677. https://doi.org/10.1371/journal.pone.0200677.
26. Nickell LT, Schucany WG, Opatowsky MJ. Kummell disease. Proc (Bayl Univ Med Cent). 2013;26(3):300–1.
27. Freedman BA, Heller JG. Kummel disease: a not-so-rare complication of osteoporotic vertebral compression fractures. J Am Board Fam Med. 2009;22(1):75–8. https://doi.org/10.3122/jabfm.2009.01.080100.
28. Morishita K, Kasai Y, Uchida A. Clinical symptoms of patients with intervertebral vacuum phenomenon. Neurologist. 2008;14(1):37–9. https://doi.org/10.1097/NRL.0b013e3180dc9992.
29. Peng B, Wu W, Hou S, Shang W, Wang X, Yang Y. The pathogenesis of Schmorl's nodes. J Bone Joint Surg. 2003;85(6):879–82.
30. Takahashi K, Miyazaki T, Ohnari H, Takino T, Tomita K. Schmorl's nodes and low-back pain. Analysis of magnetic resonance imaging findings in symptomatic and asymptomatic individuals. Eur Spine J. 1995;4(1):56–9. https://doi.org/10.1007/bf00298420.
31. Corsi A, De Maio F, Mancini F, Ippolito E, Riminucci M, Bianco P. Notochordal inclusions in the vertebral bone marrow. J Bone Miner Res. 2008;23(4):572–5. https://doi.org/10.1359/jbmr.071204.
32. Sieper J, Rudwaleit M, Baraliakos X, Brandt J, Braun J, Burgos-Vargas R, Dougados M, Hermann KG, Landewe R, Maksymowych W, van der Heijde D. The assessment of SpondyloArthritis International Society (ASAS) handbook: a guide to assess spondyloarthritis. Ann Rheum Dis. 2009;68(Suppl 2):1–44. https://doi.org/10.1136/ard.2008.104018.
33. Taurog JD, Chhabra A, Colbert RA. Ankylosing spondylitis and axial Spondyloarthritis. N Engl J Med. 2016;374(26):2563–74. https://doi.org/10.1056/NEJMra1406182.
34. Claudepierre P, Voisin MC. The entheses: histology, pathology, and pathophysiology. Joint Bone Spine. 2005;72(1):32–7. https://doi.org/10.1016/j.jbspin.2004.02.010.
35. Ranganathan V, Gracey E, Brown MA, Inman RD, Haroon N. Pathogenesis of ankylosing spondylitis – recent advances and future directions. Nat Rev Rheumatol. 2017;13(6):359–67. https://doi.org/10.1038/nrrheum.2017.56.
36. Resnick D, Niwayama G, Goergen TG. Comparison of radiographic abnormalities of the sacroiliac joint in degenerative disease and ankylosing spondylitis. AJR Am J Roentgenol. 1977;128(2):189–96. https://doi.org/10.2214/ajr.128.2.189.
37. Romanus R, Yden S. Destructive and ossifying spondylitic changes in rheumatoid ankylosing spondylitis (pelvo-spondylitis ossificans). Acta Orthop Scand. 1952;22(2):88–99.
38. Hermann K-GA, Althoff CE, Schneider U, Zühlsdorf S, Lembcke A, Hamm B, Bollow M. Spinal changes in patients with spondyloarthritis: comparison of mr imaging and

radiographic appearances. RadioGraphics. 2005;25(3):559–69. https://doi.org/10.1148/rg.253045117.
39. Ostergaard M, Lambert RGW. Imaging in ankylosing spondylitis. Ther Adv Musculoskelet Dis. 2012;4(4):301–11. https://doi.org/10.1177/1759720X11436240.
40. Jurik AG. Imaging the spine in arthritis-a pictorial review. Insights Imaging. 2011;2(2):177–91. https://doi.org/10.1007/s13244-010-0061-4.
41. Bron JL, de Vries MK, Snieders MN, van der Horst-Bruinsma IE, van Royen BJ. Discovertebral (Andersson) lesions of the spine in ankylosing spondylitis revisited. Clin Rheumatol. 2009;28(8):883–92. https://doi.org/10.1007/s10067-009-1151-x.
42. Shah NG, Keraliya A, Nunez DB, Schoenfeld A, Harris MB, Bono CM, Khurana B. Injuries to the rigid spine: what the spine surgeon wants to know. Radiographics. 2019;39(2):449–66. https://doi.org/10.1148/rg.2019180125.
43. Wang Y-F, Teng MM-H, Chang C-Y, Wu H-T, Wang S-T. Imaging manifestations of spinal fractures in ankylosing spondylitis. Am J Neuroradiol. 2005;26(8):2067–76.
44. Mandl P, Navarro-Compán V, Terslev L, Aegerter P, van der Heijde D, D'Agostino MA, Baraliakos X, Pedersen SJ, Jurik AG, Naredo E, Schueller-Weidekamm C, Weber U, Wick MC, Bakker PAC, Filippucci E, Conaghan PG, Rudwaleit M, Schett G, Sieper J, Tarp S, Marzo-Ortega H, Østergaard M. EULAR recommendations for the use of imaging in the diagnosis and management of spondyloarthritis in clinical practice. Ann Rhem Dis. 2015;74(7):1327–39. https://doi.org/10.1136/annrheumdis-2014-206971%J.
45. Hermann K-GA, Baraliakos X, van der Heijde DM, Jurik A-G, Landewé R, Marzo-Ortega H, Østergaard M, Rudwaleit M, Sieper J, Braun J. Descriptions of spinal MRI lesions and definition of a positive MRI of the spine in axial spondyloarthritis: a consensual approach by the ASAS/OMERACT MRI study group. Ann Rhem Dis. 2012;71(8):1278–88. https://doi.org/10.1136/ard.2011.150680%J.
46. Bennett AN, Rehman A, Hensor EM, Marzo-Ortega H, Emery P, McGonagle D. The fatty Romanus lesion: a non-inflammatory spinal MRI lesion specific for axial spondyloarthropathy. Ann Rheum Dis. 2010;69(5):891–4. https://doi.org/10.1136/ard.2009.112094.
47. Bennett AN, McGonagle D, O'Connor P, Hensor EMA, Sivera F, Coates LC, Emery P, Marzo-Ortega H. Severity of baseline magnetic resonance imaging–evident sacroiliitis and HLA–B27 status in early inflammatory back pain predict radiographically evident ankylosing spondylitis at eight years. Arthritis Rheum. 2008;58(11):3413–8. https://doi.org/10.1002/art.24024.
48. Truong SL, Saad NF, Robinson PC, Cowderoy G, Lim I, Schachna L, Stebbings S, Stuckey S, Taylor AL, Whittle SL, Zochling J, Bird P, Brown MA. Consensus statements on the imaging of axial spondyloarthritis in Australia and New Zealand. Am Med Imag Rad Oncol. 2017;61(1):58–69. https://doi.org/10.1111/1754-9485.12573.
49. Wilson FC, Icen M, Crowson CS, McEvoy MT, Gabriel SE, Kremers HM. Incidence and clinical predictors of psoriatic arthritis in patients with psoriasis: a population-based study. Arthritis Rheum. 2009;61(2):233–9. https://doi.org/10.1002/art.24172.
50. Chandran V, Barrett J, Schentag CT, Farewell VT, Gladman DD. Axial psoriatic arthritis: update on a longterm prospective study. J Rheumatol. 2009;36(12):2744–50. https://doi.org/10.3899/jrheum.090412.
51. Canella C, Schau B, Ribeiro E, Sbaffi B, Marchiori E. MRI in seronegative Spondyloarthritis: imaging features and differential diagnosis in the spine and sacroiliac joints. Am J Roentgenol. 2013;200(1):149–57. https://doi.org/10.2214/AJR.12.8858.
52. Mester AR, Mako EK, Karlinger K, Gyorke T, Tarjan Z, Marton E, Kiss K. Enteropathic arthritis in the sacroiliac joint. Imaging and differential diagnosis. Eur J Radiol. 2000;35(3):199–208.
53. Kwon J-W, Hyun S-J, Han S-H, Kim K-J, Jahng T-A. Pyogenic vertebral osteomyelitis: clinical features, diagnosis, and treatment. Korean J Spine. 2017;14(2):27–34. https://doi.org/10.14245/kjs.2017.14.2.27.
54. Lew DP, Waldvogel FA. Osteomyelitis. Lancet. 2004;364(9431):369–79. https://doi.org/10.1016/s0140-6736(04)16727-5.
55. Cottle L, Riordan T. Infectious spondylodiscitis. J Infect. 2008;56(6):401–12. https://doi.org/10.1016/j.jinf.2008.02.005.

56. Cahill DW, Love LC, Rechtine GR. Pyogenic osteomyelitis of the spine in the elderly. J Neurosurg. 1991;74(6):878–86. https://doi.org/10.3171/jns.1991.74.6.0878.
57. Ramadani N, Dedushi K, Kabashi S, Mucaj S. Radiologic diagnosis of spondylodiscitis, role of magnetic resonance. Acta Inform Med. 2017;25(1):54–7. https://doi.org/10.5455/aim.2017.25.54-57.
58. Mavrogenis AF, Megaloikonomos PD, Igoumenou VG, Panagopoulos GN, Giannitsioti E, Papadopoulos A, Papagelopoulos PJ. Spondylodiscitis revisited. EFORT Open Rev. 2017;2(11):447–61. https://doi.org/10.1302/2058-5241.2.160062.
59. Varma R, Lander P, Assaf A. Imaging of pyogenic infectious spondylodiskitis. Radiol Clin N Am. 2001;39(2):203–13.
60. De Vuyst D, Vanhoenacker F, Gielen J, Bernaerts A, De Schepper AM. Imaging features of musculoskeletal tuberculosis. Eur Radiol. 2003;13(8):1809–19. https://doi.org/10.1007/s00330-002-1609-6.
61. Ledermann HP, Schweitzer ME, Morrison WB, Carrino JA. MR imaging findings in spinal infections: rules or myths? Radiology. 2003;228(2):506–14. https://doi.org/10.1148/radiol.2282020752.
62. Patel KB, Poplawski MM, Pawha PS, Naidich TP, Tanenbaum LN. Diffusion-weighted MRI "claw sign" improves differentiation of infectious from degenerative modic type 1 signal changes of the spine. AJNR Am J Neuroradiol. 2014;35(8):1647–52. https://doi.org/10.3174/ajnr.A3948.
63. Kiss E, Keusch G, Zanetti M, Jung T, Schwarz A, Schocke M, Jaschke W, Czermak BV. Dialysis-related amyloidosis revisited. AJR Am J Roentgenol. 2005;185(6):1460–7. https://doi.org/10.2214/ajr.04.1309.
64. Yueniwati Y, Widhiasi DE. Role of magnetic resonance imaging in differentiating spondylitis from vertebral metastasis. Asian Spine J. 2015;9(5):776–82. https://doi.org/10.4184/asj.2015.9.5.776.
65. Resnick D, Niwayama G. Subchondral resorption of bone in renal osteodystrophy. Radiology. 1976;118(2):315–21. https://doi.org/10.1148/118.2.315.
66. Khalatbari MR, Moharamzad Y. Brown tumor of the spine in patients with primary hyperparathyroidism. Spine (Phila Pa 1976). 2014;39(18):E1073–9. https://doi.org/10.1097/brs.0000000000000455.
67. Forrester DM. Infectious spondylitis. Semin Ultrasound CT MR. 2004;25(6):461–73.
68. Omoumi P, Zufferey P, Malghem J, So A. Imaging in gout and other crystal-related arthropathies. Rheum Dis Clin N Am. 2016;42(4):621–44. https://doi.org/10.1016/j.rdc.2016.07.005.
69. Vohra R, Kang HS, Dogra S, Saggar RR, Sharma R. Tuberculous osteomyelitis. J Bone Joint Surg. 1997;79(4):562–6.
70. Hodgson SP, Ormerod LP. Ten-year experience of bone and joint tuberculosis in Blackburn 1978–1987. J R Coll Surg Edinb. 1990;35(4):259–62.
71. Engin G, Acunas B, Acunas G, Tunaci M. Imaging of extrapulmonary tuberculosis. Radiographics. 2000;20(2):471–88.; ; quiz 529–430, 532. https://doi.org/10.1148/radiographics.20.2.g00mc07471.
72. Polley P, Dunn R. Noncontiguous spinal tuberculosis: incidence and management. Eur Spine J. 2009;18(8):1096–101. https://doi.org/10.1007/s00586-009-0966-0.
73. Garg RK, Somvanshi DS. Spinal tuberculosis: a review. J Spinal Cord Med. 2011;34(5):440–54. https://doi.org/10.1179/2045772311Y.0000000023.
74. Rivas-Garcia A, Sarria-Estrada S, Torrents-Odin C, Casas-Gomila L, Franquet E. Imaging findings of Pott's disease. Eur Spine J. 2013;22(Suppl 4):567–78. https://doi.org/10.1007/s00586-012-2333-9.
75. Lee KY. Comparison of pyogenic spondylitis and tuberculous spondylitis. Asian Spine J. 2014;8(2):216–23. https://doi.org/10.4184/asj.2014.8.2.216.
76. Wolansky LJ, Heary RF, Patterson T, Friedenberg JS, Tholany J, Chen JK, Patel N, Doddakashi S. Pseudosparing of the endplate: a potential pitfall in using MR imaging to diagnose infectious spondylitis. AJR Am J Roentgenol. 1999;172(3):777–80. https://doi.org/10.2214/ajr.172.3.10063881.

77. Kim CW, Perry A, Currier B, Yaszemski M, Garfin SR. Fungal infections of the spine. Clin Orthop Relat Res. 2006;444:92–9. https://doi.org/10.1097/01.blo.0000203451.36522.4c.
78. Williams RL, Fukui MB, Cidis Meltzer C, Swarnkar A, Johnson DW, Welch W. Fungal spinal osteomyelitis in the immunocompromised patient: MR findings in three cases. 1999;20(3):381–5.
79. Hadjipavlou AG, Mader JT, Nauta HJ, Necessary JT, Chaljub G, Adesokan A. Blastomycosis of the lumbar spine: case report and review of the literature, with emphasis on diagnostic laboratory tools and management. Eur Spine J. 1998;7(5):416–21. https://doi.org/10.1007/s005860050100.
80. Sethi S, Siraj F, Kalra K, Chopra P. Aspergillus vertebral osteomyelitis in immunocompetent patients. Indian J Orthop. 2012;46(2):246–50. https://doi.org/10.4103/0019-5413.93693.
81. Bosilkovski M, Dimzova M, Grozdanovski K. Natural history of brucellosis in an endemic region in different time periods. Acta Clin Croat. 2009;48(1):41–6.
82. Li T, Liu T, Jiang Z, Cui X, Sun J. Diagnosing pyogenic, brucella and tuberculous spondylitis using histopathology and MRI: a retrospective study. Exp Ther Med. 2016;12(4):2069–77. https://doi.org/10.3892/etm.2016.3602.
83. Chanchairujira K, Chung CB, Kim JY, Papakonstantinou O, Lee MH, Clopton P, Resnick D. Intervertebral disk calcification of the spine in an elderly population: radiographic prevalence, location, and distribution and correlation with spinal degeneration. Radiology. 2004;230(2):499–503. https://doi.org/10.1148/radiol.2302011842.
84. Moshrif A, Laredo JD, Bassiouni H, Abdelkareem M, Richette P, Rigon MR, Bardin T. Spinal involvement with calcium pyrophosphate deposition disease in an academic rheumatology center: a series of 37 patients. Semin Arthritis Rheum. 2019;48(6):1113–26. https://doi.org/10.1016/j.semarthrit.2018.10.009.
85. Koyfman A, Yaffe D. Crowned dens syndrome. A case report. Neuroradiol J. 2014;27(4):495–7. https://doi.org/10.15274/NRJ-2014-10056.
86. Chakraverty JK, Lawson TM, Herdman G. Not just simple degenerative disc disease (alkaptonuria). Spine J. 2013;13(8):985–6. https://doi.org/10.1016/j.spinee.2013.03.007.
87. Gil JA, Wawrzynski J, Waryasz GR. Orthopedic manifestations of ochronosis: pathophysiology, presentation, diagnosis, and management. Am J Med. 2016;129(5):536.e531–6. https://doi.org/10.1016/j.amjmed.2016.01.010.
88. Olivieri I, D'Angelo S, Palazzi C, Padula A, Mader R, Khan MA. Diffuse idiopathic skeletal hyperostosis: differentiation from ankylosing spondylitis. Curr Rheumatol Rep. 2009;11(5):321. https://doi.org/10.1007/s11926-009-0046-9.
89. Arad U, Elkayam O, Eshed I. Magnetic resonance imaging in diffuse idiopathic skeletal hyperostosis: similarities to axial spondyloarthritis. Clin Rheumatol. 2017;36(7):1545–9. https://doi.org/10.1007/s10067-017-3617-6.
90. Yamashita Y, Takahashi M, Matsuno Y, Sakamoto Y, Yoshizumi K, Oguni T, Kojima R. Spinal cord compression due to ossification of ligaments: MR imaging. Radiology. 1990;175(3):843–8. https://doi.org/10.1148/radiology.175.3.2111569.
91. Saetia K, Cho D, Lee S, Kim DH, Kim SD. Ossification of the posterior longitudinal ligament: a review. Neurosurg Focus. 2011;30(3):E1. https://doi.org/10.3171/2010.11.Focus10276.

# Clinical Examination and History Taking in Patients with Suspected Degenerative Disc Disease

3

Stephanie M. Robert, Ramana Gorepati, Arian Boylan, and Michele H. Johnson

## 3.1 Introduction

Degenerative disc disease (DDD) is a common age-related condition that develops as the discs separating the vertebral bodies of the spinal column breakdown over time. Age-related degeneration and disc dehydration, combined with the normal downward forces experienced by the spinal column, cause discs to develop tears and lose height. The outer portion of the disc, the annulus fibrosus, weakens, further damaging the structural integrity of the spine. This disc damage and resulting loss of height is accompanied by many secondary degenerative changes, including disc herniation, weakening and buckling of the longitudinal ligaments along the anterior and posterior walls of the vertebral bodies, and bone spur/osteophyte development, all of which can lead to spinal canal and foraminal stenosis. Compression of the spinal canal and nerve roots by degenerative spinal stenosis may cause classic symptoms of neck or back pain, neurogenic claudication, and/or radiculopathy in a subset of patients. Localized back pain may also be caused by inflammatory changes in the endplates associated with Modic changes or Schmorl's nodes, as well as uncovertebral or facet arthropathy and other common conditions.

The workup and diagnosis of DDD in patients presenting with back/neck pain or symptoms of neurogenic claudication or radiculopathy should entail a detailed history of present illness (HPI), physical exam, and, if warranted, spinal imaging. Given the significant prevalence of back pain and the numerous etiologies that can cause this common symptom, it is important to first elucidate a thorough

S. M. Robert · R. Gorepati · A. Boylan
Department of Neurosurgery, Yale University School of Medicine, New Haven, CT, USA

M. H. Johnson (✉)
Department of Radiology and Biomedical Imaging, Yale University School of Medicine, New Haven, CT, USA
e-mail: michele.h.johnson@yale.edu



L. Manfrè, J. Van Goethem (eds.), *The Disc and Degenerative Disc Disease*, New Procedures in Spinal Interventional Neuroradiology,
https://doi.org/10.1007/978-3-030-03715-4_3

understanding of the patient's complaints, timeline of symptoms, and if any neurological deficits are present. Spinal imaging should then be used to rule out more serious pathologies, clarify diagnosis, and guide further treatment and follow-up.

## 3.2 Pathophysiology of Degenerative Disc Disease

The structure and function of intervertebral discs are similar in the cervical, thoracic, and lumbar spine. However, the differences that do exist are, in part, due to the unique features associated with axial loading, bending, and rotation of the regional spinal segments. The majority of this discussion will focus on lumbar disc anatomy and pathology; however, regional differences will be highlighted and discussed.

Intervertebral discs consist of a central nucleus pulposus surrounded by a firm outer annulus fibrosus. Superiorly and inferiorly, the disc is lined with cartilage and attaches to the endplates of the surrounding vertebral bodies. Intervertebral discs are designed to distribute mechanical loading evenly throughout the vertebral bodies of the spine and function to provide tensile strength and resist compressive loading. The center of the disc, the nucleus pulposus, consists of proteoglycans, large molecules with sugar subunits that have a strong attraction to water, held together loosely by type II collagen and elastin fibers. The outer annulus is made of type I collagen fibers running obliquely in alternating directions [1, 2].

Interestingly, intervertebral discs are avascular and therefore have to derive nutrition from the vessels within the bone of the endplate through passive diffusion. With aging, the disc composition changes, with loss of proteoglycans, increased cross-linking of collagen, and decreased water content. As a result, the disc becomes unable to distribute forces evenly across its surface. Thus, weight-bearing shifts from the nucleus to the annulus, causing further cross-linking of collagen fibers leading to the disc becoming increasingly brittle over time. This degeneration combined with the lack of inherent blood supply in the disc results in slow and inefficient repair of damaged intervertebral discs. As the integrity of the discs degrade, they begin to bulge circumferentially, causing loss of disc height and further disc bulging and leading to increased mechanical forces on surrounding bony structures and secondary growth of osteophytes and osteoarthritis [1].

Although similar in design and function, cervical intervertebral discs have specific properties that make their physiology and pathology unique enough to warrant a separate discussion. In the cervical spine, the nucleus pulposus is proportionally larger than in the lumbar spine and has a higher collagen content. Throughout development, more fibrocartilage deposits, and the nucleus becomes more fibrous. In the cervical spine, the annulus fibrosus is crescent-shaped, composed of thick collagen anteriorly which tapers laterally toward the uncinate processes. It is thin posteriorly and the fibers are oriented in a longitudinal direction, rather than obliquely as they are in the lumbar spine. The ventral and dorsal components of cervical discs are designed as such to give support as well as to limit the range of motion introduced by the uncovertebral and zygapophyseal joints. Further, supporting the more complex bending and axial movements capable in the cervical spine, the anterolateral capsular ligaments maintain contact with the facets, and the anterior annulus creates a pivot point. Anterior and posterior longitudinal ligaments, which surround the anterior and posterior disc space, respectively, also significantly contribute to stability and force bearing in the cervical spine. Over time, the cervical disc breaks down and degenerates as do the lumbar discs, leading to similar pathologies and symptoms due to bony overgrowth and nerve and/or spinal cord compression [3, 4].

Thoracic intervertebral discs are also similar in structure and function; however, it is important to recognize a few distinct differences in the thoracic spine. Compared to the cervical and lumbar spine, the thoracic spine is functionally rigid. This difference is due to the interaction and stability of the adjoined ribcage. Further contributing to a rigid section is the orientation of the facet joints and the presence of thinner intervertebral discs. The vertebral canal of both the cervical and thoracic region is also typically narrow, making disc herniation and bony overgrowth more likely to cause cord damage and result in neurological deficits [5].

## 3.3 Evaluation of a Patient with Suspected Degenerative Disc Disease

The incidence of neck and back pain across the population is high, and lifetime incidence is estimated to reach over 70% [6]. For most patients, pain is "axial," or arising from along or around the spinal column. Although the specific etiology remains undetermined, this type of pain is typically ascribed to mechanical issues, and surrounding muscle and/or joint sprains. Discogenic pain is also common and occurs when nociceptors in the annulus fibrosus perceive pain. Inflammation and response to bony degeneration also precipitate sensation of pain in patients [2]. For these types of axial and discogenic back or neck pain, nonoperative management and treatment is preferred. Many patients will experience relief or resolution of their symptoms over time with conservative therapy in the form of pain control, exercise, physical therapy, epidural steroid injections, and anti-inflammatory medications.

The first step in evaluating a patient presenting with complaints of neck or back pain is a thorough understanding of the symptoms. Specific details of the patient's presenting complaints can be revealing regarding underlying pathology and may indicate the need for imaging and inform treatment decisions. Myelopathy and radiculopathy cause pain related to compression or irritation of the exiting nerve roots or spinal cord and typically indicate the presence of a structural abnormality caused by trauma, or degenerative processes. Vascular compromise secondary to venous compression with reduced blood flow and/or reduced oxygenation is often a contributing cause of cervical myelopathy in the setting of cervical spondylosis. Radicular symptoms are caused by compression of the nerve roots exiting the spinal canal through the neuroforamen on either side, typically referred to as foraminal stenosis. The foramen may be compromised by disc herniations, degenerative discs, facet arthropathy, and/or uncovertebral degenerative arthropathy in the case of the cervical spine. Myelopathy is due to compression or injury to the spinal cord.

Non-compressive etiologies of myelopathy, including medical causes such as multiple sclerosis, vascular, autoimmune, vitamin deficiencies, must be differentiated from surgical compressive disease when a patient presents with symptoms of myelopathy [6].

Although most neck and back pain is benign and can be managed, at least initially, by conservative, nonoperative treatments, and there are certain "red flag" symptoms that should be addressed with greater urgency. These include motor weakness, significant sensory changes, loss of bowel/bladder control, and saddle anesthesia. Furthermore, given the possibility of non-central nervous system etiology of symptoms, it is important to rule out underlying joint problems (shoulder, hip, sacroiliac), as well as peripheral nerve pathologies. Similarly, more concerning symptoms or history, such as night sweats, weight loss, cancer diagnosis, diabetes, or intravenous drug abuse (IVDA), will change the workup and require further investigation into underlying pathologies beyond DDD.

## 3.4 Cervical Spine Degenerative Disc Disease

Degenerative cervical spine disease is common and often benign; however, it can become severe and debilitating, with the development of neurological symptoms as it progresses. Specifically, for cervical spine pathology, myelopathic signs and symptoms are important to uncover if present, as this finding necessitates earlier consideration of surgical management [7].

### 3.4.1 History of Presentation

Cervical spinal stenosis commonly presents with complaints of neck pain, radiculopathy, myelopathy, numbness, parasthesias, and coordination issues including difficulty with buttons, zippers, jewelry clasps, dropping things, and even handwriting changes. Symptom details such as time of onset, severity, location/distribution, and progressiveness are also important, as well as alleviating and aggravating factors.

The distribution of pain and symptoms is paramount, and can be axial, radicular, or myelopathic. Axial pain typically presents as long-standing, dull, diffuse neck pain and is more likely due to multilevel disc degeneration, facet, or paraspinal muscle sprain than a structural lesion such as disc herniation or neuroforaminal stenosis which would present with more discrete localizing symptoms [8]. More acute symptoms consistent with a radiculopathy occur in a specific distribution served by a spinal nerve root and indicate a structural lesion causing compression or irritation [9] (i.e., pain radiating into the shoulder suggesting C4/5 disc herniation and compression of the C5 nerve root). Myelopathy, in additional to neck pain, presents as gait instability, loss of fine motor control, weakness, and, if severe, urinary incontinence [10, 11].

Although nerve root irritation, or radicular pain, is not always dermatomal, a dermatomal distribution of pain is important to elucidate, as steroids (typically medrol) and/or medications such as gabapentin may be effective for symptom control. Conversely, pain that appears more axial than dermatomal typically indicates a need for dynamic imaging, specifically flexion/extension X-rays, to ensure no instability is present with movement. MRI dynamic imaging can be employed in selected difficult cases.

The duration/chronicity of the patient's symptoms can help to determine the urgency and type of imaging indicated. If the pain is chronic and/or improving, routinely scheduled X-rays may be appropriate, conversely if the pain started after a recent traumatic event and/or is significantly worsening, X-rays at time of the visit would be indicated and possibly more urgent CT or MRI may be needed depending on additional findings such as bowel or bladder incontinence or neurological deficit on exam and in accordance with trauma imaging guidelines.

### 3.4.2 Physical Exam

Complementary to a thorough patient history, a complete but focused neurological exam is important to guide diagnosis, imaging, and management decisions. Testing extremities for weakness and numbness may allow localization of a neurological deficit or radiculopathy to a specific spinal level. These findings can then be confirmed on imaging studies. If any urinary symptoms or perineal numbness are present, a rectal exam is indicated as well. Loss of rectal tone or any history of bowel incontinence requires immediate MRI to rule out pathology needing emergent surgical management.

Reflex examination is one of the most objective parts of a neurological exam and can be helpful especially when the symptoms and participation-dependent exam (i.e., strength and sensory testing) are unclear. Given that most descending pathways in the spinal cord relay a tonic inhibitory effect on reflexes, damage to these tracts results in hyperactive reflexes. Upper extremity hyperreflexia indicates possible cervical spine injury/compression. Hoffman's reflex is specifically useful, as it is a sign of cervical cord compression, especially in patients with complaints and symptoms that correspond with cervical myelopathy. Hoffman's reflex is tested by loosely holding the middle finger of the hand and flicking downward on the nail bed, with a positive test resulting contraction of the thumb of the same hand. The brachioradialis reflex involves the C5 and C6 nerve roots and is elicited by briskly tapping the muscle–tendon interface. A positive test occurs with finger flexion or slight elbow extension [12]. Additionally, although not a reflex rest, the Spurling compression test uses lateral bending and axial compression of the cervical spine to reproduce the patient's symptoms [13] and indicate positive findings that can be helpful clinically.

Asymmetric reflexes are also an indication of pathology and location. Abnormal reflexes deserve consideration of cranial and peripheral nerve pathology, especially if present in both upper and lower extremities, and can typically be further evaluated based on the patient's history and motor/sensory exam. Consider a detailed neurology (independent-nonsurgical) evaluation, if any concern for cortical or peripheral nerve etiology of hyper- or hyporeflexia, for workup of a nonsurgical pathology. Furthermore, if pain or paresthesias are present in a strictly median or ulnar nerve distribution, peripheral nerve tests such as Tinel and Phalen can help identify a likely compressive peripheral nerve pathology that may respond to conservative therapy or require surgical decompression of the entrapped nerve.

Specifically, for cervical spine pathology, myelopathic signs and symptoms are important to uncover if present, as the presence of myelopathy necessitates early consideration of surgical management. The presence of Hoffman's reflex, possibly in conjunction with Babinski and/or clonus, difficulty with tandem gait, and complains of numbness, coordination issues, grip weakness, and bowel/bladder issues point toward myelopathy due to underlying damage to and/or compression of the cervical spinal cord. These patients typically do not respond well to conservative therapy, and many patients will progress without surgical intervention.

Sensation should be tested in a dermatomal pattern to identify specific distributions of numbness, pain, and paresthesias. Axial pain that is reproducible with palpation should be first imaged with upright X-rays, then either with CT or MRI depending on the X-ray findings. If shoulder pain can be elicited during exam, consider appropriate imaging and referral to either physiatry or orthopedics for management of non-neurosurgical etiology of pain and symptoms.

### 3.4.3 Imaging

Cervical imaging is often needed to diagnose specific pathologies causing a patient's pain and symptoms. Plain (anteroposterior and lateral views ± oblique images) and dynamic radiographs, when instability is suspected (i.e., flexion and extension views), are useful initial studies to determine the alignment of the cervical vertebrae and can diagnose conditions such as cervical kyphosis, ossification of the posterior longitudinal ligament (OPLL), diffuse idiopathic skeletal hyperostosis (DISH), or the presence of posterior osteophytes that may be contributing to stenosis. Plain X-rays are also useful to assess the sequelae of past trauma or surgical intervention. If there are persistent radicular complaints, neurological deficits, or symptoms of myelopathy, an MRI of the cervical spine is indicated to better evaluate the neural foramina and neural elements, ligaments, discs, and spinal cord [14].

CT or MRI of the cervical spine is obtained to better evaluate the underlying boney structures and soft-tissue components to aid in treatment decisions, especially if surgical management is being considered. CT (non-contrast) is particularly useful for surgical planning as the bony structural details are needed to determine the type and location of the surgical treatment. MRI is best for visualization of the integrity and pathology of the intervertebral discs, ligaments, and neural elements. Degenerative disc disease (DDD), disc herniation, and adjacent segment disease are better evaluated with MRI. In many situations, CT and MRI are complementary and both may be required for effective surgical treatment planning.

## 3.5 Lumbar Spine Degenerative Disc Disease

### 3.5.1 History of Presentation

Patients with degenerative disc disease in the lumbar spine commonly present with back pain and/or radicular symptoms. Symptoms consistent with axial back pain present as pain in the low back region that may become chronic. Nerve root irritation typically presents as sharp or burning pain down the leg, with the exact location determined by the nerve root involved. This radicular lumbar back pain is most common in the L4, L5, and/or S1 dermatomal distributions. Other neurological symptoms may also be present, including weakness (corresponding to the affected nerve roots), numbness, or paresthesias.

Neurogenic claudication, due to central canal stenosis from extruded disc or ligamentous hypertrophy, is classically described as lower back pain and pain, discomfort, numbness, or weakness in the legs bilaterally. It is typically exacerbated by walking and prolonged standing, with relief by siting or bending forward. These patients describe what is referred to as the "shopping cart sign," where bending over and leaning on a shopping cart relieves symptoms as it serves to widen the spinal canal temporarily. Patients with spinal stenosis do not typically present with acutely worsening neurological symptoms [6].

### 3.5.2 Physical Exam

In many cases, the description of the patient's symptoms gives significant insight into the etiology of the pain; however, physical exam is important to further clarify the pathology as well to exclude additional pathology. Pain with palpation of the center of the back suggests vertebral origin, whereas pain more laterally likely originates from the facet joints or paraspinal musculature. The straight leg test is a common provocative test that can elicit pain on the affected side by extending the leg greater than 60°. Pain radiating down the leg suggests radiculopathy.

Reflexes can also be helpful for lumbar pathology (Table 3.1), with L4 involvement (and some L3), the patellar reflex can be affected, medial hamstring with L5, and Achilles with S1 pathology [6]. Pain radiating below the knee is common for lower lumbar stenosis, with L4 radiating down the anterior lower leg, L5 composing the lateral lower leg, and S1 radiating into the posterior calf. Of note, lower

**Table 3.1** Lumbar and sacral nerve roots motor, sensory, and reflexes [6, 15]

| | Motor | Sensory | Reflex |
|---|---|---|---|
| L2 | Hip flexion, thigh adduction | Upper thigh | |
| L3 | Quadriceps, knee extension | Anterolateral thigh | (patellar) |
| L4 | Knee extensors, foot dorsiflexion | Anteriomedial calf | Patellar |
| L5 | Foot and toe dorsiflexion | Lateral calf, dorsum of foot | Medial hamstring |
| S1, 2 | Foot and toe plantar flexions | Lateral foot, sole of foot | Achilles |
| S2–5 | Sphincters | Perianal and saddle regions | Bulbocavernosus |

extremity hyperreflexia is a sign of thoracic cord compression, warranting at minimum thoracic MRI imaging.

A large lumbar disc herniation which causes cauda equina compression can be a surgical emergency. In addition to back pain, cauda equina pathology presents with urinary retention and bowel incontinence. Sensory and motor deficits as well as saddle anesthesia are typically present, and patient has diminished rectal tone. If symptoms appear acutely, immediate imaging is necessary with MRI to identify both etiology and extent of disease, as the patient may need urgent surgical decompression [15].

### 3.5.3 Imaging

Lumbar imaging is useful when the history and physical exam do not clearly define the diagnosis, or when operative intervention is being considered. More urgent imaging is needed when there are neurological symptoms, especially weakness or symptoms concerning for cauda equina. Other "red flag" symptoms that need more urgent imaging include fever, unexpected weight loss, or history of immunosuppression. If only radicular symptoms are present, conservative management without imaging beyond plain X-rays can be appropriate with follow up to determine if any improvement has occurred. Persistent chronic symptoms or development of new neurological symptoms are indications for MRI with or without CT imaging to assess location and extent of disease.

Plain (anteroposterior and lateral views) and dynamic radiographs (i.e., flexion and extension views) can be useful initial studies to determine the alignment of the lumbar spine, diagnose fractures and other common pathologies. When certain patient movements exacerbate symptoms leading the surgeon to suspect mechanical instability, flexion extension films are often performed. Plain X-rays are also useful to determine if any complications exist from previous surgical intervention, especially if hardware was placed. CT imaging is useful to detect bony changes and alignment and better evaluate any possible complications with existing hardware. If concerns exist for pathology of the intervertebral disc, spinal canal or nerve root, or surrounding soft tissue, MR-imaging is needed. Furthermore, if patients are initially evaluated with only an MRI and the patient is in need of surgical management, a non-contrast CT scan is often needed for preoperative planning [16, 17].

## 3.6 Case Presentations

### 3.6.1 Case 1

*History of presentation*: 72-year-old female presenting with lower extremity heaviness with ambulation which is limiting activity. She describes paresthesias in feet when she walks more than one block. Her lower extremity symptoms resolve when she sits down but are not relieved with flexion or extension. She also has some urinary urgency when she transitions from seated to standing position but acknowledges urge to void and denies incontinence or saddle anesthesia. Of note, she sustained a mechanical fall 2 weeks prior to presentation and has some increased back pain.

*Physical exam*: She has mild tenderness to palpation on exam with full motor strength, intact sensation, and 2+ reflexes at patellar tendon bilaterally.

*Imaging*: Routine X-ray lumbar spine AP/lateral are ordered to look for compression fracture as well as MRI lumbar spine to asses for structural basis of her clinical neurogenic claudication. On imaging, no fracture was noted; however, she had Grade 1 anterolisthesis of L4 on L5 with moderate-to-severe stenosis L2–5 (Fig. 3.1a–c).

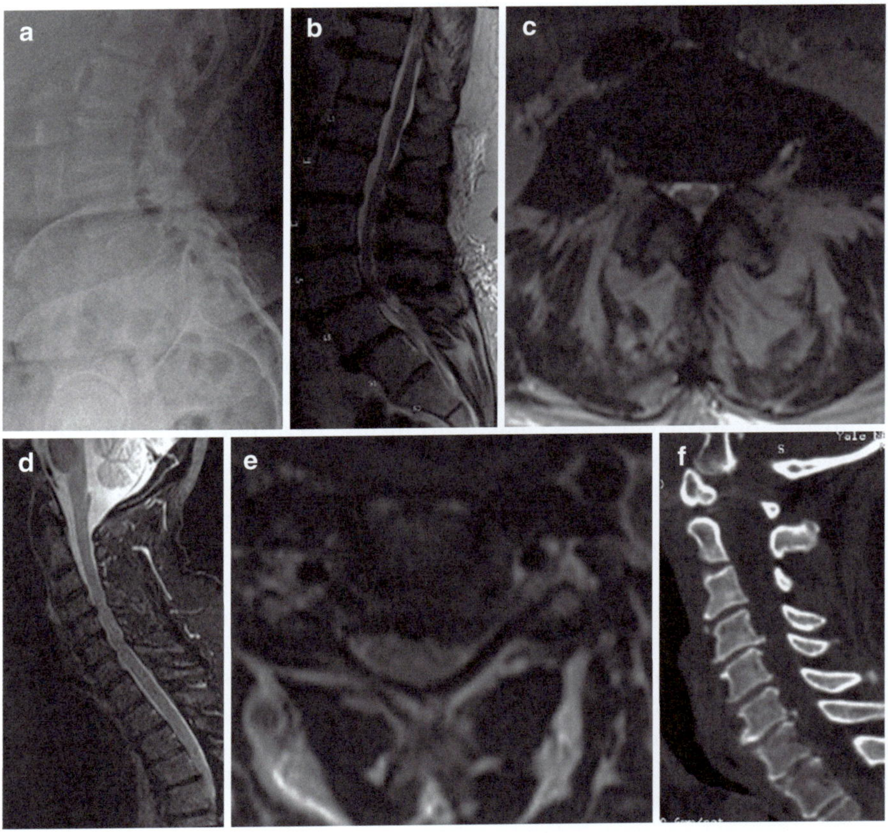


**Fig. 3.1** (**a–c**) Lumbar imaging. Lateral X-ray and sagittal STIR. Grade I anterolisthesis of L4 on L5 and degenerative spinal stenosis L2–L5. Axial T2 at L4–5 with bulging annulus and facet and ligamentous hypertrophy. (**d–f**) Cervical Imaging. Sagittal STIR demonstrates degenerative spinal stenosis from C3–C6. Axial T2 at C5–6 demonstrates uncovertebral degenerative disease with posterior osteophytes and foraminal and canal stenosis. Sagittal CT demonstrates the disc space narrowing and posterior osteophytes to better advantage

*Return clinic visit*: She follows up to clinic after imaging completed. Imaging was reviewed and her back pain has improved. Of note, during this follow-up visit she describes new paresthesias in her hands including all the fingers which is worse at night. She also notes some increasing clumsiness in her hands specifically with buttons, zippers, and jewelry clasps. She is finding it increasingly difficult to stand with her eyes closed in the shower and has had another fall.

*Physical exam*: On exam, she has negative Tinel and Phalen tests at wrist and elbow. She has negative Spurlings and is full strength. Brachioradialis is 3+ and she has positive Hoffman's bilaterally. She has difficulty with tandem gait. This constellation of exam findings are not consistent with peripheral neuropathy and most consistent with cervical myelopathy.

*Imaging*: MRI cervical spine without contrast was ordered to evaluate her cervical myelopathy for location and extent of disease. MRI shows severe cervical stenosis most prominent at C5–6. (Fig. 3.1d, f).

*Treatment plan*: She follows up to clinic after imaging completed, and after reviewing the imaging and discussing possible surgical intervention for cervical degenerative spinal stenosis with patient, a CT scan of cervical spine is ordered for surgical planning (Fig. 3.1f).

### 3.6.2 Case 2

*History of presentation*: 60-year-old man presents with worsening back pain and leg heaviness/paresthesias which improve with flexion and sitting. Stationary bike is comfortable for him but walking is very limited. He denies frank bowel or bladder symptoms but has more urgency and difficulty getting to restroom in time secondary to pain. He had a prior L3–4 laminotomy for disc 10 years ago when he had right leg pain which has resolved.

*Physical exam*: Motor and sensory functions are intact, but he has markedly antalgic gait. Patellar tendon reflex muted on right. Negative straight leg raise test. Prior incision is well-healed. Clinical diagnosis is central canal stenosis with claudication.

*Imaging*: Routine MRI was ordered which revealed multilevel degenerative changes with varying degrees of central and foraminal stenosis worse at L2–3. Hypertrophied facets containing fluid are noted at the prior laminotomy site. There was significant lateral recess stenosis at multiple levels resulting in clumping of nerve roots and disc degeneration with various degrees of bulging. Flexion/extension X-rays are ordered which show no instability or listhesis, given fluid in facets and prior surgery. CT lumbar spine ordered which showed prior surgical site and overgrown facets without pars defect (Fig. 3.2a–f).

*Treatment plan*: Patient undergoes course of physical therapy without improvement. He had facet injections which briefly helped with his back pain but his leg symptoms were unchanged. Patient queried intraspinous devices and was advised this would be less likely to help patient than decompression, given degree of nerve root clumping due to lateral recess stenosis and disc bulging contributing to stenosis. Plans were made for patient to undergo surgical decompression from L2 to L5

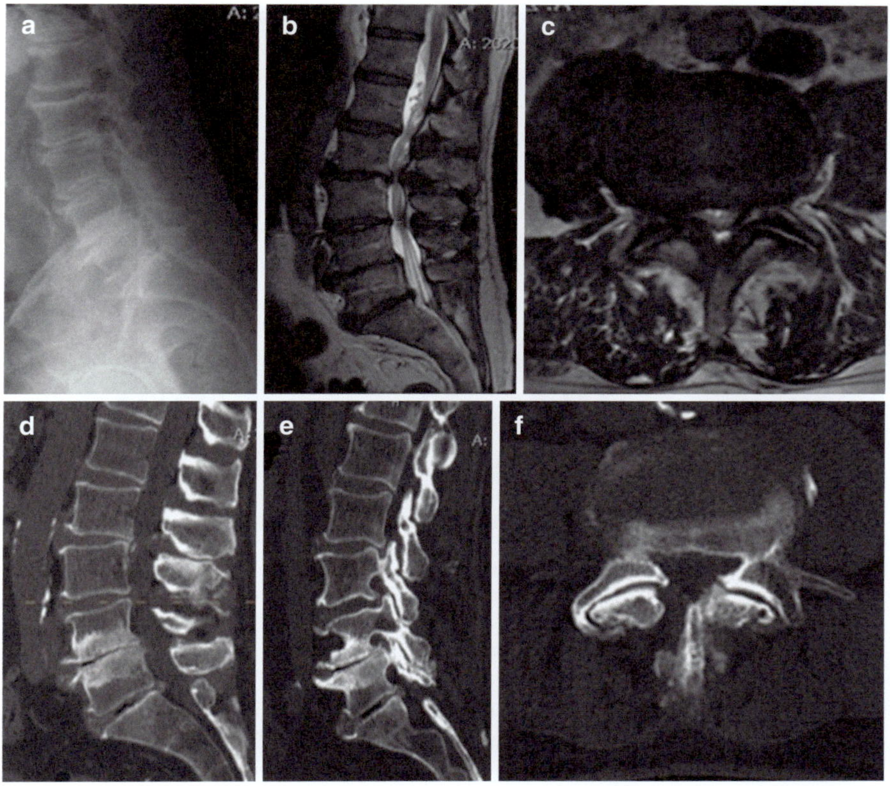


**Fig. 3.2** (**a–c**) Lumbar imaging. Lateral X-ray and sagittal STIR demonstrate degenerative spinal stenosis L2-5 with degenerated discs, posterior osteophytes, and annular bulges. Axial T2 at L3–4 shows bulging annulus, facet, and ligamentous hypertrophy with severe bilateral foraminal stenosis. (**d–f**) Lumbar imaging. Midline and left lateral CT sagittal reconstructions demonstrate severe disc space narrowing, vacuum disc phenomenon, endplate sclerosis, facet hypertrophy, and severe foraminal stenosis on the left. On the axial CT, note the facet hypertrophy, canal stenosis, and the right laminotomy defect

with medial facetectomies and foraminotomies without fusion since no instability was noted.

### 3.6.3 Case 3

*History of presentation*: 66-year-old man presents with long-standing intermittent back pain. Avid hiker and cyclist, he finds that cannot hike anymore because legs get too heavy and feels like he cannot lift legs. This resolves after sitting for 5–10 min. Biking helps his symptoms and he finds leaning forward like on a shopping cart makes the symptoms more tolerable. No bowel or bladder symptoms, radicular pain, or numbness.

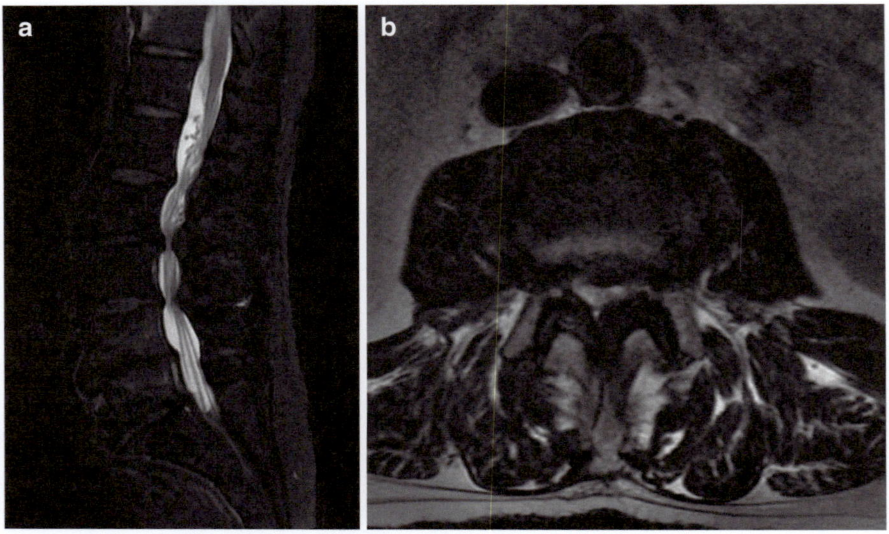


**Fig. 3.3** (**a**, **b**) Lumbar imaging. Sagittal midline STIR image demonstrates multilevel degenerative spinal stenosis, most severe at L2–3 and L3–4. Note endplate changes and decreased disc space height at L4–5 and L5-S1. Axial T2 at L3–4 demonstrates bulging annulus, facet, ligamentous hypertrophy, and central canal stenosis

*Physical exam*: On exam, he is full strength and sensation intact to light touch. Symmetric 1+ reflexes at patellar tendon and Achilles tendon exam. Gait is within normal limits but he starts to lean forward as he ambulates across room.

*Imaging*: Routine MRI was ordered which revealed severe lumbar central stenosis L2–5 with clumping nerve roots and fluid in facets at multiple levels without spondylolisthesis. There are Modic type I changes at L4–5 which may be contributing to the patient's back pain. (Fig. 3.3a, b).

*Treatment plan*: The patient returned to clinic. He is eager to avoid surgery. He is advised there is no injection which will be helpful for his back pain, given the lack of radicular symptoms. He elects to trial physical therapy. After 6 weeks, he returns with improving strength and mobility. He is followed conservatively over time.

## 3.7 Conclusion

Degenerative disc disease is common. Although many patients can be treated conservatively without surgery, it is important to gain a full understanding of the symptoms and pathology to ensure that there are no underlying etiologies present that require more urgent treatment. The most important initial evaluation of a patient presenting with symptoms of cervical or lumbar disc disease is a thorough but focused history and physical exam. A patient's description of symptoms, timing, chronicity, and distribution, alleviation and aggravation, combined with findings on physical exam can guide imaging and treatment. Chronic, long-standing axial pain would warrant plain X-rays in clinic, more recent but not improving radicular pain would suggest the need for a non-urgent MRI to be scheduled, and acute onset of severe sensory symptoms, weakness, or bowel/bladder issues would require emergent MR-imaging to rule out pathology needing urgent surgical management. Through a detailed understanding of the patient's symptoms and physical exam findings, the most effective and appropriate imaging modalities and treatment can be determined to expeditiously address the underlying etiology of the patient's disease process.

## References

1. Adams, M.A. 2015. Intervertebral disc tissues. In: Derby B. and Akhtar, R. eds. Mechanical properties of aging soft tissues. Engineering materials and processes. Cham: Springer, pp. 7–35.
2. Choi Y-S. Pathophysiology of degenerative disc disease. Asian Spine J. 2009;3(1):39–44.
3. Mercer S, Bogduk N. The ligaments and annulus fibrosus of human adult cervical intervertebral discs. Spine. 1999;24(7):619–26. discussion 627
4. Tonetti J, Potton L, Riboud R, Peoc'h M, Passagia JG, Chirossel JP. Morphological cervical disc analysis applied to traumatic and degenerative lesions. Surg Radiol Anat. 2005;27(3):192–200.
5. Waxenbaum JA, Futterman B. Anatomy, back, thoracic vertebrae. Treasure Island, FL: StatPearls Publishing; 2018.
6. Patel EA, Perloff MD. Radicular pain syndromes: cervical, lumbar, and spinal stenosis. Semin Neurol. 2018;38(6):634–9.
7. Nouri A, Cheng JS, Davies B, Kotter M, Schaller K, Tessitore E. Degenerative cervical myelopathy: a brief review of past perspectives, present developments, and future directions. J Clin Med. 2020;9(2):535.
8. Jones TR, Rao R. Pathophysiology of axial low back pain. Sem Spine Surg. 2008;20(2):78–86.
9. Govind J. Lumbar radicular pain. Aust Fam Physician. 2004;33(6):409–12.
10. Donnally CJ III, Hanna A, Odom CK. Cervical myelopathy. Treasure Island, FL: StatPearls Publishing; 2020.
11. de Oliveira Vilaça C, Orsini M, Leite MAA, de Freitas MRG, Davidovich E, Fiorelli R, Fiorelli S, Fiorelli C, Oliveira AB, Pessoa BL. Cervical spondylotic myelopathy: what the neurologist should know. Neurol Int. 2016;8(4):6330.
12. Cao T, Tadi P. Brachioradialis reflex. Treasure Island, FL: Stat Pearls Publishing; 2020.
13. Anekstein Y, Blecher R, Smorgick Y, Mirovsky Y. What is the best way to apply the Spurling test for cervical radiculopathy? Clin Orthop Relat Res. 2012;470(9):2566–72.
14. Todd AG. Cervical spine: degenerative conditions. Curr Rev Musculoskelet Med. 2011;4(4):168–74.
15. Lavy C, James A, Wilson-MacDonald J, Fairbank J. Cauda equina syndrome. BMJ. 2009;338:b936.
16. Balagué F, Mannion AF, Pellisé F, Cedraschi C. Clinical update: low back pain. Lancet. 2007;369(9563):726–8.
17. Chou R, Qaseem A, Snow V, Casey D, Cross JT, Shekelle P, Owens DK, Clinical Efficacy Assessment Subcommittee of the American College of Physicians, American College of Physicians and American Pain Society Low Back Pain Guidelines Panel. Diagnosis and treatment of low back pain: a joint clinical practice guideline from the American College of Physicians and the American pain society. Ann Intern Med. 2007;147(7):478–91.

# Conventional Neuroradiology of Degenerative Disc Disease

# 4

Majda M. Thurnher and Johan Van Goethem

## 4.1 Anatomy

The intervertebral disc is an avascular structure consisting of three parts: (a) the *nucleus pulposus*; (b) the *annulus fibrosus*; and (c) the *vertebral endplate*.

The nucleus pulposus consists of 70–90% water and the remaining percentage are cells that are largely chondrocytes, as well as a matrix of proteoglycans, collagen fibers, other non-collagenous proteins, and elastin. The nucleus pulposus is avascular and its nutrition is achieved through diffusion.

The annulus fibrosus is composed of collagen fibers tightly arranged in 10–12 sheets called lamellae. The lamellae are arranged in concentric rings (like an onion) around the central nucleus pulposus. The direction of the fibers differs from one lamina to the other. The thinnest part of the annulus is posterolateral and contains more vertical fibers and a greater amount of disorganized collagen bundles. This feature makes the posterolateral area the weakest part of the disc and accounts for a high rate of disc herniation. The inner layers have neither innervation nor blood supply and receive nutrition via diffusion. The outer fibers of the annulus fibrosus receive blood supply from adjacent vessels in the endplate and are innervated by the sinuvertebral nerves that arise from the dorsal root ganglia.

Both the nucleus and the annulus contain collagen, with type I collagen mostly in the nucleus and type II collagen in the annulus.

M. M. Thurnher (✉)
Department of Biomedical Imaging and Image-Guided Therapy, Medical University Vienna, Vienna, Austria
e-mail: majda.thurnher@meduniwien.ac.at

J. Van Goethem
Department of Radiology, AZ Nikolaas, Sint-Niklaas, Belgium

University of Antwerp, Antwerp, Belgium



L. Manfrè, J. Van Goethem (eds.), *The Disc and Degenerative Disc Disease*, New Procedures in Spinal Interventional Neuroradiology,
https://doi.org/10.1007/978-3-030-03715-4_4

There is no distinct differentiation between the central gelatinous nucleus pulposus and the fibrous outer ring annulus fibrosus (this area is termed the *transitional zone*).

The vertebral endplates are thin layers of cartilage that cover the vertebral body and are encircled by the ring apophysis. The endplates are strongly attached to the annulus fibrosus (the outer *articular zone* consisting of fibrocartilage), but rather weakly attached to the vertebral bodies (the inner *growth zone* consisting of hyaline cartilage).

The vertebral endplates play a key role in the metabolism of the avascular intervertebral disc in adults.

The innervation of the disc occurs mainly via the sinuvertebral nerve from the ventral rami and the sympathetic chain, and in a normal disc, this nerve penetrates only the outer lamellae [1].

## 4.2 Aging of the Disc

The structure of the intervertebral disc changes dramatically with age. Interindividual differences in age-related changes exist between sexes because of confounding effects (sport). With advanced age, the water content of the disc decreases, and it becomes more fibrous. The nucleus pulposus demonstrates the most prominent changes due to the loss of water as it changes from a fluid body into a more solid and dry mass. The border between the nucleus pulposus and annulus fibrosus becomes blurred and indistinguishable. Tears are characteristic of aging of the annulus fibrosus and are a precondition for disc protrusions. Vertebral endplates become thinner, and focal areas of degeneration may progress to become full-thickness defects. Finally, the vertebral endplate may calcify and be replaced by bone. Spondylosis deformans, with ventral and lateral spondylophytes, is considered to be age-related, whereas posterior spondylophytes are considered pathological [2, 3].

## 4.3 Disc Degeneration

Disc degeneration is caused by several factors: mechanical loading; biochemical; nutritional; traumatic; and genetic.

Degenerative changes of the disc refer to a decrease of hydration (desiccation) and the elasticity of the nucleus pulposus and annulus fibrosus. Loss of water-holding proteoglycans occur in the nucleus pulposus, and type II collagen increases in the annulus fibrosus. Following these changes, the annulus fibrosus becomes prone to fissures (tears) and progressive structural degradation. Degeneration of the endplates leads to defects and sclerosis.

## 4.4 Epidemiology

Imaging features of spine degeneration are common in symptomatic and asymptomatic individuals. Disc protrusions in asymptomatic adults have been reported from 10% to 30% in different studies, with the prevalence increasing with age. Disc extrusions are rarely seen in an asymptomatic population (0–4%) and are much more common in symptomatic patients (5–10%). Disc bulge has been found in 6% of asymptomatic and 43% of the symptomatic population.

In one recently published meta-analysis of MR imaging, the evidence of disc bulge, degeneration, extrusion, protrusion, Modic 1 changes, and spondylolysis were found to be more prevalent in adults 50 years of age or younger with back pain compared to asymptomatic individuals [4]. The percentage of disc abnormalities found in the meta-analysis suggests that there is no direct causative association between the disc degeneration and pain [4].

## 4.5 Conventional Radiography

Radiography with anteroposterior (AP) and lateral views is the first diagnostic step in providing baseline information regarding spinal disorders. The major advantages of radiography are the wide availability and low cost. Radiography is effective at showing narrowed spinal channels, fractures, bone spurs (osteophytes), or osteoarthritis (Fig 4.1).

## 4.6 Computed Tomography (CT)

CT has the highest exposure of ionizing radiation of all the spinal imaging modalities. It is optimal for assessing osseous structures, especially as the first-line assessment in the emergency department setting following acute traumatic injuries.

Computed tomography myelography is used to assess compression of the neural elements when MRI cannot be performed.

In one recently published study, myelography and CT myelography were helpful in unclear cases of degenerative disorders of the cervical spine, particularly for multilevel stenosis [5]. Myelography and MCT added relevant information for therapeutic decisions in more than a quarter of the patients in comparison with MRI as the sole diagnostic modality and also changed therapeutic strategies. However, a significant part of the information drawn from myelography and MCT can be obtained with noninvasive examinations (unenhanced CT and radiographs) [5].

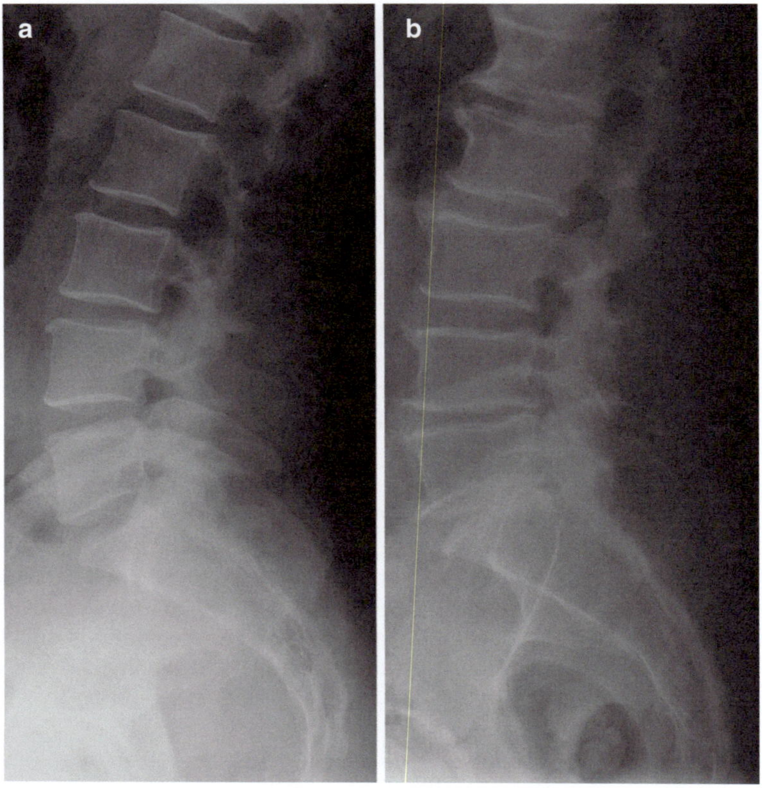


**Fig. 4.1** Radiography (lateral view) in two patients presenting with back pain. (**a**) 51-year-old female patient with subtle ventral bone spurs (spondylophytes) at vertebral bodies L3 and L4 and (**b**) A 79-year-old male patient with large ventral spondylophytes at L1–S1, sclerosis of the vertebral endplates, and narrowing of the disc spaces.

## 4.7 Magnetic Resonance Imaging (MRI)

Magnetic resonance imaging (MRI) is the most commonly used imaging modality for the evaluation and diagnosis of degenerative disc disease.

### 4.7.1 MRI Protocol

The standard MRI protocol for degenerative disc disease typically includes two-dimensional (2D) sagittal T1-weighted (T1w) fast spin-echo (FSE), sagittal T2-weighted (T2w) FSE, and axial T2w FSE images. A short tau inversion recovery (STIR) sequence, a gradient echo sequence (in the cervical spine), and a coronal proton-density-weighted (PDw), T2w, or T1w sequence should be added.

Contrast-enhanced T1w images are used in the postoperative setting, mainly to differentiate between epidural fibrosis and disc tissue. In epidural fibrosis/granulation tissue, diffuse enhancement will be observed, whereas rim enhancement will be detected in disc tissue. Further, partially healed chronic annular tears may demonstrate enhancement due to the presence of granulation tissue, not identified on normal T2w non-contrast MR images.

### 4.7.2 MRI Findings

## 4.8 Nomenclature

The nucleus pulposus is T1-hypointense compared to the vertebral bodies and T2-hyperintense due to its high water and proteoglycan content. The annulus fibrosus has a lower signal on both T1w and T2w images. In young adults (>30 years), in the center of the disc, a transverse band of hypointense signal is often visible on T2w images and is called the *intranuclear cleft,* and represents a fibrous plate [6, 7] (Fig. 4.2).

The vertebral endplates are well defined and smooth with an intact covering of cortical bone. They demonstrate low signal on T2-weighted images and cannot be clearly differentiated from the bony endplate. Due to its vascularization, enhancement can be noted on post-contrast T1w images.

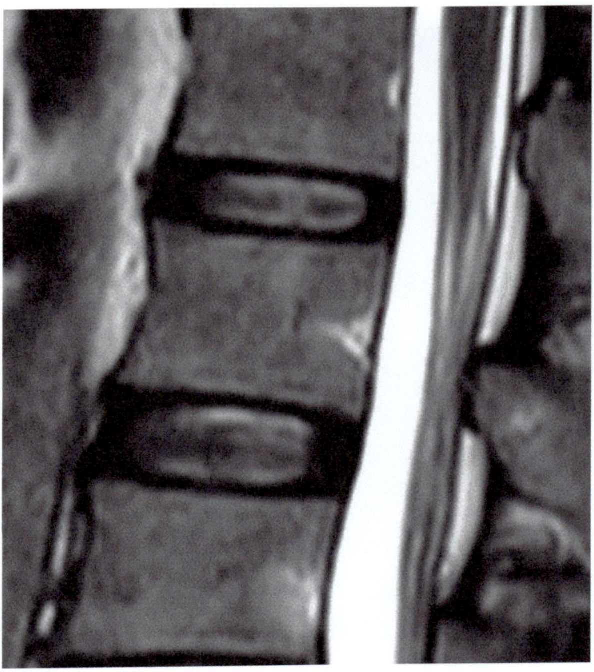

**Fig. 4.2** On sagittal T2w images of the lumbar spine, high-signal-intensity discs with a central linear hypointensity (intranuclear cleft) are easily recognized.

### 4.8.1 Degenerative Disc Disease (DDD)

Degeneration of the nucleus pulposus includes a decrease of proteoglycan and type II collagen and an increase of type I collagen. These processes lead to fissures, fibrosis, the appearance of cell clusters, and a loss of notochordal cells with the appearance of chondrocyte-like cells. Degeneration of the annulus fibrosis is demonstrated by the cross-linking of collagen fibers followed by disruption of the lamella, fissure, vascularization, and innervation.

The decrease of proteoglycan in the cartilage endplate leads to microfractures and sclerosis of the subchondral bone, as well as thinning and a reduction in the number of vascular channels [8, 9].

#### 4.8.1.1 Grading Methods

Various grading methods have been proposed for disc degeneration [10].

The Dallas classification uses post-discography CT observations of the integrity of the interior of the disc [11]. A five-category grading scheme for assessing the gross morphology of midsagittal sections of the human lumbar intervertebral disc was developed by Thompson et al., in 1990 [12]. The Thompson score uses disc height and disc signal intensity on T2-weighted MR images (Table 4.1, Fig. 4.3).

Another grading system for DDD proposed by Pffirmann et al. [13] uses five grades (Table 4.2).

#### 4.8.1.2 I Annulus Fibrosus Tears (Annular Fissures)

There are three types of annular tears/fissures: "concentric;" "radial;" and "transverse." They can be recognized on MRI as a T2 high-signal-intensity disruption of the annulus fibrosus (Fig. 4.4). According to the new lumbar disc nomenclature, the term "fissure" is favored rather than "tear." Most annular fissures are asymptomatic;

**Table 4.1** Macroscopic grading of lumbar disc degeneration on sagittal sections proposed by Thompson et al. [12]

| | Nucleus | Annulus | Endplate | Vertebral body |
|---|---|---|---|---|
| I | Bulging gel | Discrete fibrous lamellas | Hyaline, uniformly thick | Margins rounded |
| II | White fibrous tissue | Mucinous material between lamellas | Irregular thickness | Margins pointed |
| III | Consolidated fibrous tissue | Extensive mucinous infiltration | Focal defects in cartilage | Osteophytes at margins |
| IV | Horizontal clefts parallel to endplate | Focal disruptions | Fibrocartilage extending from subchondral bone, irregularity and focal sclerosis in subchondral bone | Osteophytes <2 mm |
| V | Clefts extended through nucleus and annulus | | Diffuse sclerosis | Osteophytes >2 mm |

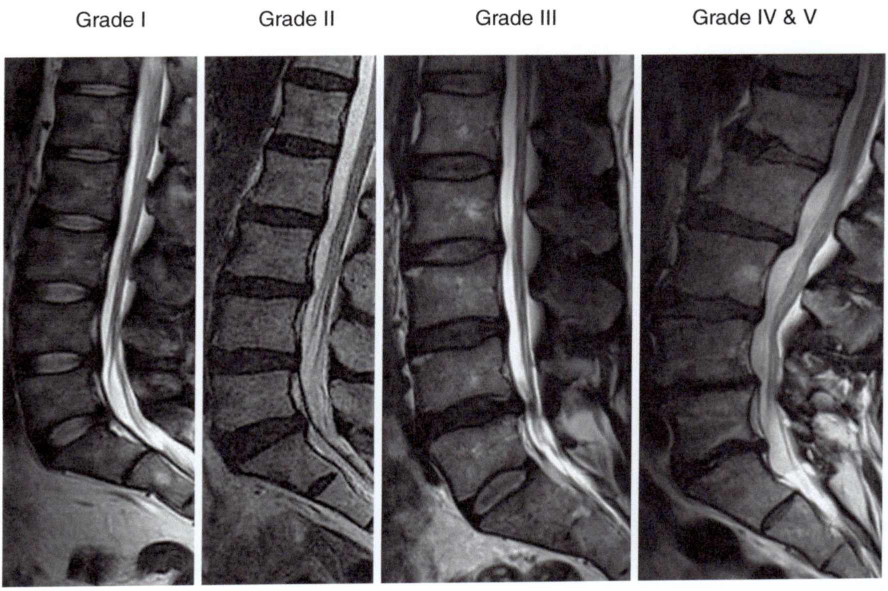


**Fig. 4.3** Sagittal T2w images of the lumbar spine at the different stages of degenerative disc disease

**Table 4.2** Disk degenerative disease in five stages based on Pffirmann et al. [13].

| | Height | T2 signal intensity | |
|---|---|---|---|
| I | Normal | Homogeneously bright | 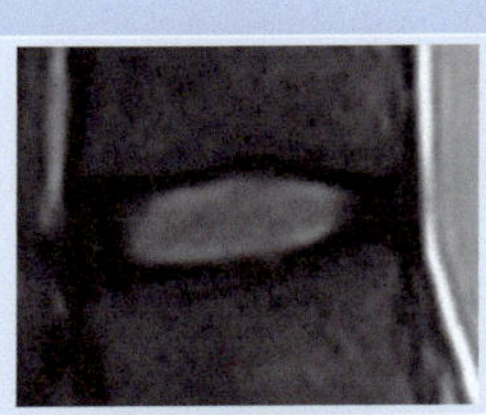 |
| II | Normal | Inhomogeneous hyperintense disc and clear differentiation between nucleus and annulus | 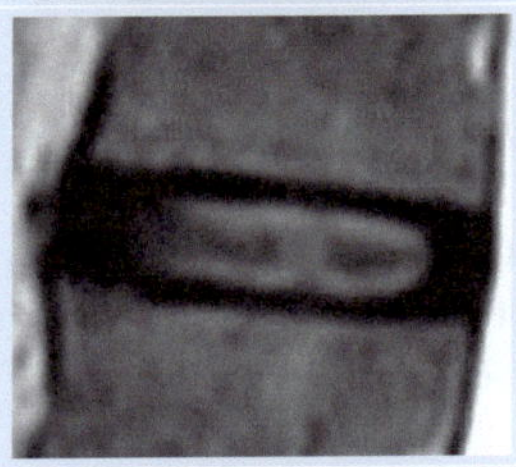 |
| III | Normal or slightly decreased | Inhomogeneous, intermediately gray disc, and unclear distinction between nucleus and annulus | 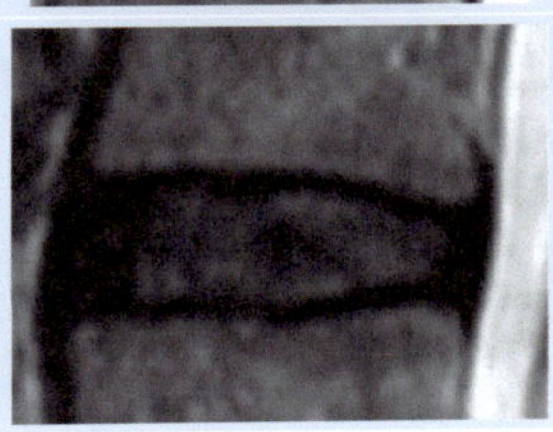 |

(continued)

**Table 4.2** (continued)

| | Height | T2 signal intensity | |
|---|---|---|---|
| IV | Normal to moderately decreased | Inhomogeneous, hypointense dark gray disc, and lost distinction between nucleus and annulus | 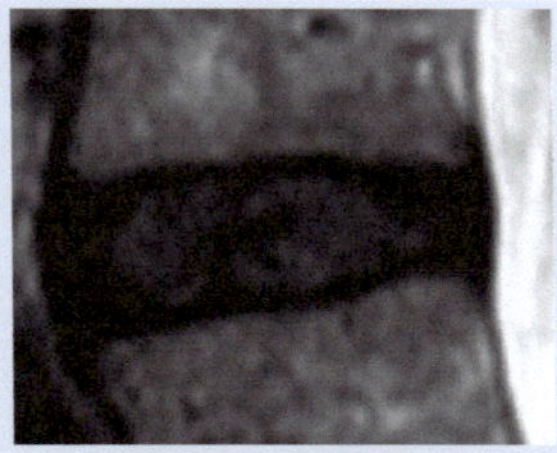 |
| V | Collapsed disc space | inhomogeneous, hypointense black disc, and lost distinction between nucleus and annulus | 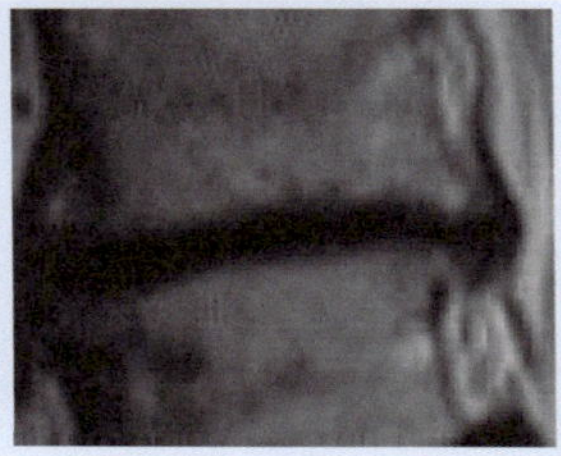 |

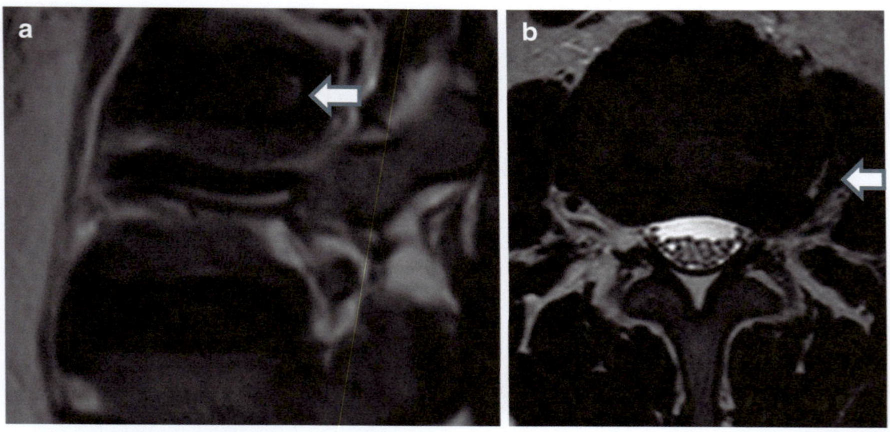


**Fig. 4.4** On sagittal T2w image (**a**) of the lumbar spine, a high-signal-intensity area is detected on the lateral part of the disc (arrow). Axial T2w image (**b**) shows linear hyperintensity at the lateral left circumference of the disc (arrow)

however, some are painful. The defects allow ingrowth of nerve endings and granulation tissue.

#### 4.8.1.3 High-Intensity Zone (HIZ)

The high-intensity zone was first described in 1992 and is defined as a deep radial tear of the annulus fibrosus. It is believed to represent fluid and/or granulation tissue that may enhance on post-contrast images. On MRI, the T2-hyperintensity is usually detected at the dorsal circumference of the disc (Fig. 4.5).

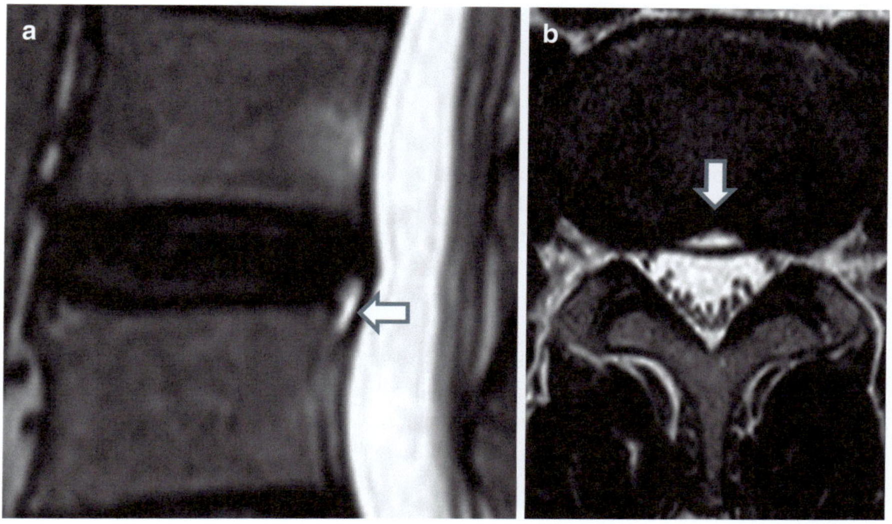


**Fig. 4.5** On sagittal T2w image (**a**) linear hyperintensity is visible on the dorsal caudal part of the disc (arrow). Axial T2w image (**b**) shows linear hyperintensity at the dorsal posterior circumference of the disc (arrow)

HIZs detected on T2 and T1w images (dual HIZs) represent calcified tissue [14, 15].

The high-intensity zone is classified based on location as (a) anterior and (b) posterior and based on morphology as (a) round, (b) fissure, (c) vertical, (d) rim, and (e) giant type.

The presence of an HIZ does not imply a traumatic etiology or that the disc is a source of pain, as it has been found in symptomatic and asymptomatic individuals. Whether HIZs are symptomatic is under continued debate. The percentage of an HIZ in the general population is reportedly around 11%, with 9.5% in asymptomatic and 10.4% in symptomatic subjects [16]. One large-scale population-based study has shown that multilevel homogeneous HIZs of the lumbar spine were significantly and independently associated with prolonged severe LBP and sciatica [17].

#### 4.8.1.4 II Disc Bulging

A disc bulge is a circumferential prolapse of the intervertebral disc (>25% of the circumference of the disc), with an intact annulus fibrosus. It will often be detected in asymptomatic people (Fig. 4.6).

#### 4.8.1.5 III Disc Herniations

A disc herniation is a localized or focal displacement of the disc material beyond the normal margins of the disc space, but involves less than 25% of the periphery of the disc on the axial plane (Fig 4.6). Displacement of the disc material occurs through the disruption of the annulus. Herniations are classified based on the shape of the displaced material as a protrusion or an extrusion. Herniated disc material is termed "contained," if located wholly within an intact annulus and/or posterior longitudinal ligament (PLL). In cases where PLL is not intact, the disc material is considered "uncontained."

#### 4.8.1.6 Disc Protrusion

Disc protrusion is diagnosed when the protruded disc material extends <50% of the disc circumference and if the size of the base/neck of the protruded material exceeds the maximal length of the protruded material (Fig 4.6). It can be *focal* or *broad-based.* The annulus fibrosus is usually not completely disrupted in a protrusion, as some intact fibers will be found at surgery.

#### 4.8.1.7 Disc Extrusion

Disc extrusion refers to a situation in which the size of the base/neck of the protruded material is less than the maximal length of the protruded material. In extrusion, the annulus fibrosis is focally disrupted (defect in the annulus fibrosus). Extrusion may be located anterior (subligamentous extrusion) (Fig. 4.7) or posterior to the posterior longitudinal ligament (PLL).

#### 4.8.1.8 Sequestration

A "free disc" fragment or "sequestrated" fragment is defined as a piece of disc that is separated from the original disc (Fig 4.6). The fragment may migrate ("migrated")

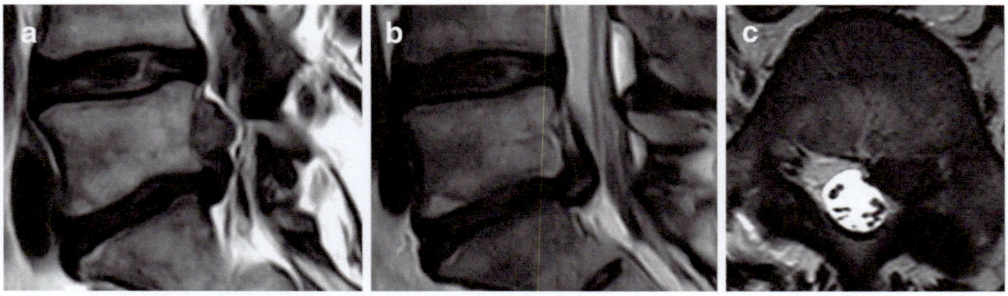


**Fig. 4.6** Different types of disc pathology: (**a**) disc bulging; (**b**) protrusion; (**c**) extrusion; and (**d**) sequestration

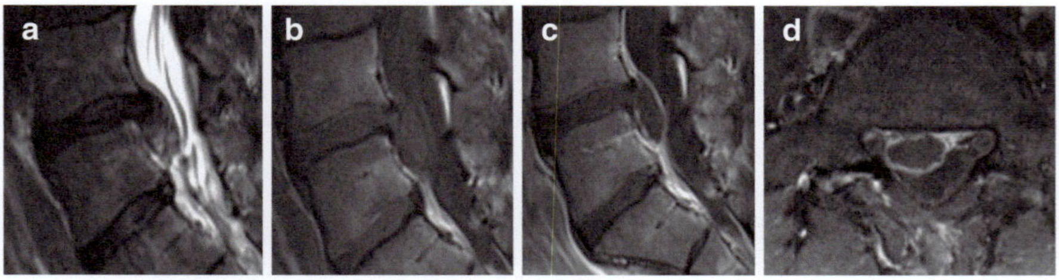


**Fig. 4.7** On a sagittal T2w image (**a**) of the lumbar spine, narrowing of the disc space, and T2 low-signal-intensity disc and disc herniation with cranial migration is detected. On sagittal T2w image (**b**) an intact posterior longitudinal ligament is clearly visible covering the herniated disc material. The axial T2w image shows a mediolateral location of the disc extrusion

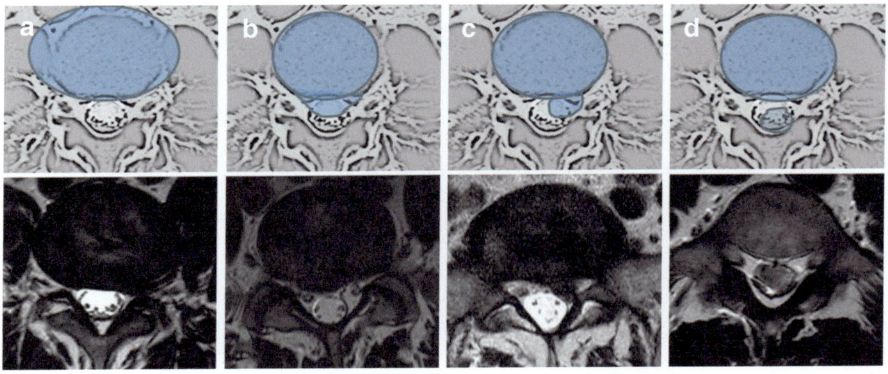


**Fig. 4.8** On a sagittal T2w image (**a**) of the lumbar spine, T2 low-signal-intensity disc with herniation and caudal migration are shown. Sagittal pre- (**b**) and post-contrast T1w image (**c**) demonstrates ring-like enhancing, sequestrated disc material. (**d**) Post-contrast axial T1w image shows mediolateral right location of the free fragment of the disc

superiorly or inferiorly with respect to the disc space and rarely may be located in the thecal sac (intradural) (Fig 4.8) [18].

According to the location of the disc herniation in the axial plane, these zones can be distinguished: (a) median/central; (b) paracentral/recessal; (c) foraminal; and (d) extraforaminal (Fig. 4.9). Large-size disc herniation may occupy more than one zone.

In the sagittal plane, disc herniations can be: (a) at the disc level; (b) extend to the suprapedicular zone; and (c) extend to the pedicular zone.

In relation to a recessal nerve root irritation, Pfirrmann et al. [13] proposed a classification for the lumbar spine: (a) grade 1 describes contact with the nerve root without displacement or compression; (b) grade 2 refers to nerve root displacement by disc material; and (c) grade 3 encompasses nerve root compression. This grading system has been shown to be reliable with a good inter-reader agreement for the higher grades (comparing grades I–III), but was slightly less reliable in distinguishing normal roots versus grade I (contact).

The *vacuum phenomenon* describes gas (nitrogen) that occurs in the disc due to negative pressure produced by abnormal spaces [19]. On radiography and CT, it will be recognized as a radiolucency, and on MRI, as an area of signal void [20]. Differential diagnosis includes infections with intradiscal and intraosseous gas collections [21].

#### 4.8.1.9 Disc Calcification

Calcification of the intervertebral disc is commonly seen in the elderly, especially in the annulus fibrosus and lower thoracic spine. The prevalence increases with age and extent of disc space loss [22].

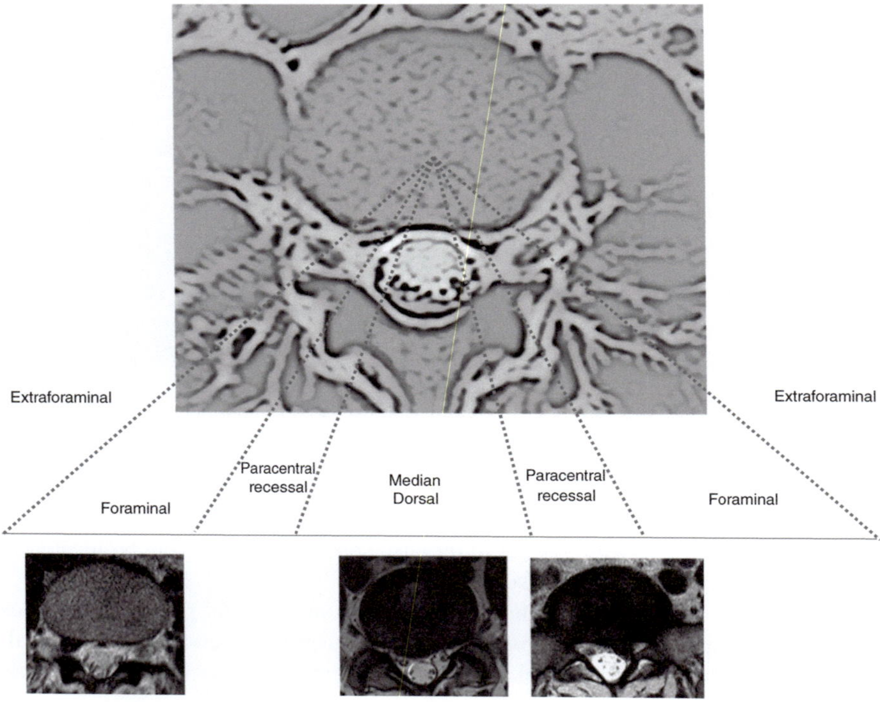


**Fig. 4.9** Locations of the disc herniation in the axial plane

#### 4.8.1.10 Vertebral Endplates

The most commonly used score for degenerative endplate changes was initially proposed in the 1980s by Modic et al. [23]. Modic type I changes represent bone marrow edema and inflammation (subchondral fractures and vascularized fibrous tissue replacing the hematopoietic bone marrow), Modic type II changes represent bone marrow conversion into fatty marrow as a result of marrow ischemia, and Modic type III changes represent subchondral bony sclerosis (Table 4.3). Modic type I and III changes are more often associated with back pain [24].

One possible pathophysiological explanation for disc degeneration is initial endplate damage that leads to decreased disc nutrition. Rajasekaran et al. introduced an endplate damage score in 2008 based on five visibly distinguishable diffusion patterns observed in serial post-contrast MRI [25] (Table 4.4).

#### 4.8.1.11 Schmorl Nodes

Schmorl nodes are common in the spine in an elderly population, with a frequency similar to that in a younger population. They are associated with moderate, but not advanced, degenerative changes [26]. The etiology is complex, and multifactorial origins, including embryological and genetic origins, as well as an autoimmune process are possible. Schmorl nodes usually show the same signal characteristics as the

**Table 4.3** Modic classification of vertebral body endplate changes [23]

| | T1 | | T2 | | STIR | |
|---|---|---|---|---|---|---|
| Modic I | Low | 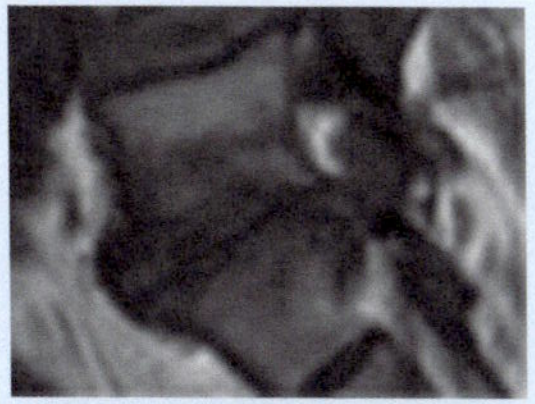 | High | 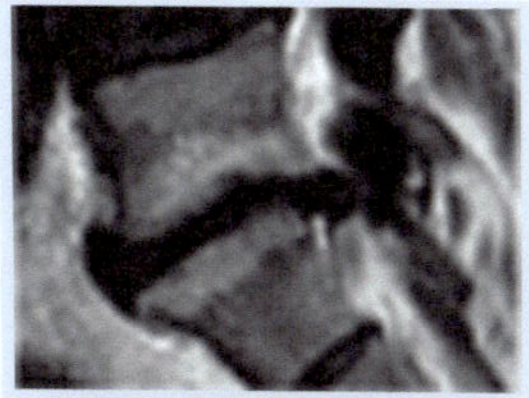 | High | 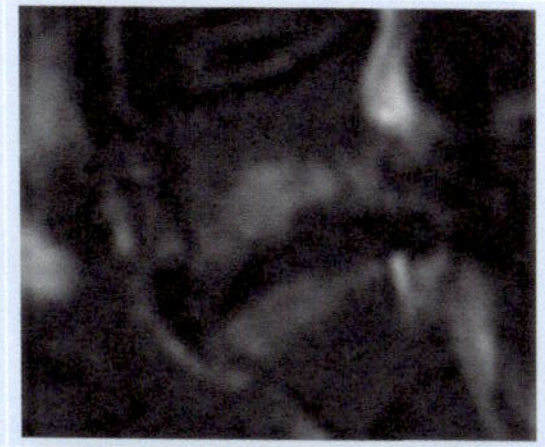 |
| Modic II | High | 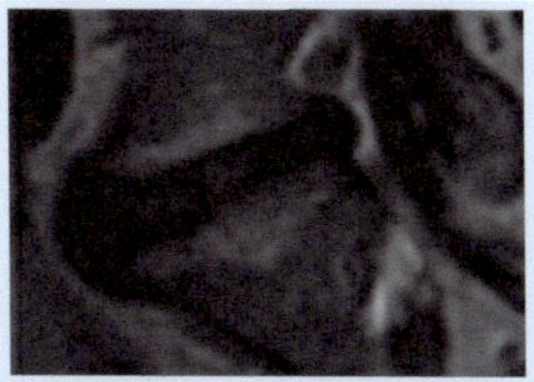 | Iso-high | 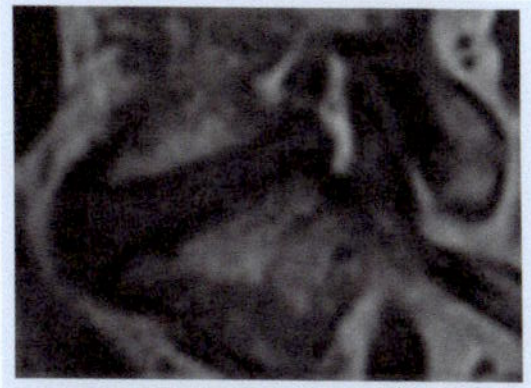 | Low | 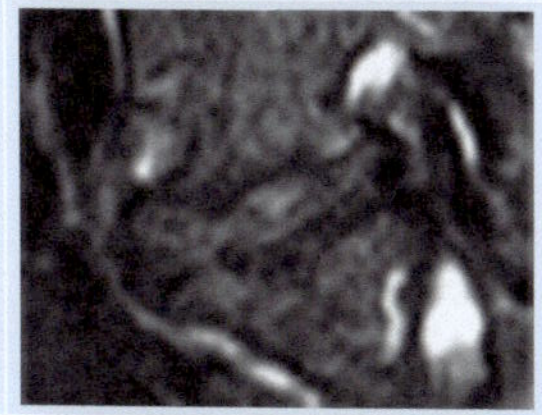 |
| Modic III | Low | 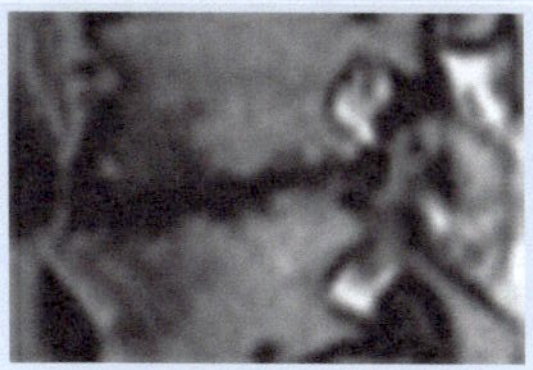 | Low | 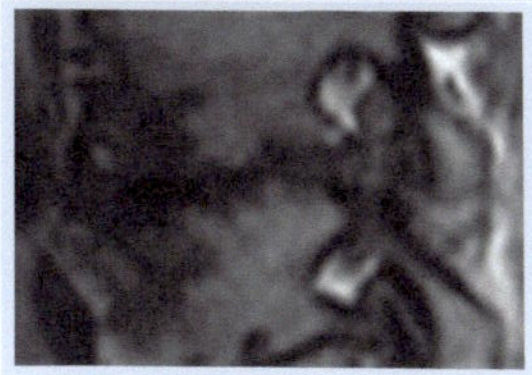 | | 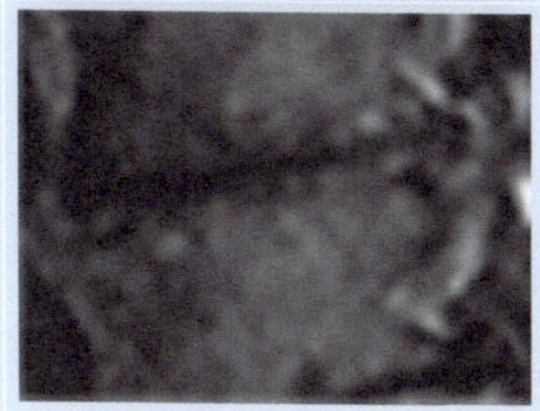 |

**Table 4.4** Vertebral endplate damage score from A–F on T1w images [25].

| | Vertebral endplate | T1wi |
|---|---|---|
| A | Normal, no interruption | 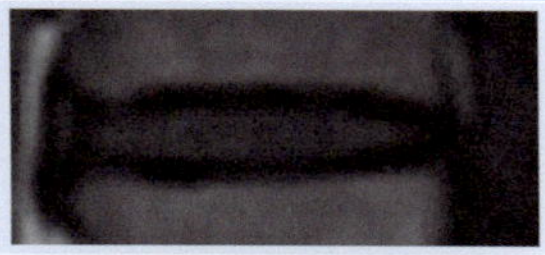 |
| B | Thinning, but no interruption |  |
| C | Focal defect with involvement of the subchondral bone | 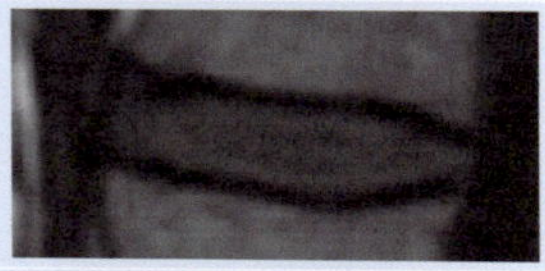 |
| D | Focal defect <25% of the endplate area | 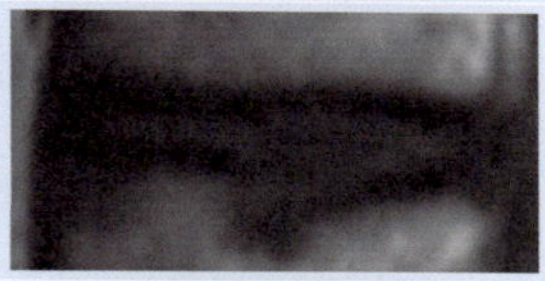 |
| E | Focal defect >50% of the endplate area | 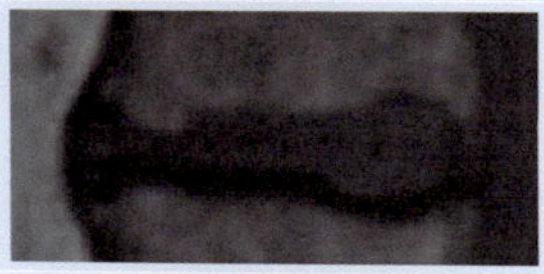 |
| F | Extensively damaged endplate | 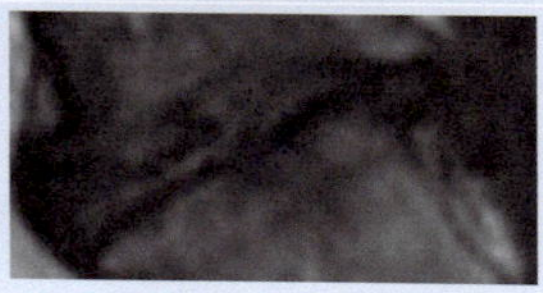 |

adjacent disc, with a thin rim of sclerosis at the margins. Acute herniation can demonstrate surrounding bone marrow edema and peripheral enhancement (Fig. 4.10).

#### 4.8.1.12 Spondylosis Deformans

Spondylosis deformans refers to the growth of bone spurs (osteophytes) or bony bridges around a degenerating intervertebral disc in the spine. When the desiccation of the nucleus pulposus and the degeneration of the annulus fibrosis occur, the disc becomes unable to withstand the stresses of axial loading, causing bulging. Over time, this bulging of the annulus on the vertebral edge leads to formation of an osteophyte at the osseous site of attachment to the annulus (Sharpey's fibers).

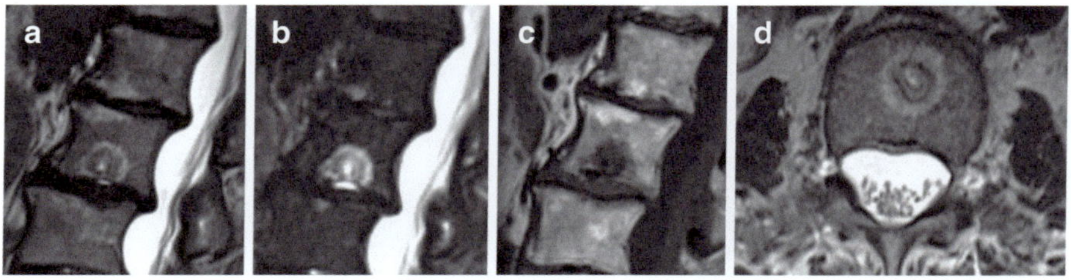


**Fig. 4.10** Sagittal T2w image (**a**) and STIR sequence (**b**) show a round, well-defined lesion in the vertebral body close to the inferior endplate. On T1w image (**c**) the lesion shows a low signal and a defect of the endplate

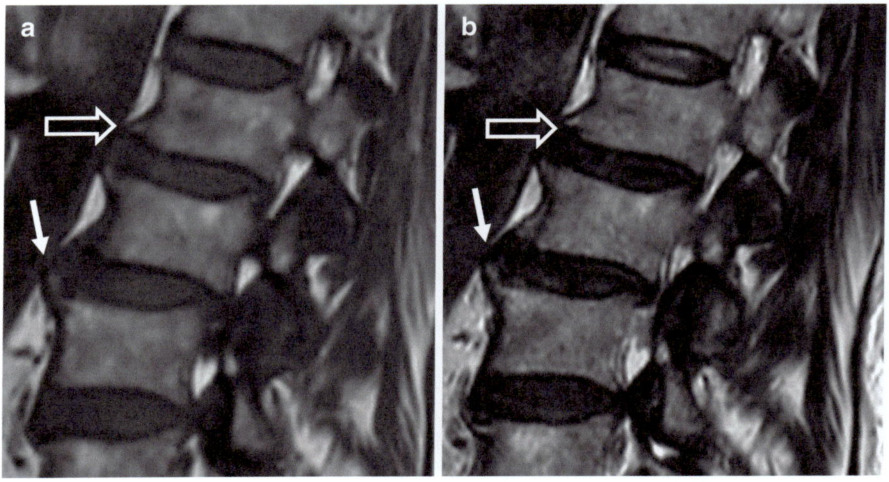


**Fig. 4.11** Sagittal T1 (**a**) and T2 (**b**) show "traction" (open arrow) and "claw" osteophytes (arrow)

Small osteophytes that are parallel to the endplate are called *traction osteophytes*. Osteophytes that are large, curved, and even bridging two adjacent vertebrae are known as *claw osteophytes* (Figs. 4.11 and 4.12).

The levels most commonly affected by degenerative changes in the cervical spine are C5–6 and C6–7, and these frequently affect young adults in their early 30s. The cervical intervertebral discs have lower T2-signal intensity compared to the lumbar spine; thus, low T2 signal should not be interpreted as disc degeneration. Disc herniations are rare in the thoracic spine and are usually seen at the lowest thoracic levels (Th11–12 and Th12–L1). DDD of lumbar spine is most often observed at the L4/5 and L5/S1 level.

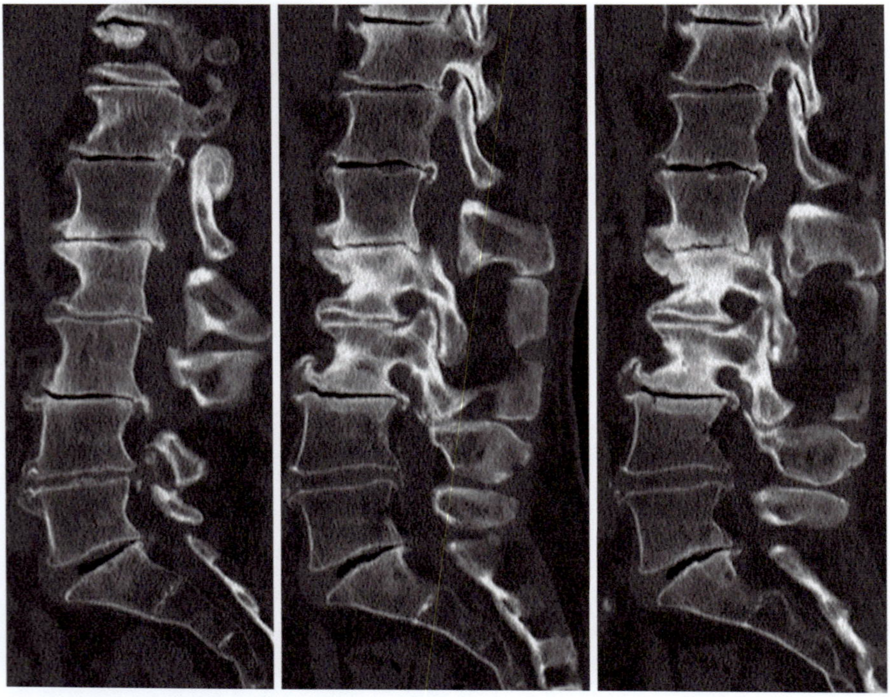

**Fig. 4.12** Bone window CT demonstrates extensive sclerotic changes of the vertebral endplates of the L1–2, L2–3, and L3–4 lumbar segments and large ventral osteophytes (Courtesy of Merhemic Zulejha)

## 4.9 Correlation

To promote consistency in the use of spinal terminology, a lumbar disc nomenclature was published in 2001 by Fardon et al. [27]. In 2014, the authors published changes based on current concepts in radiologic and clinical care [28]. In the new version of the nomenclature (lumbar disc nomenclature 2.0), the diagnostic categories are based on pathology. Lumbar discs can be classified into the following diagnostic categories: normal; congenital/developmental variation; degeneration; trauma; infection/inflammation; neoplasia; and/or morphologic variant of uncertain significance. In each category, different degrees can be specified as "possible," "probable," or "definite."

Recently, a new classification scheme (Michigan State University classification) was described by Mysliwiec et al. [29]. This classification separated lumbar disc disease into different zones based purely on location. Furthermore, the classification scheme was applied to 100 patients and microdiscectomies were performed on only those with disc disease in Zones 2 and 3 (larger and more extensive). All these nomenclatures and grading scores have undergone improvements and adaptations [30].

## 4.10 Correlation of Imaging Findings and Clinical Presentation

The main issue in the management of patients with lumbar disc disease is the correlation of imaging findings with clinical presentation and symptomatology to guide treatment and intervention. The main pain generators are the intervertebral disc, facet joint, sacroiliac joint, and spine muscles. Pain generators might coexist in the same patient, causing mixed pain types and referral patterns with multiple mechanisms and pathways [31].

It is estimated that only <30% of lumbar back pain is due to nerve root compression [32]. The most frequent cause of nonspecific lumbar axial spinal pain is believed to be the discogenic pain due to internal disruption of the disc and endplate changes [33]. In degenerative disc disease, a cascade of events causes fissures in the annulus fibrosus, water leaks, decreasing intradiscal pressure, inflammation, neovascularization, and ingrowth of free nerve endings to the nucleus pulposus.

The data from a recently published study of 975 individuals suggest that disc degeneration alone is not associated with low back pain. By contrast, the combination of disc degeneration and endplate changes was highly associated with low back pain [34]. Similar findings were reported by another large MRI study on Modic changes, where Modic changes were associated with both disc degeneration and the presence and severity of low back pain [35].

## 4.11 Progression of DDD

The reported rates of annual progression of DDD in adults varies from 0.42% to 76% in population-based epidemiological studies, although in a majority of those studies, no uniform cohort was investigated. A recently published study that used a uniform cohort for age and nationality (617 subjects were followed for more than 4 years as part of the Wakayama Spine Study) demonstrated that DDD progression per year (based on MRI) in the entire lumbar spine was 13.0% and 15.1% in Japanese men and women, respectively [36]. The female sex and diabetes mellitus were the risk factors for DDD progression in the upper lumbar spine.

In the presence of new symptoms, it is certainly justified to repeat diagnostic imaging before surgery. The results of a recently conducted study showed that routine reimaging prior to surgery, simply because the existing MRI was 6–12 months old, may not be beneficial [37]. Furthermore, the study also indicated that, in a subset of patients, preoperative CT myelography reduces revision rates.

## 4.12 Differential Diagnosis

Spine abnormalities are associated with axial spondyloarthritis (axSpa) on radiographs and MRI mimic degenerative lesions. Bone marrow edema of the endplates will also be present in patients with spondyloarthritis. On radiographs, syndesmophytes and spondylophytes are both bony spurs arising from the corner of vertebral bodies and are distinguished by the angle that they form with the vertebra [38].

## References


1. Edgar MA. The nerve supply of the lumbar intervertebral disc. J Bone Jt Surg. 2007;89:1135–9.
2. Modic MT, Ross JS. Lumbar degenerative disk disease. Radiology. 2007;245(1):43–61.
3. Nathan H, Islael J. Osteophytes of the vertebral column: an anatomical study of their development according to age, race, and sex with consideration as to their etiology and significance. J Bone Joint Surg Am. 1962;44(2):243–68.
4. Brinjikji W, Diehn FE, Jarvik JG, et al. MRI findings of disc degeneration are more prevalent in adults with low back pain than in asymptomatic controls: a systematic review and meta-analysis. AJNR Am J Neuroradiol. 2015;36:2394–9.
5. Westermaier T, Doerr C, Stetter C, et al. Influence of myelography and postmyelographic CT on therapeutic decisions in degenerative diseases of the cervical spine. Clin Spine Surg. 2017;30(5):E656–61.
6. Lundon K, Bolton K. Structure and function of the lumbar intervertebral disk in health, aging, and pathologic conditions. J Orthop Sports Phys Ther. 2001;31:291–306.
7. Aguila LAL, Piraino DWD, Modic MTM, et al. The intranuclear cleft of the intervertebral disk: magnetic resonance imaging. Radiology. 1985;155:155–8.
8. Sive JI, Baird P, Jeziorsk M, Watkins A, Hoyland JA, Freemont AJ. Expression of chondrocyte markers by cells of normal and degenerate intervertebral discs. Mol Pathol. 2002;55:91–7.
9. Oichi T, Taniguchi Y, Oshima Y, Tanak S, Saito T. Pathomechanism of intervertebral disc degeneration. JOR Spine. 2020;3:1076.
10. Kettler A, Wilke HJ. Review of exisrting grading systems for cervical or lumbar disc and facet joint degeneration. Eur Spine J. 2006;15:705–18.
11. Sachs BL, Vanharanta H, Spivey MA, et al. Dallas discogram description. A new classification of CT/discography in low-back disorders. Spine. 1987;12:287–94.
12. Thompson JP, Pearce RH, Schlechter MT, et al. Preliminary evaluation of a scheme for grading the gross morphology of the human intervertebral disc. Spine (Phila Pa 1976). 1990;15(5):411–5.
13. Pfirrmann CW, Metzdorf A, Zanetti M, Hodler J, Boos N. Magnetic resonance classification of lumbar intervertebral disc degeneration. Spine. 2001;26(17):1873–8.
14. Shan Z, Chen H, Liu J, et al. Does the high-intensity zone (HIZ) or lumbar intervertebral discs always represent an annular fissure? Eur Radiol. 2017;27:1267–76.
15. Cheung JPY, Luk KDK. The relevance of high-intensity zone in degenerative disc disease. Int Orthop. 2019 Apr;43(4):861–7.
16. Campos M, Vial R, Castro J, Urrutia J. Prevalence of lumbar high-intensity zone: assessment using a screening tool independent of spinal symptoms. Acta Orthop Belg. 2019;85:47–53.
17. Teraguchi M, Cheung JPY, Karppinen J, et al. Lumbar high-intensity zones on MRI: imaging biomarkers for severe, prolonged low back pain and sciatica in a population-based cohort. Spine J. 2020;20(7):1025–34.
18. Theodorou DJ, Theodorou SJ, Kakitsubata Y, Papanastasiou EI, Gelalis ID. Posterior and anterior epidural and intradural migration of the sequestered intervertebral disc: three cases and review of the literature. J Spinal Cord Med. 2020;4:1–6.

19. Knutsson F. The vacuum phenomenon in the intervertebral discs. Acta Radiol. 1942;23:173–9.
20. Grenier N, Grossman RI, Schiebler ML, Yeager BA, Goldberg HI, Kressel HY. Degenerative lumbar disk disease: pitfalls and usefulness of MR imaging in detection of vacuum phenomenon. Radiology. 1987;164(3):861–5.
21. Bielecki DK, Sartoris D, Resnick D, Van Lom K, Fierer J, Haghighi P. Intraosseous and intradiscal gas in association with spinal infection: report of three cases. AJR Am J Roentgenol. 1986;147(1):83–6.
22. Chanchairujira K, Chung CB, Kim JY, et al. Intervertebral disk calcification of the spine in an elderly population: radiographic prevalence, location, and distribution and correlation with spinal degeneration. Radiology. 2004;230:499–503.
23. Modic MT, Steinberg PM, Ross JS, et al. Degenerative disk disease: assessment of changes in vertebral body marrow with MR imaging. Radiology. 1988;166(1):193–9.
24. Toyone T, Takahashi K, Kitahara H, et al. Vertebral bone-marrow changes in degenerative lumbar disc disease. An MRI study of 74 patients with low back pain. J Bone Jt Surg Br. 1994;46:757–64.
25. Rajasekaran S, Venkatadass K, Naresh Babu J, Ganesh K, Shetty AP. Pharmacological enhancement of disc diffusion and differentiation of healthy, ageing and degenerated discs. Eur Spine J. 2008;17:626–43.
26. Pfirrmann CW, Resnick D. Schmorl nodes of the thoracic and lumbar spine: radiographic-pathologic study of prevalence, characterization, and correlation with degenerative changes of 1,650 spinal levels in 100 cadavers. Radiology. 2001;219:368–74.
27. Fardon DF, Milette PC. Nomenclature and classification of lumbar disc pathology: recommendations of the combined task forces of the North American Spine Society, the American Society of Spine Radiology and the American Society of Neuroradiology. Spine. 2001;26:E93–113.
28. Fardon DF, Williams AL, Dohring EJ, Murtagh FR, Gabriel Rothman SL, Sze GK. Lumbar disc nomenclature: version 2.0: recommendations of the combined task forces of the North American Spine Society, the American Society of Spine Radiology and the American Society of Neuroradiology. Spine J. 2014;14(11):2525–45.
29. Mysliwiec LW, Cholewicki J, Winkelpleck MD, Eis GP. MSU classification for herniated lumbar discs on MRI: toward developing objective criteria for surgical selection. Eur Spine J. 2010;19:1087–93.
30. Li Y, Fredrickson V, Resnick DK. How should we grade lumbar disc herniation and nerve root compression? A systematic review. Clin Orthop Relat Res. 2015;473:1896–902.
31. Izzo R, Popolizio T, D'Aprile P, Muto M. Spinal pain. Eur J Radiol. 2015;84:746–56.
32. Mooney V. Where is the pain coming from? Spine. 1987;12:754–9.
33. Schwarzer AC, Aprill CN, Derby R, et al. The prevalence and clinical features of internal disc disruption in patients with chronic low back pain. Spine. 1995;20:1878–83.
34. Teraguchi M, Yoshimura N, Hashizume H, et al. The association of combination of disc degeneration, endplate signal change, and Schmorl node with low back pain in a large population study: the Wakayama spine study. Spine J. 2015;15:622–8.
35. Mok FP, Samartzis D, Karppinen J, Fong DY, Luk KD, Cheung KM. Modic changes of the lumbar spine: prevalence, risk factors, and association with disc degeneration and low back pain in a large-scale population-based cohort. Spine J. 2016;16:32–41.
36. Teraguchi M, Yoshimura N, Hashizume H, et al. Progression, incidence, and risk factors for intervertebral disc degeneration in a longitudinal population-based cohort: the Wakayama Spine Study. Osteoarthr Cartil. 2017 Jul;25(7):1122–31.
37. Ries ZG, Glassman SD, Vasilyev I, et al. Updates imaging does not affect revision rates in adults undergoing spine surgery for lumbar degenerative disease. J Neurosurg Spine. 2019;30:228–33.
38. De Bruin F, Treyvaud MO, Feydy A, et al. Prevalence of degenerative changes and overlap with spondyloarthritis-associated lesions in the spine of patients from the DESIR cohort. MD Open. 2018;4:e000657.

# 5 Advanced Imaging: DWI, DTI, PWI, and MR-Spectroscopy of the Disc

Johan Van Goethem, Caro De Weerdt, Stephan Becker, John P. Claude, and Jeffrey Lotz

## 5.1 Technical Challenges

### 5.1.1 Anatomical

The normal human intervertebral disc is relatively small. Disc height is minimum at the Th4–Th5 level. The thickest disc is found at L4–L5, the longest disc at L5–S1. The thickness of the discs varies from 4.5 to 9.0 mm, with the middle disc height approximately 25% greater than the anterior and posterior disc height [1, 2]. The L5–S1 nucleus pulposus is the longest at 21.6 ± 3.1 mm [2].

The cross-sectional area increases from superior to inferior. Cervical discs tend to have an elliptical cross-sectional shape, thoracic discs are more circular, and lumbar discs tend to have an elliptical cross-section flattened posteriorly [3].

J. Van Goethem (✉)
Department of Radiology, AZ Nikolaas, Sint-Niklaas, Belgium

University of Antwerp, Antwerp, Belgium
e-mail: johan.vangoethem@uantwerpen.be

C. De Weerdt
University of Antwerp, Antwerpen, Belgium

S. Becker
Vitalzentrum, Salzburg - Grödig, Austria
e-mail: stephan.becker@vitazen.at

J. P. Claude
Nocimed Inc., San Mateo, CA, USA

J. Lotz
University of California, San Francisco (UCSF), San Francisco, CA, USA



L. Manfrè, J. Van Goethem (eds.), *The Disc and Degenerative Disc Disease*, New Procedures in Spinal Interventional Neuroradiology,
https://doi.org/10.1007/978-3-030-03715-4_5

The anterior annulus fibrosus occupies 20.5% of the L4–L5 disc length, which is significantly greater than that of the posterior annulus fibrosus (15.6%). At L5–S1, the anterior and posterior annulus fibrosus are similar in length (14.1% and 13.6% of the disc, respectively) [2].

## 5.2 Artifacts

### 5.2.1 CSF-Pulsation Artifacts

Arterial blood entering the skull vault at systole pushes CSF downward into the spinal canal while the reverse movement happens at diastole. This CSF flow is turbulent and causes CSF-pulsation artifacts. These can be seen as areas of signal loss in the CSF, especially at longer echo times and may also result in phase-encoding artifacts. Several modifications may reduce CSF-pulsation artifacts, including cardiac gating, even-echo rephasing, changing the phase-encoding direction from anteroposterior to head feet (Fig. 5.1), averaging of excitations, and flow compensation.

### 5.2.2 Swallowing, Breathing, and Movement Artifacts

Clear patient instructions are the easiest and most effective way to reduce these artifacts. Swallowing and coughing can be avoided by good patient preparation. Breathing artifacts can be reduced by instructing the patient to use thoracic rather than abdominal breathing. In general, a well prepared and relaxed patient will do much better. Technical modifications to reduce these artifacts include averaging of

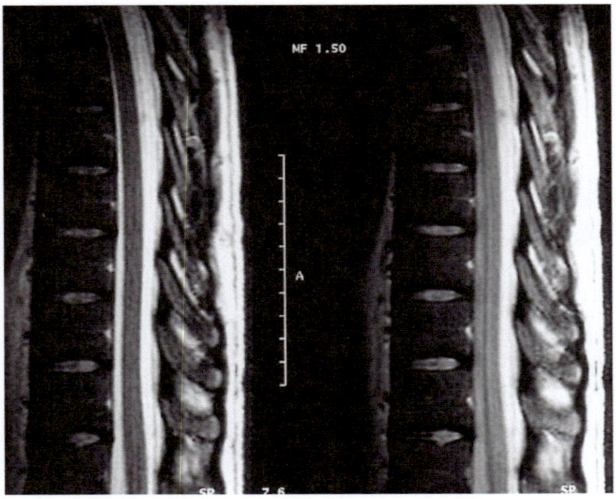


**Fig. 5.1** Reduction of CSF-pulsation artifacts by swapping the phase-encoding direction to head-feet (left) from anteroposterior (right). This simple technical modification should be considered for all thoracic and lumbar MR imaging

excitations, judicious use of saturation zones, and changing the phase-encoding direction from anteroposterior to head-feet.

### 5.2.3 Magnetic Susceptibility Artifacts

The intervertebral disc is surrounded mainly by cartilage, bone, and fat. Moreover, in the cervical and thoracic region, air is nearby too. This mixture of tissues leads to an environment with a very heterogeneous magnetic susceptibility. This in turn causes inhomogeneities in the linear magnetic gradients used in MRI, giving bright and dark areas at the border of tissues or substances with different magnetic susceptibility. Turbo spin-echo sequences are less susceptible than basic spin echo sequences because of the use of many refocusing pulses. Gradient echo sequences that do not use refocusing pulses are most susceptible to this artifact. This is the reason why cervical foramina look narrower than they really are on gradient echo images. A shorter echo time and a higher bandwidth also reduce this kind of artifact.

## 5.3 Diffusion-Weighted Imaging, Diffusion Tensor Imaging, and Diffusion Kurtosis Imaging

In the intervertebral disc, water molecules are scattered in the extracellular matrix. When an intervertebral disc degenerates, the movement of these free water molecules decreases, the distribution of water molecules in the matrix changes, and the water content declines. In addition to these functional alterations, the biochemical composition of the tissue also changes, affecting the diffusion of water molecules. Diffusion-weighted (DW) MRI is very sensitive in detecting these early changes, particularly in detecting the diffusion movement and the distribution and quantity of free water molecules. Using DW-MRI, it is possible to evaluate the degree of intervertebral disc degeneration by analyzing changes in apparent diffusion coefficient (ADC) values. DW-MRI and diffusion tensor imaging (DTI) reflect microstructural changes in tissue by describing the diffusion of water molecules. ADC and fractional anisotropy (FA) are the two most important quantitative units of measurement that are very sensitive to this. The diffusion of water molecules is divided into isotropic and anisotropic types. First, isotropic diffusion is proportional to the average ADC values in each direction. In addition, FA values reflect the ratio of anisotropic diffusion within the total diffusion tensor. DW-MRI, on the one hand, is used to detect the ability of water diffusion and generate ADC images for contrast. DTI, on the other hand, describes the directional characteristics of water diffusion and produces FA images.

The ADC values of both the nucleus pulposus and the annulus fibrosus decrease with age [4]. Disturbance in the metabolism of the center of the intervertebral disc, i.e., the nucleus pulposus, occurs at a very early pathological stage [4]. This results in a gradual loss of proteoglycans, damage to collagen fibers, and a reduced amount of water. It is very important to realize that these biochemical changes occur before

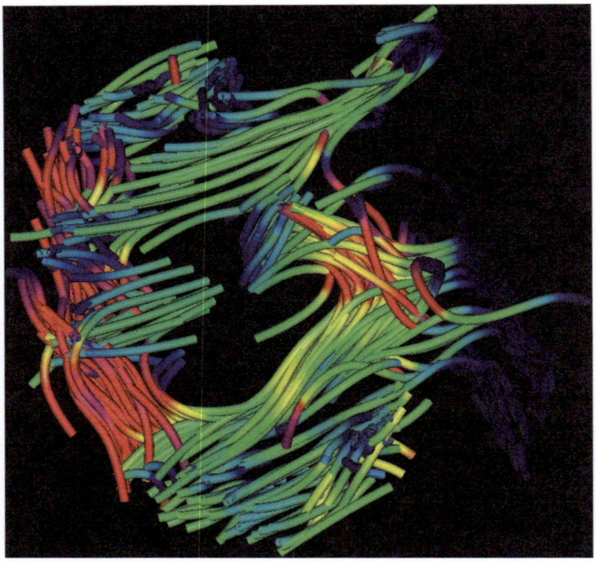

**Fig. 5.2** In vivo DTI of a normal intervertebral disc in an asymptomatic volunteer. Colored areas represent voxels with high FA and their respective preferred direction of diffusion of water molecules (green: anterior-posterior, red: left-right and blue: up-down). This image demonstrates the direction of movement along the orientation of the intact lamella of the annulus fibrosus. Compare with the absence of signal in the center of the disc, i.e. at the level of the nucleus pulposus, due to isotropic water diffusion (Image courtesy Johan Van Goethem)

morphological and clinical signs appear. The healthy annulus fibrosus consists of concentric laminates of fiber bundles. Water molecules diffuse more readily parallel to these laminae than moving through them. The combination of DTI with fiber tracking results in an image showing the integrity of the annulus fibrosus, allowing to visualize this structure of the annulus fibrosus. A DTI scan of a healthy annulus fibrosus shows a multilayered fiber bundle composed of successive regular rings (Fig. 5.2). A DTI scan of a degenerated annulus fibrosus, on the contrary, shows an irregular, disordered, and much thinner structure [5] (Fig. 5.3).

Both the nucleus pulposus and annulus fibrosus undergo structural and morphological changes throughout the various stages of development and aging, in which these two areas become more fibrous, and the sharp distinction between them is lost. Significant age-related changes are seen in elderly, with a decrease of mean diffusivity (MD) (11%) and an increase of FA (20%) [6]. FA increases during the transition from young to elderly age groups, consistent with the developing fibrous nature and an overall increased microstructural complexity of the intervertebral disc. Interestingly, in the elderly group, the FA tended to increase more rapidly with age, possibly reflecting that the ongoing process of disc degeneration becomes accelerated during this age range, which is in agreement with postmortem studies [6]. Meanwhile, MD decreasing with age is probably associated with the changes in the disc water content and shrinkage of the disc volume. By visual inspection of the image, the nucleus pulposus and annulus fibrosus in intervertebral discs can be distinctively separable on FA and MD maps, while they are identical on T2-weighted images. This demonstrates that the degenerative-related changes taking place in the intervertebral discs through aging can be quantitatively accessed by DTI-derived metrics, while these changes are difficult to identify on conventional T2-weighted images [6].

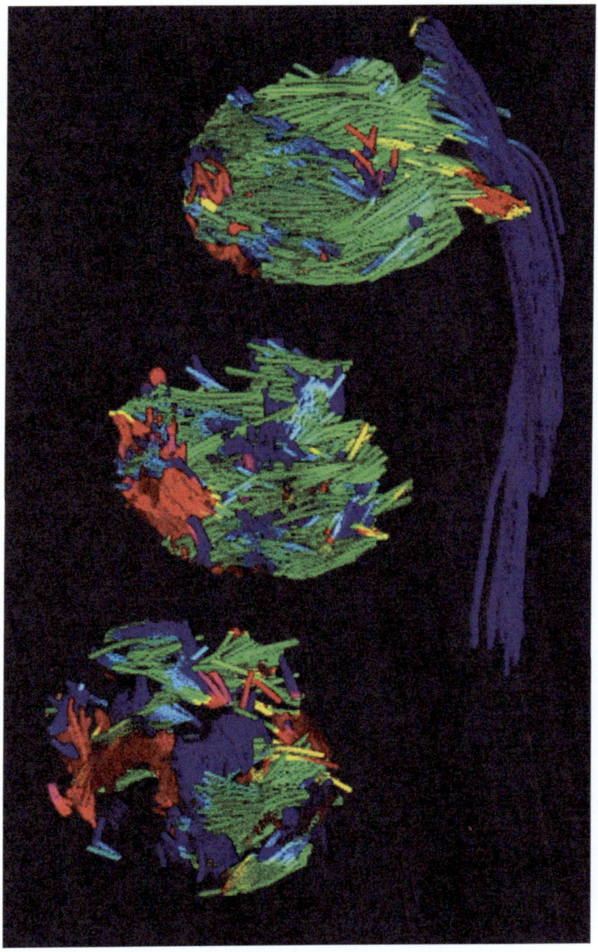

**Fig. 5.3** In vivo DTI of three consecutive thoracolumbar discs in a volunteer. Colored areas represent voxels with high FA and their respective preferred direction of diffusion of water molecules (green: anterior-posterior, red: left-right and blue: up-down). Compare the normal pattern in the L1–L2 disc (top) to the more random pattern in the degenerative L3–L4 disc (bottom). Note the signal in the nerve roots of the cauda equina (blue) (Image courtesy Johan Van Goethem)

In collagenous tissues, such as the annulus fibrosus, DTI provides information about the direction and degree of collagen fiber alignment. The noninvasive, non-irradiating nature of DTI means, it provides a promising technique to explore the functional microarchitecture of the annulus fibrosus. Since water is one of the main constituents of the annulus fibrosus and the biomechanics of the intervertebral disc are reliant upon both the movement and the entrapment of the water molecules during different loading modes and conditions, the biomechanical behavior of the annulus fibrosus is intimately related to the movement of water molecules within the tissue. By permitting a more detailed understanding of the morphology of the annulus fibrosus to be developed in the context of diffusion of water molecules, both in the unloaded tissue and during/following mechanical loading, DTI provides a tool to monitor changes in microstructure with different loading scenarios. During loading the disc shows clear changes in diffusivity, indicating the tissue becomes more anisotropic [7]. It is proposed that this increase in fractional anisotropy is due to loading-induced modification of collagen fiber alignment. During axial compression collagen fibers reorient within the anulus fibrosus, becoming more consistently aligned parallel to the plane of the endplates [7].

Diffusion kurtosis imaging (DKI) is a newer MR-technique measuring diffusion of water molecules based on a probability distribution function. Mean kurtosis (MK) is the main extra parameter that is derived from this technique. It represents the statistical difference from a normal/random distribution (of water movement). DKI is a noninvasive technique to evaluate intervertebral discs [8]. MK increases with disc degeneration grade and is more sensitive than other techniques [9].

## 5.4 Perfusion-Weighted Imaging

Arterial blood reaches the vertebral bodies by small penetrating arteries. Vascular supply is regionally organized in three horizontal networks: superior, central, and inferior. The superior and inferior networks provide a capillary bed near the superior and inferior vertebral endplates. Also, blood vessels are found in the peripheral annulus and endplates of healthy adult intervertebral discs. The normal intervertebral nucleus pulposus has no blood vessels. Although few, it does contain cells and those have a metabolic need. Due to a concentration gradient, small molecules such as oxygen and glucose diffuse from the vertebral endplates to the disc. Larger molecules are transported by convection: they are pushed out of the disc under loading and they are drawn into the disc by unloading. These mechanisms work inefficient and oxygen levels in the disc are much lower than in other tissues. Therefore, cells in the nucleus pulposus rely on glycolysis, a form on anaerobic metabolism.

Perfusion can be studied in vivo by dynamic contrast enhancement (DCE) MRI. In this technique fast sequential T1-WI are obtained after bolus contrast administration. Temporal changes in signal intensities reflect changes in contrast concentration and allow construction of time–concentration curves for each voxel. Several parameters can be studied: in the first minute(s), contrast will be mainly intravascular and DCE-perfusion will show tissue perfusion. Later, contrast also enters the extravascular space and other parameters such as vascular permeability and extravasular/intravascular space ratio can be derived.

### 5.4.1 EndPlate Perfusion

It has been hypothesized that impaired nutrition of the endplates may lead to (accelerated) disc degeneration. The vertebral endplate is the main route of intravascular solute transport into the nucleus pulposus of intervertebral discs, and inhibition of endplate perfusion causes inhibited solute transport into the disc intranuclear tissue [10]. Other studies observed with MR-angiography showed that impairment of lumbar arterial flow is associated with decreased diffusion of blood to the lumbar intervertebral disks and may act as a promoter of disk degeneration [11].

Dynamic contrast-enhanced (DCE) perfusion is the best technique to study endplate perfusion and shows less susceptibility artifacts in this region with a mixture of bone and fat.

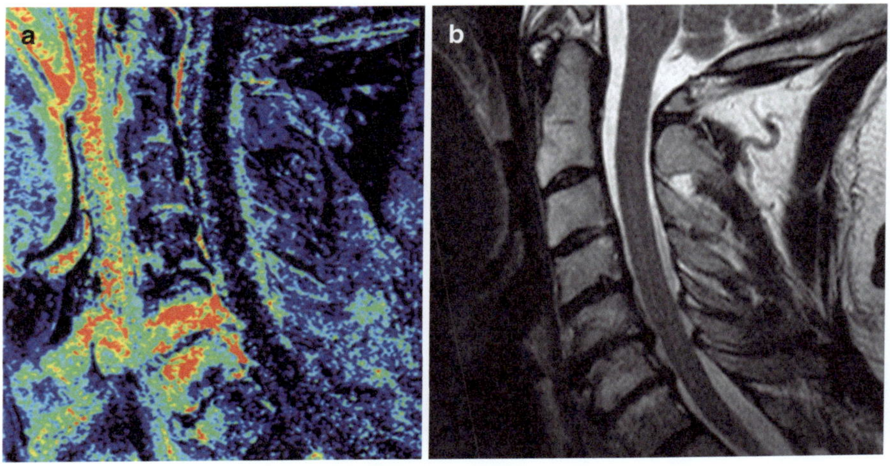

**Fig. 5.4** (**a**) DCE-perfusion and (**b**) T2-WI in a patient with cervical degenerative disc disease. There is a clear elevated perfusion at the endplates C5–C6 representing inflammatory changes at an active degenerative level. On the corresponding T2-WI, the discs and endplates C5–C6 and C6–C7 are almost identical. This demonstrates the superior sensitivity of MR-perfusion for active inflammatory and possible painful endplate changes, in cases of degenerative disease (Image courtesy Johan Van Goethem)

Studies have shown conflicting results on the association between disc degeneration and endplate perfusion. Several studies have indicated increased enhancement in the endplates adjoining degenerative intervertebral discs, which might be an indication of ongoing damage in these tissues [12, 13]. Other studies showed an increase in time-to-peak (TTP) values in endplates at degenerative lumbar levels [14]. Increased perfusion is mainly seen in the early stages of disc degeneration and usually corresponds to Modic type I changes in the adjoining endplates. Indeed, Modic type I changes reflect vascular granulation tissue adjacent to the endplates with resulting bone marrow edema [15] (Fig. 5.4).

On the other hand, in more chronic degenerative disc disease, as represented by Modic type II changes, red bone marrow is replaced by metabolic less active fatty bone marrow and, in general perfusion, is inversely related to marrow fat content [16]. Lumbar vertebral marrow perfusion is shown to be less in the vertebral body marrow between two degenerated disks than in vertebral marrow between two normal disks [17].

### 5.4.2 Disc Perfusion

In healthy intervertebral discs, there are no intrinsic blood vessels within the normal nucleus pulposus and a paucity of vessels in the annulus fibrosus. Therefore, MR perfusion depending on transport of marker molecules by larger blood vessels will show no signal in the normal disc. The very slow process of diffusion of gadolinium into intervertebral discs can be observed with nonionic components after several hours. Contrast diffusion peaks after 10 min in the subchondral bone and vertebral

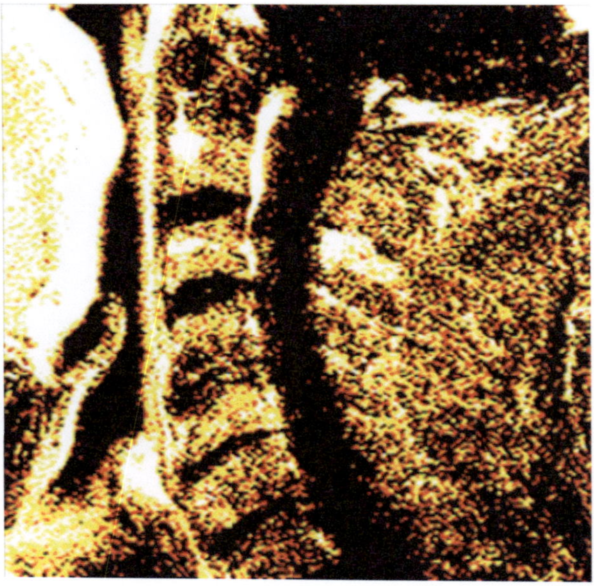

**Fig. 5.5** DCE-perfusion in a patient with cervical degenerative disc disease (different patient than Fig. 5.4). In this patient, there is abnormal perfusion of the disc at level C4–C5. Note that all other discs are "dark," i.e., showing no perfusion, which is the expected normal pattern. Elevated (present) disc perfusion can be associated with ingrowth of nerve endings and might be associated with a painful disc (Image courtesy Johan Van Goethem)

body, at 2 h in the vertebral endplates, and at 6 h in the intervertebral disc [18]. In general, diffusion seems to be less in degenerative discs than in normal discs [19]. But in mildly degenerative discs diffusion can be enhanced [20].

Degenerative changes however allow vessels to grow inward. The density of blood vessels increases with the grade of disc degeneration [21, 22]. Blood vessels are seen in fissures and cracks, which are areas with low proteoglycan [15]. Moreover, nerve and blood vessel ingrowth into the annulus fibrosis is strongly associated with proteoglycan depletion [23]. In healthy discs, nerve fibers can be seen in the outer one-third of the annulus fibrosus and sometimes even in the middle one-third. In patients with chronic low back pain, nerve fibers are also seen in the inner one-third of the annulus fibrosus [24]. Nerves are usually, but not always, associated with blood vessels. Sometimes vascularization is associated with discogenic pain [15], maybe because of the association with nerve fibers (Fig. 5.5).

## 5.5 MR Spectroscopy

### 5.5.1 Introduction

Magnetic resonance spectroscopy (MRS), formerly known as nuclear magnetic resonance (NMR) spectroscopy, is based on a quantum physics principle that enables researchers to determine the chemical composition of tissue containing hydrogen atoms. MRS evolved to become magnetic resonance imaging (MRI) which generates images of tissues based on hydrogen protons in water and lipid. As MRI technology improved, so did the ability to resolve and identify additional chemical components in tissue. Chemical shift imaging (CSI), a hybrid of MRI and MRS, generates chemical "maps" across regions of tissue.

An MR spectral plot contains multiple spectral peaks that correspond to the chemicals present. The chemicals are identified by their chemical shift (CS) measured in parts per million (PPM). The concentration of a chemical is indicated by the area under the curve (AUC) of the spectral peak (Fig. 5.6).

Peaks that are commonly measured in physiological tissues are shown in Table 5.1.

Given the ability to measure a wide range of biochemical markers, MRS has been used in many clinical applications including MRS of the brain (stroke, tumors, Alzheimer's, seizures, depression) [25, 26], the prostate [27], and the liver [28]. MRS has also been used to determine muscle metabolism by measuring intracellular lipid content.

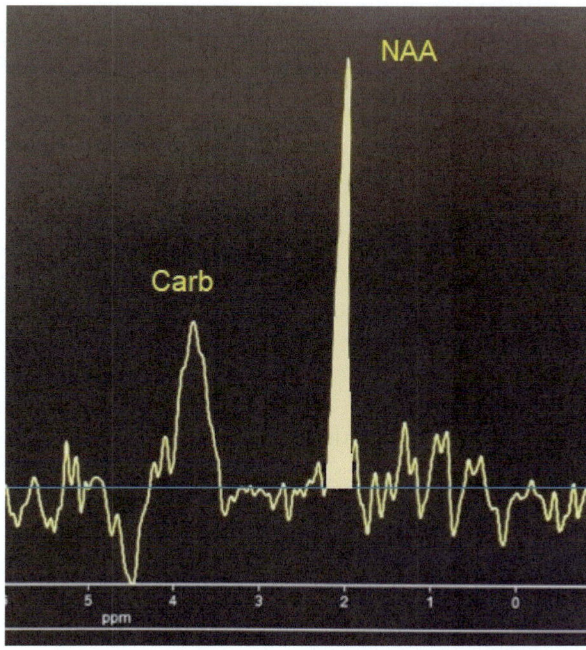


**Fig. 5.6** Area under curve (AUC) for proteoglycan peak

**Table 5.1** Most commonly measured peaks in MRS [31]

| | |
|---|---|
| Lactate | 1.3 ppm |
| Lipids | 1.3 ppm |
| Alanine | 1.48 ppm |
| Proteoglycan | 2.1 ppm |
| Glutamine/glutamate | 2.2–2.4 ppm |
| GABA | 2.2–2.4 ppm |
| 2-Hydroxyglutarate | 2.25 ppm |
| Citrate | 2.6 ppm |
| Creatine | 3.0 ppm |
| Choline | 3.2 ppm |
| Myo-inositol | 3.5 ppm |
| Water | 4.7 ppm |

The ability of MRS to differentiate the aforementioned biomarkers is directly proportional to the magnetic field strength and magnetic field homogeneity (B0). In vivo clinical measurements of metabolites become accurate at 1 T and improve at higher field strengths. High precision MRS is performed in vitro on 7 and 11 T magnets.

For those suffering from chronic low back pain (CLBP), not responding to conservative therapy and/or whose lumbar MRI does not present any findings suggestive for a pain generator (e.g., Modic type I changes, inflammatory facet joints), provocative discography (PD) may be used in helping to diagnose a painful disc. During PD, a needle is inserted into the lumbar disc of a mildly sedated patient. A dye which can be observed on fluoroscopy is injected to identify fissures in the disc. During the procedure, the patient is asked to grade the resulting pain level on a scale of 1–10. A disc that scores 6 or more is considered painful. There is an ongoing debate in the literature on the accuracy and value of PD and its safety and diagnostic accuracy are contended. Therefore, the ability of MRS to perform a noninvasive diagnostic test to identify painful discs is compelling.

### 5.5.2 Lumbar Disc Biomarkers

The primary component of the lumbar disc is proteoglycan (PG). Proteoglycan is a molecule consisting of various glycosaminoglycans that contain the NAA compound that has a chemical shift of 2.1 ppm (Fig. 5.7). Proteoglycans are the molecules that bind water in the nucleus of the disc which in turn generates the disc's cushioning effect.

When proteoglycans breakdown, they lose their ability to retain water. On T2-WI, a low water disc appears darker than a normal disc. In addition to

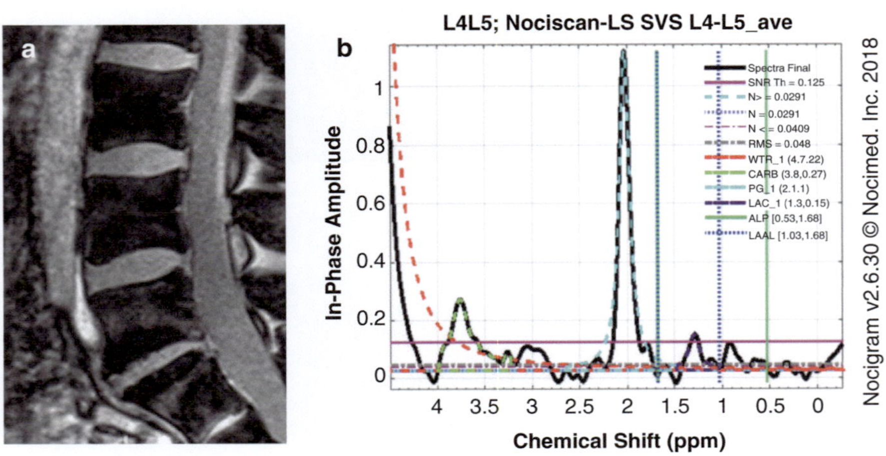


**Fig. 5.7** (**a**) MRI image of a spine and (**b**) corresponding MR spectral plot of the L4–L5 lumbar disc

retaining water, proteoglycans also inhibit the ingress of nerves that may emanate from the vertebral endplate. The lumbar disc is not vascularized and thus nutrients and oxygen require passive diffusion. The metabolic activity of the nerves generates an anaerobic environment which results in the production of lactic acid which in turns irritates the nerve endings resulting in lumbar disc pain. As such lactic acid and other acidic components are pain biomarkers. The chemical assay of the lumbar disc may thus be used in conjunction with the MRI image to diagnose the state of the disc and differentiate dark discs that are painful from those that are not.

## 5.6 The NOCISCAN-LS "Virtual Discography" Exam and System

### 5.6.1 Introduction

NOCISCAN-LS™ (Lumbar Spine) (Nocimed Inc.) is the only CE and FDA approved system currently available and clinically proven for MRS of the lumbar disc. It is a software as a service (SaaS) application that runs in the cloud. The NOCISCAN-LS exam study data is sent from the MR to the NOCISCAN-LS application. A NOCIGRAM-LS report is generated and returned to the original study in the PACS. The report may also be viewed on the NociWeb portal using a web browser.

The NOCISCAN-LS exam should be performed on a mid- or high-field MRI system (1.5 or 3 T) using standard spine coils. The NOCISCAN-LS exam protocol uses standard MRS pulse sequences typically used in spectroscopy of the brain, the breast, or the prostate. The parameters are optimized for spectroscopy of lumbar discs and organized in an exam protocol with optimized exam workflow.

### 5.6.2 Voxel Prescription

Localizer images are based on the location of water. However, the chemical shift effect of lipid in the vertebral endplates shifts the actual voxel image down and to the right. This requires biasing the voxel towards the inferior vertebral endplate resulting in the voxel "sitting" on the endplate. Sufficient gap must be provided between the voxel and the superior vertebral endplate (Fig. 5.8). Proper voxel placement is required to avoid lipid contamination which can invalidate an acquisition. To address this issue, Nocimed has developed *Autovox*™, an automatic voxel prescription function that segments the vertebral endplates and the lumbar disc within the scanner's coordinate space and optimizes the placement of the voxel volume within the disc. While currently not used in real time on a scanner, it can be used as quality assurance to assess correct voxel location.

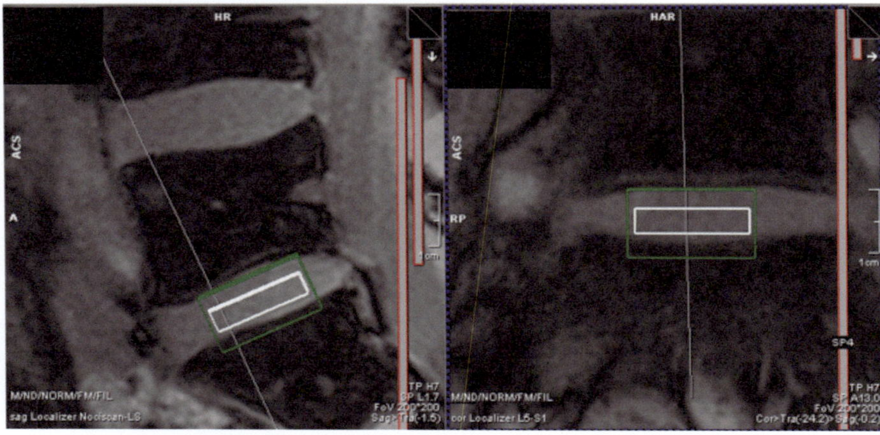


**Fig. 5.8** Sagittal and coronal L5–S1 voxel prescription. The outer green box is the adjustment or shimming volume. The white box is the voxel. Proper voxel placement is required to avoid lipid contamination which can invalidate an acquisition. Chemical shift effect of lipid in the vertebral endplates shifts the actual voxel image down and to the right. This requires biasing the voxel towards the inferior vertebral endplate resulting in the voxel "sitting" on the endplate. A sufficient gap must be left between the voxel and the superior vertebral endplate

### 5.6.3 MRS Data Acquisition

MRS data is acquired by a point-resolved spectroscopy sequence (PRESS). PRESS is a spin-echo sequence that uses a 90°–180°–180° slice selective pulse train. The 90° radio frequency pulse rotates the spins in the xy-plane, followed by the first 180° pulse (spin rotation in the *xz*-plane) and the second 180° pulse (spin rotation in the *xy*-plane), after which the signal is measured. The junction of the three planes defines the voxel volume which generates a free inductive decay (FID) RF signal.

Water is present in tissues at concentrations 10,000 times higher than the metabolites of interest. An unprepared MR spectrum would thus be dominated by a giant water peak, while the low concentration biomarkers/metabolites would be virtually undetectable above the background noise.

To visualize the organic molecules of interest, the large water peak must be suppressed. The most common technique to accomplish this is chemical shift selective saturation (CHESS). CHESS was originally developed as a technique for fat suppression in conventional MR imaging, where it is commonly known by the generic name fatsat. By tuning the CHESS pulses to the resonant frequency of water instead of fat, water suppression may be obtained. A CHESS pulse selectively rotates water magnetization into the transverse plane where it is immediately dephazed by application of a strong crusher or spoiler gradient. For MRS, a single CHESS pulse provides insufficient water suppression, so three CHESS pulses are used in a typical clinical implementation. To ensure frequency selectivity, CHESS pulses are relatively long (20–30 ms). The optimal flip angle for each pulse depends on the interpulse spacing as well as on the local T1 and B1 effects. MR vendors offer automated water suppression procedures that iteratively evaluate and optimize flip angles based on the residual water signal. CHESS also offers the unique feature of partial water suppression. This way special signal processing techniques such as frequency error correction and frame editing can be used. A downside of CHESS is the introduction of sideband noise and transverse magnetization artifacts that reduce the signal-to-noise ratio (SNR). Advanced water suppression sequences such as VAPOR do not introduce sideband noise but leave no residual water. The CHESS and PRESS timing pulses are interleaved to create a sequence with a typical TE of approximately 30 ms and a typical TR of 1500 ms at 3 T. At 1.5 T, the TR may be reduced to 1200 ms. If the voxel volume is between 1 and 2 cc, then 160–192 FIDs can provide enough averaging to extract coherent, robust spectra.

### 5.6.4 MRS Data Processing

The original strategy used by MR spectroscopists to improve the SNR of a spectrum has been to increase the number of acquisitions or FIDs. The SNR of a given spectrum or signal increases as the square root of the number of acquisitions. To double the SNR would thus requires four times as many acquisitions, which is not a favorable solution when scanning a patient with back pain. An alternative approach is to perform a series of signal processing steps called "frame editing," which requires each FID to be analyzed for frequency shift error, full width at half maximum (FWHM), water confidence level, and phase error. FIDs that do not meet certain criteria are either corrected or eliminated. Improved coherence resulting in more robust spectra is achieved through subtraction and not addition.

The metabolite peaks for the biomarkers of interest in the resulting spectrum are automatically located and their peak amplitude, chemical shift (PPM), FWHM (Hz), and area under the curve (AUC) are determined via a Lorentzian–Gaussian curve fit. This signal processing is repeated for all the lumbar disc acquisitions, and the spectral data is placed in an array for additional analysis and classification. Each lumbar disc spectrum is analyzed for features that may disqualify it from further analysis and classification (Table 5.2).

**Table 5.2** MRS procedural failure reports

| Feature | Description |
|---|---|
| Low SNR | Acquisition disqualified due to insufficient biomarker peak amplitudes with respect to signal noise (no biomarkers present) |
| Excessive lipid | Acquisition disqualified because voxel prescription overlapped with vertebral endplate resulting in lipid contamination |
| Spectral artifact | Acquisition disqualified due to scanner acquisition artifact |
| Poor shim | Acquisition disqualified due to poor shim |
| Small voxel | Warning that voxel volume is below recommended minimum volume (1 cc) and may decrease the reliability of the interpretation |

### 5.6.5 NOCISCORE Lumbar Disc Classification

A cohort of patients with axial lumbar pain without a clear pain generator on plain MRI underwent provocative discography (PD) and NOCISCAN-LS. A database of over 300 discs with PD scores and biomarker measurements was used to develop a classification system. The classifier uses ratios of AUCs and peaks of biomarkers, including proteoglycans, lactic acid, alanine, propionic acid, and narrow band lipids that have been identified as pain generators. The ratios are summed for each disc and then normalized across discs (Fig. 5.9). The scores (total and normalized) are then plotted on an *XY* graph. Regions are then defined for NOCI+ (red) and NOCI– (green) that provide the greatest correlation to PD+ and PD– scores. A NOCI-mild region (yellow) is an indeterminant score.

Additionally, a structural integrity score (SI score) is generated (Fig. 5.10). An SI score is derived from calculations (AUC, peak, SNR) for an MRS range corresponding with proteoglycan, normalized to the highest value between discs for each

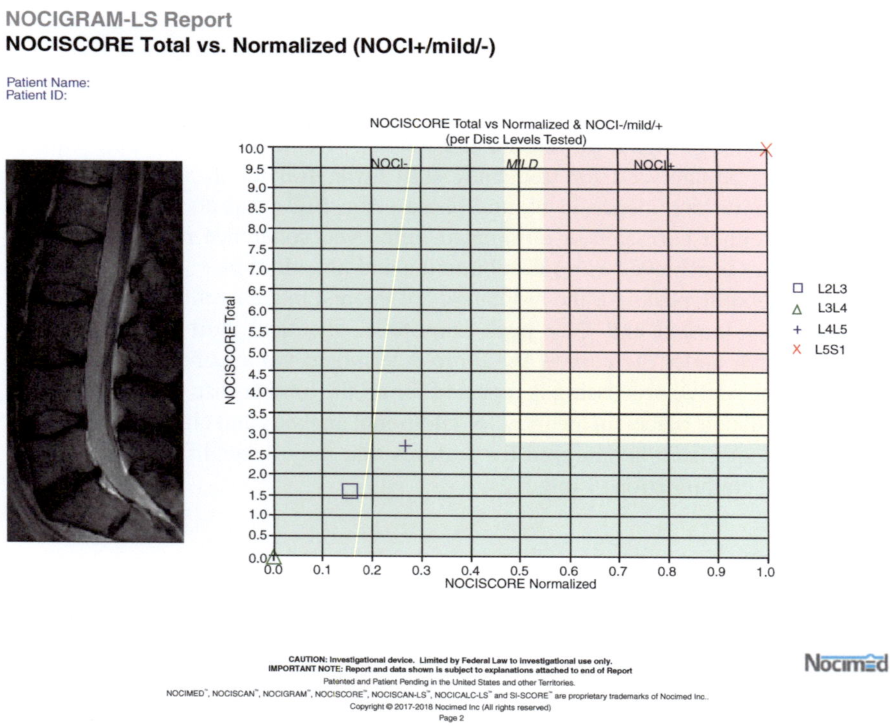


**Fig. 5.9** A typical NOCIGRAM-LS report. Negative scores for the L2–L3, L3–L4, and L4–L5 discs, a positive score for the L5–S1 disc, identified as painful

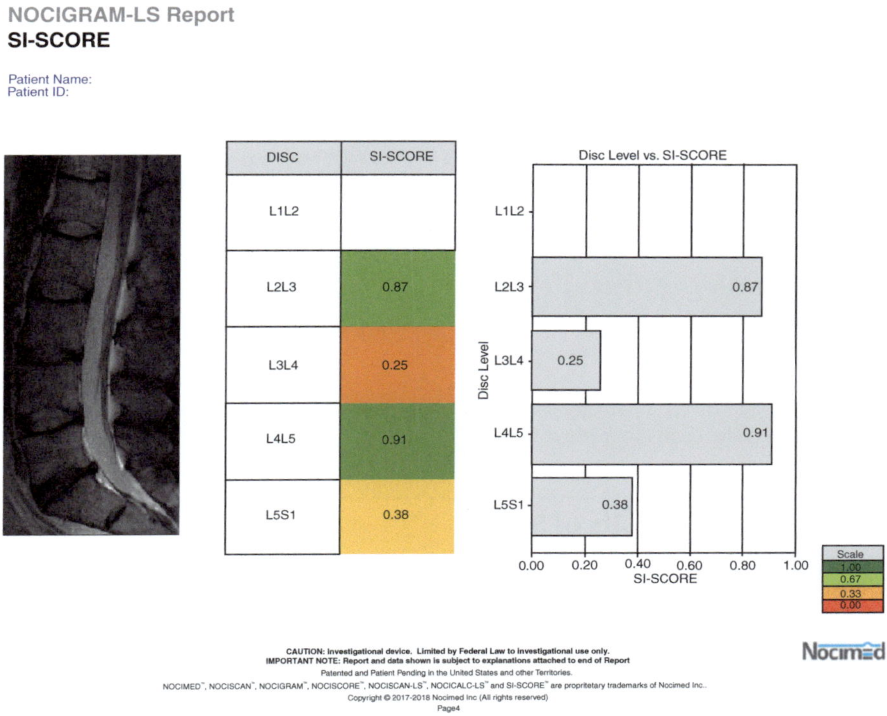


**Fig. 5.10** Structural integrity score (SI score). An SI score is derived from calculations (AUC, peak, SNR) for an MRS range corresponding to proteoglycan, normalized to the highest value between discs for each calculated parameter, and then averaged for a total SI score (maximum SI score = 1)

calculated parameter, and then averaged for a total SI score (maximum SI score = 1). SI scores are relative values comparing discs for a single exam in a single patient. Higher SI scores reflect higher relative values as compared between discs in the patient and do not necessarily reflect high structural integrity. A low SI score, corresponding to a lower structural integrity, is associated with more advanced degeneration (relative between discs).

### 5.6.6 Limitations

NOCISCAN-LS lumbar disc spectroscopy is subject to a number of limitations. Exclusion criteria are listed in Table 5.3. The exam can be performed in cases of previous surgery without implants/devices and in patients with Modic changes to the endplates.

**Table 5.3** Disc MRS exclusion criteria

| |
|---|
| Meets exclusion criteria for standard lumbar MRI exam |
| Disc height loss of more than 50% (compared to intact adjacent disc) |
| Disc height less than 4 mm |
| Implants/devices in the disc |
| Prior lumbar back surgery with total disc replacement or fusion at any lumbar level |
| Diagnosis, based on radiographic evidence, of clinically relevant lumbar vertebral abnormalities, including: |
| Spondylolisthesis with more than 2 mm of translation, or with pars fracture, at the involved level |
| Spondylolysis |
| Lumbar scoliosis with a cobb angle greater than 15° |
| Evidence of fracture or trauma |
| Lumbar kyphosis |
| Disc extrusion |
| Prior provocative discography showing evidence of grade 5 annular tear with contrast leakage |
| Motor strength deficit in lower extremities |

## 5.7 Clinical Results of MRS

Currently, MRS is CE and FDA approved for clinical diagnosis. The indications for NOCISCAN MRS are different in the US and in Europe. In the US, surgeons use the NOCISCAN as a replacement for discography in order to define the painful disc prior to fusion or total disc replacement. In Europe, the focus is on defining biomechanics (inflammation, instability) in order to regenerate the disc or treat the underlying disorder. The aim is to treat disc pathologies earlier to delay or avoid further degeneration and subsequent possible fusion or disc replacement. The different biological/regenerative techniques based on MRS as well as a comprehensive approach is described in Chap 12.

The learning curve in data acquisition and interpreting NOCISCAN MRS is steep. However, in Europe, training programs are available both for MRI-technicians and radiologists to learn data acquisition and interpretation as well as for interventional radiologists, surgeons, and pain specialists to learn disc regenerative techniques based on the MRS findings.

### 5.7.1 MRS Experience in the US

The latest and one of the most comprehensive clinical studies of MRS in the US has been published recently (Fig. 5.11) [29]. In a multicentre study, 623 discs were examined in 139 patients. In 275 discs (44.1%), a PD was used prior to the spectroscopy. The data was used to analyse disc structure (proteoglycan) and acidity (lactic acid, alanine, and propionic acid) (Fig. 5.6). Compared to PD (provocative discogram), which was considered the gold standard, MRS showed a total accuracy of

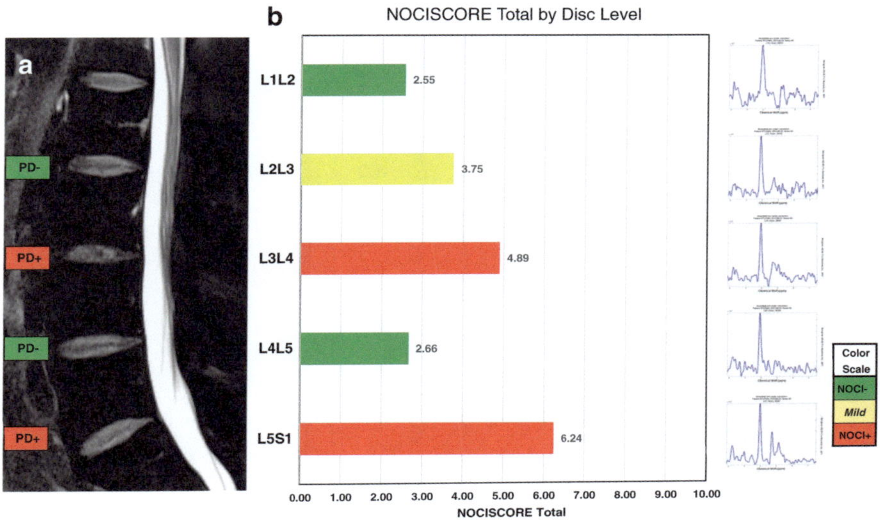


**Fig. 5.11** (**a**) results of discography (PD) and (**b**) MRS results of a 49-year-old male patient. No acute injury and chronic severe lumbar pain. Pain radiating to right buttock, hip, leg, and occasional pain to foot and ankle. Note negative discogram, but mildly elevated MRS levels on L2/L3 [29]

85%, sensitivity of 82%, and specificity of 88% in detecting painful discs. These values increased to 93%, 91%, and 93%, respectively in non-herniated discs.

Fusion surgery at the index level of disc pain as determined by discography and clinical evaluation was performed in 73 patients, independent of MRS scores. The patients with negative or only mildly elevated MRS scores at the operated level had consistently worse outcomes than patients with positive MRS spectroscopy results (treatment success, determined by ODI and VAS 55% vs. 97%). The result was similar in patients where two levels were fused. In cases where MRS showed painful discs on both levels, the clinical results were better than in patients with negative or only mildly elevated MRS scores on one or both discs. This clearly shows that clinicians cannot rely just on discography and clinical examination in order to find the painful disc level (Figs. 5.11 and 5.12).

### 5.7.2 MRS Experience in Europe

After CE approval in autumn 2017, the first EU MRS on patients was performed in November 2017 in Austria. In a first set of 30 patients, technical issues were resolved, existing routines from the US were adapted, and further exam

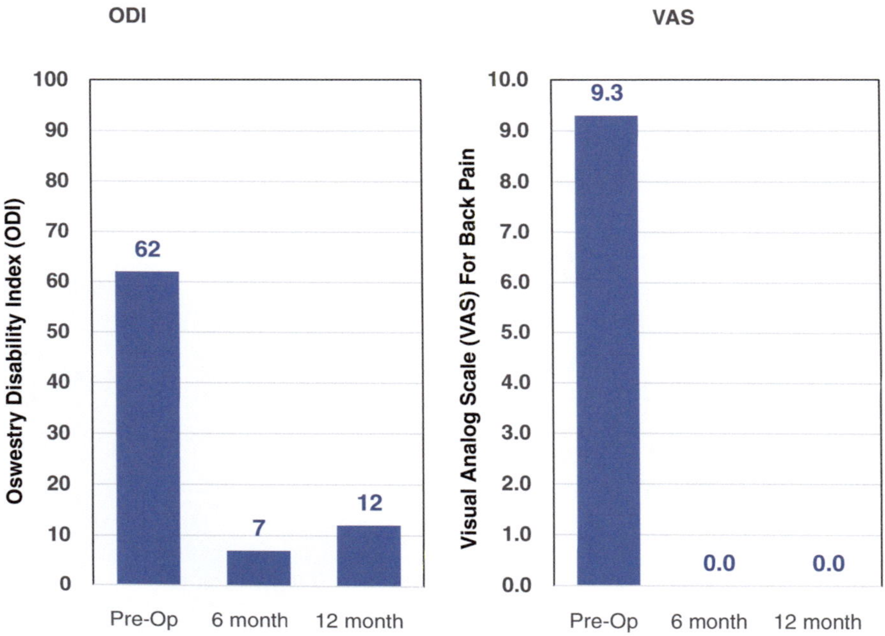


**Fig. 5.12** Good clinical results after fusion L3/L4 and L5/S1 [29]. However, the mildly elevated biomarker levels at L2/L3 may indicate an early failure of this disc in the future (see Fig. 5.11)

workflows were developed. This first group is still under follow-up regarding clinical outcome after a variety of disc preserving minimal-invasive or conservative treatments. After completing these first 30 cases, MRS continues at our site since February 2018. Further MRS sites were opened in 2018 and 2019 in Germany, Italy, and Austria.

The experience of the first 30 patients in Austria led to the development of a tentative treatment scheme based not only on pain generators but also on disc degeneration (Pfirrmann grade). This first feasibility analysis in Austria involved 30 patients (17 male and 13 female) with suspected discogenic pain. In order to get experience with all types of intradiscal lesions, seven patients with prior intradiscal therapy such as platelet-rich plasma injection (PRP), ozone therapy, nucleoplasty, and microdiscectomy were included. MRS confirmed the clinical suspicion in 26 cases and showed clear signs of discogenic pain with elevated biomarkers. The MRS was also very helpful in the MRS-negative patients, as the treatment could be adapted accordingly by considering other possible sources of pain. Interestingly, it came as a sort of a positive surprise and actually did ease the burden on the MRS-negative patients in realizing that their discs were normal and not the cause of back pain.

The patients were treated accordingly to the algorithm shown in chapter 13 (13, Fig. 8). This led to surgery in eight patients and conservative treatment in 24 patients. The patients that had surgical treatment showed significant improvement in their symptoms after 6 weeks and 3 months in seven out of eight cases and in all cases at 6 months (pre-op VAS 7.6, ODI 56.7, 6 weeks VAS 2.6, ODI 34.7, 3 months VAS 1.9, ODI 16; 6 months VAS 1.8; ODI 16).

A targeted conservative therapy considering the biochemical conditions in the intervertebral disc showed a significant improvement in 15 out of 16 patients (two patients lost in follow-up; pretreatment VAS 5.6; ODI 36.5 6 weeks VAS 1.8; ODI 12, 3 months VAS 1.2; ODI 8.3, 6 months VAS 1.1; ODI 8).

### 5.7.3 Clinical Examples of Patients Treated Before MRS Acquisition

These examples show a variety of cases with standard treatments without prior MRS acquisition (Figs. 5.13, 5.14, 5.15, and 5.16). All patients were examined at the same site (1.5 T Siemens Aera, regular Nocimed protocol). These examples demonstrate findings that can be expected in patients where the decision-making was not performed on prior MRS studies.

Examples with previously untreated patients where the course of treatment was defined after MRS acquisition, and the course of treatment/decision-making is discussed in detail in Chap. 12.

### 5.7.4 Implications

Over the last decades, the surgical community has been under scrutiny for high operation rates, unnecessary operations, high surgical morbidity, and various other issues in low back surgery. Improvements by using more biologic approaches, biotechnologies, biomaterials, and minimal-invasive techniques may make gross instrumented fusion and cage/screw approaches as well as the use of artificial discs more obsolete.

Previous to MRS, there was no proper imaging technique to accurately describe the biochemical state of a lumbar disc. Knowing the biochemical state of a disc and finding the origin of back pain offers a whole new line of approach focusing on regenerating and restoring the disc or at least slowing the degeneration and thus

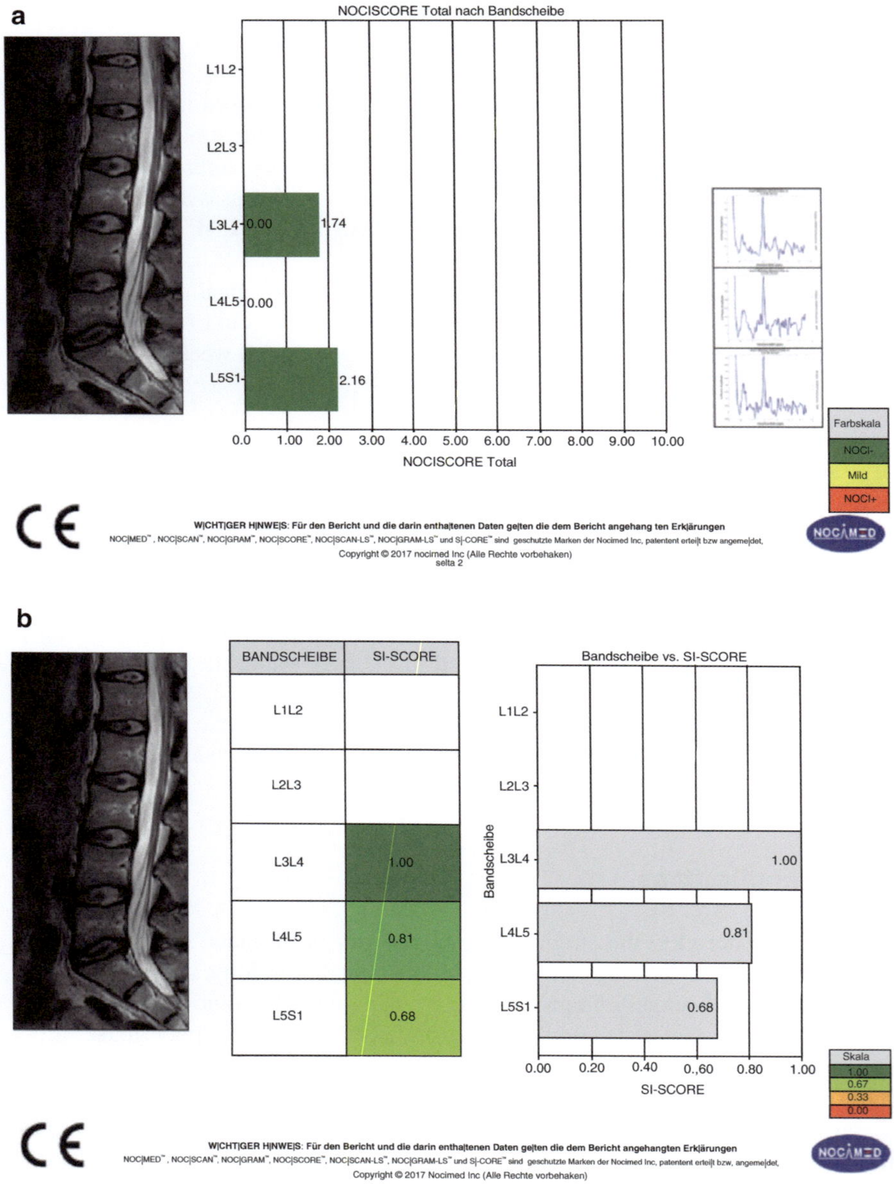


**Fig. 5.13** Follow-up 1 year after platelet-rich plasma (PRP) injection into the L5–S1 disc after a positive discography in a 27-year-old woman. Preoperative lumbar pain improved significantly after PRP injection, there is no radicular pain. Afterwards, she started to complain about sacroiliac (SI) joint pain on the left. MRS shows a normal biochemistry of the lumbar disc (**a**). The proteoglycan content was slightly decreased in L5–S1, but within normal limits (**b**). Renewed clinical analysis confirmed SI joint instability on the left side, which was successfully treated with SI fusion. Note that a score of 0.00 corresponds to no measurable pain biomarkers

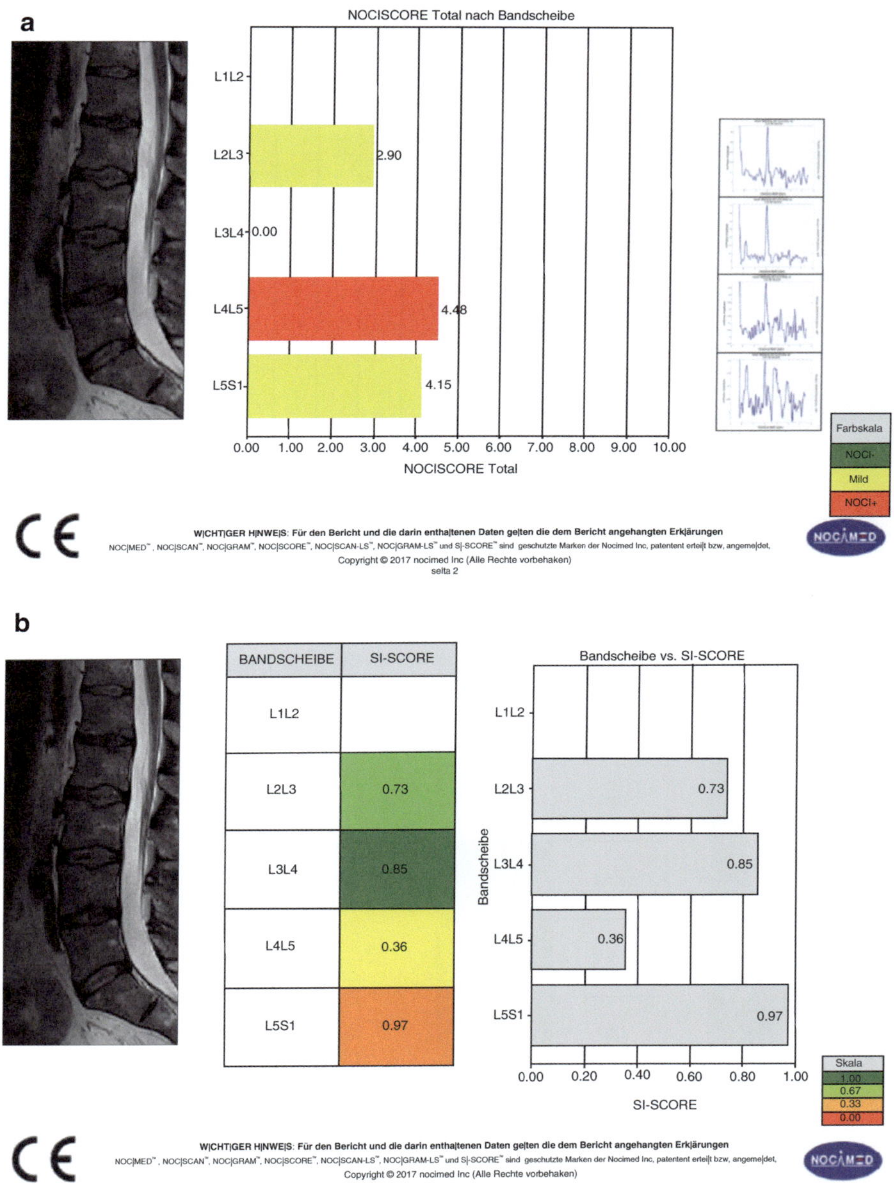


**Fig. 5.14** Fifty-one-year-old man with low back pain and a positive discogram at L4–L5. The patient received a PRP injection at L4–L5 in 2017 and slowly improved over the next 6 months (VAS 4–VAS 2). At that time, MRS was performed as treatment control showing increased acidity (pain) biomarkers at L4–L5 and mildly increased biomarkers at L5–S1 and L2–L3 (**a**). Only L4–L5 shows significantly decreased proteoglycan content (**b**)

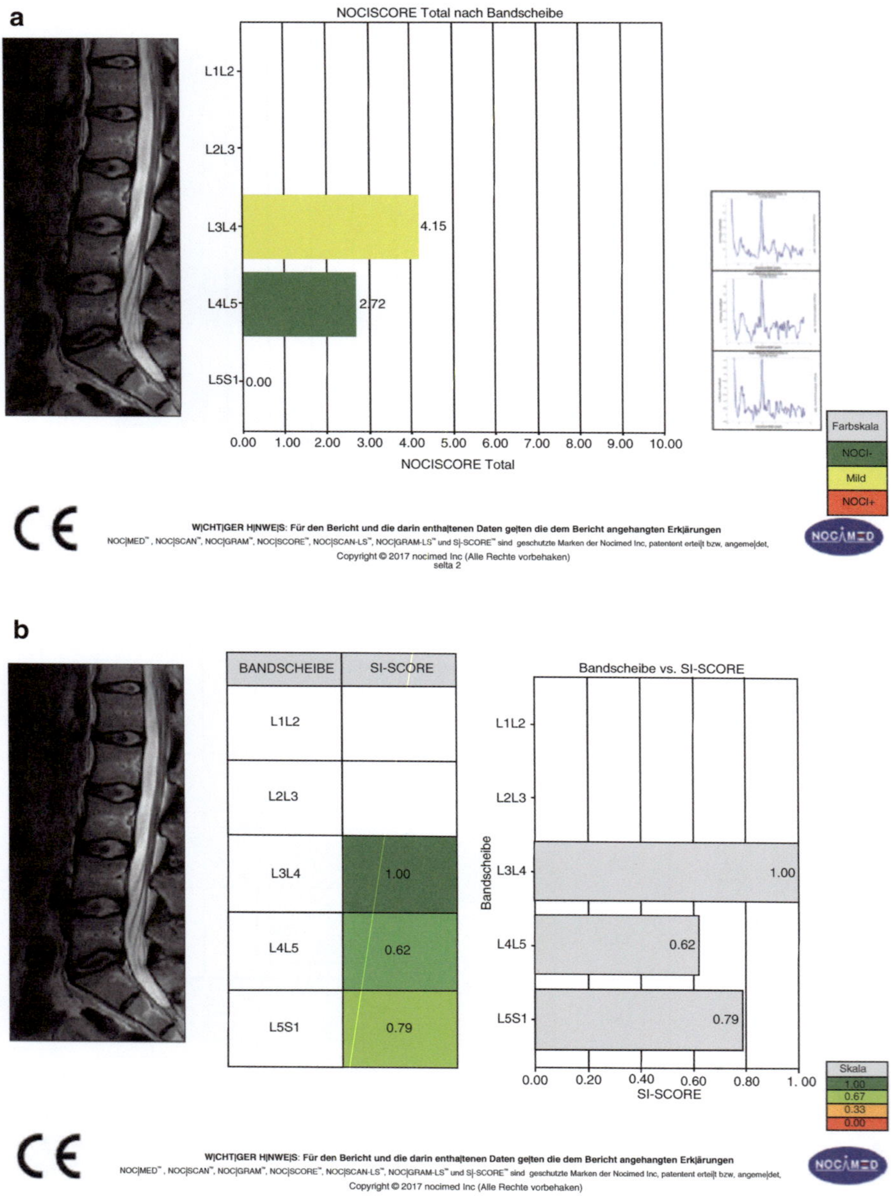


**Fig. 5.15** Sixty-six-year-old woman with a history of herniectomy at L5–S1 in 2015. Currently she has no back pain, but the patient opted for an MRS to check the health status of her intervertebral discs. Mildly increased biomarkers at L3–L4 (**a**). Normal result at the L4–L5 and L5–S1 discs. All discs show a normal proteoglycan content (**b**). This case shows the potential of disc healing without any medical intervention

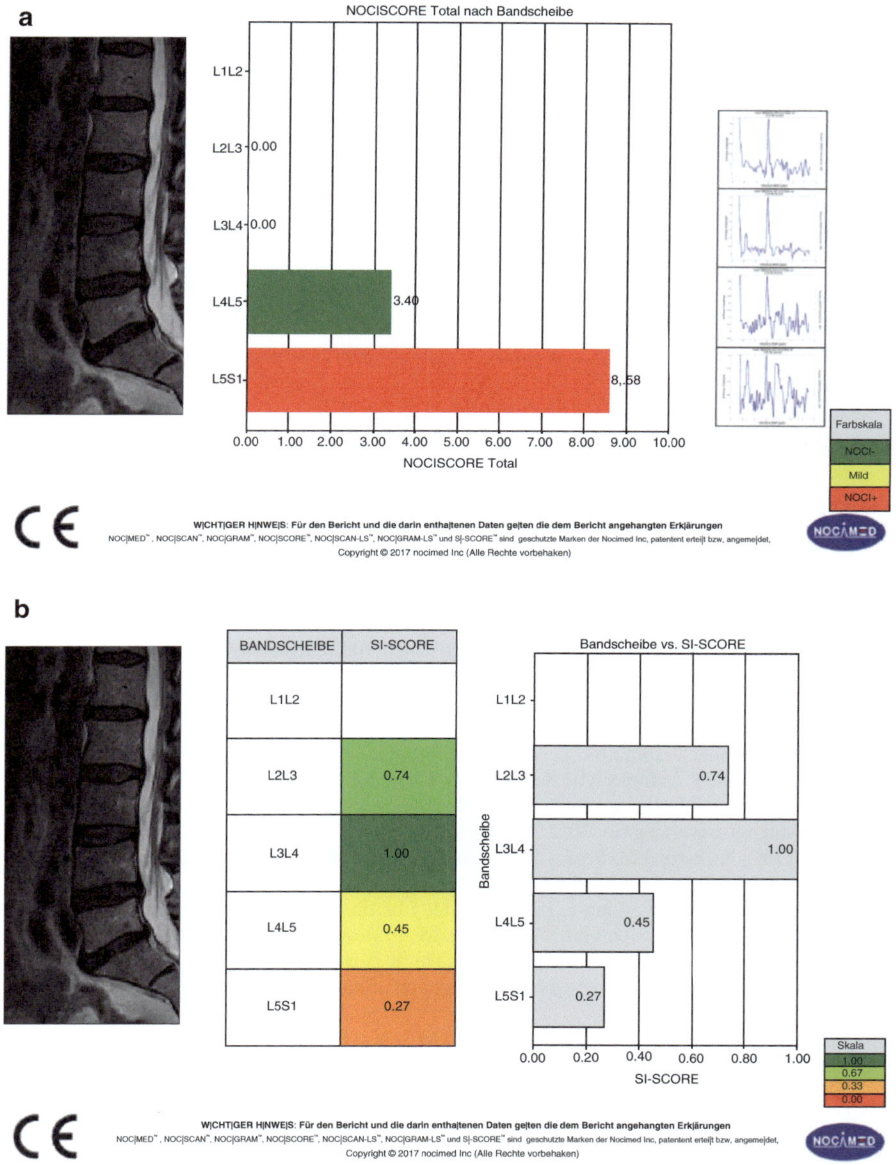


**Fig. 5.16** (**a**, **b**) 49-year-old man after surgery at the level L4–L5 and L5–S1, including sequestrectomy in 2014 at L4–L5 and microdiscectomy in 2016 at L5–S1 complicated with a CSF leak for which a surgical revision at that level was needed. Afterwards he suffers from chronic low back pain. MRS 21 months after last operation shows increased biomarkers at L5–S1 and normal biomarkers at L2–L3, L3–L4, and L4–L5 (**a**). Proteoglycan levels were abnormally low at L5–S1 and reduced at L4–L5 (**b**). In literature [30], no difference between the surgical outcome after sequestrectomy and microdiscectomy was found, but this case suggests otherwise. After a microdiscectomy/revision at the level L5–S1, the disc obviously remained acidic, while a sequestrectomy did not interfere with disc healing. This example demonstrates that MRS is able to discern and objectively evaluate the result of surgical treatment and accurately assess microdiscectomy as a cause of failed back surgery syndrome

avoiding major "destructive" surgery. For the first time, we have a better understanding of disc biology and can decide whether a patient is at risk for an increased rate of degeneration and pain and intervene proactively much earlier than until now. By assessing the disc biology, we should be able to reduce disc replacement/fusion rates in degenerative disc disease. Restoration and protective measurements will be of high interest to all pain physicians, interventional radiologists, and spine surgeons seeking to maintain and not replace the disc.

MRS is also very valuable for researchers looking at disc biology, as well as for clinicians looking for long-term surveillance of conservative treatments schemes (see Chap. 12).

## References

1. Kunkel ME, Herkommer A, Reinehr M, Böckers TM, Wilke HJ. Morphometric analysis of the relationships between intervertebral disc and vertebral body heights: an anatomical and radiographic study of the human thoracic spine. J Anat. 2011;219(3):375–87.
2. Zhong W, Driscoll SJ, Wu M, Wang S, Liu Z, Cha TD, Wood KB, Li G. In vivo morphological features of human lumbar discs. Medicine (Baltimore). 2014;93(28):e333.
3. Pooni JS, Hukins DW, Harris PF, Hilton RC, Davies KE. Comparison of the structure of human intervertebral discs in the cervical, thoracic and lumbar regions of the spine. Surg Radiol Anat. 1986;8(3):175–82.
4. Li LY, Wu XL, Roman RJ, Fan F, Qiu CS, Chen BH. Diffusion-weighted 7.0T magnetic resonance imaging in assessment of intervertebral disc degeneration in rats. Chin Med J. 2018;131(1):63–8.
5. JinYan Z, NingYang J, ChenGuang W. Diffusion tensor imaging of lumbar intervertebral disc. Joint Bone Spine. 2015;82:64.
6. Zhang Z, Chan Q, Anthony MP, Samartzis D, Cheung KMC, Khong PL, Kim M. Age-related diffusion patterns in human lumbar intervertebral discs: a pilot study in asymptomatic subjects. Magn Reson Imaging. 2012;30:181.
7. Tourell MC, Kirkwood M, Pearcy MJ, Momot KI, Little JP. Load-induced changes in the diffusion tensor of ovine anulus fibrosus: a pilot MRI study. J Magn Reson Imaging. 2017;4:5.
8. Li L, Zhu W, Chen W, Fang J, Li J. The study of the intervertebral disc microstructure in matured rats with diffusion kurtosis imaging. Magn Reson Imaging. 2017 Oct;42:101–6.
9. Zeng F, Zha Y, Li L, Xing D, Gong W, Hu L, Fan Y. A comparative study of diffusion kurtosis imaging and T2* mapping in quantitative detection of lumbar intervertebral disk degeneration. Eur Spine J. 2019;28:2169.
10. van der Werf M, Lezuo P, Maissen O, van Donkelaar C, Ito K. Inhibition of vertebral endplate perfusion results in decreased intervertebral disc intranuclear diffusive transport. J Anat. 2007;211:769–74.
11. Kurunlahti M, Kerttula L, Jauhiainen J, et al. Correlation of diffusion in lumbar intervertebral disks with occlusion of lumbar arteries: a study in adult volunteers. Radiology. 2001;221:779–86.
12. Arpinar VE, Rand SD, Klein AP, Maiman DJ, Muftuler LT. Changes in perfusion and diffusion in the endplate regions of degenerating intervertebral discs: a DCE-MRI study. Eur Spine J. 2015;24(11):2458–67.
13. Muftuler LT, Jarman JP, Yu HJ, Gardner VO, Maiman DJ, Arpinar VE. Association between intervertebral disc degeneration and endplate perfusion studied by DCE-MRI. Eur Spine J. 2015;24(4):679–85.
14. Savvopoulou V, Maris TG, Koureas A, Gouliamos A, Moulopoulos LA. Degenerative endplate changes of the lumbosacral spine: dynamic contrast-enhanced MRI profiles related to age, sex, and spinal level. J Magn Reson Imaging. 2011;33(2):382–9.

15. Modic MT, Steinberg PM, Ross JS, Masaryk TJ, Carter JR. Degenerative disk disease: assessment of changes in vertebral body marrow with MR imaging. Radiology. 1988;166:193–9.
16. Bluemke DA, Petri M, Zerhouni EA. Femoral head perfusion and composition: MR imaging and spectroscopic evaluation of patients with systemic lupus erythematosus and at risk for avascular necrosis. Radiology. 1995;197:433–8.
17. Liu YJ, Huang GS, Juan CJ, Yao MS, Ho WP, Chan WP. Intervertebral disk degeneration related to reduced vertebral marrow perfusion at dynamic contrast-enhanced MRI. AJR. 2009;192:974–9.
18. Rajasekaran S, Babu JN, Arun R, Armstrong BR, Shetty AP, Mu-Rugan S. ISSLS Prize Winner: a study of diffusion in human lumbar discs: a serial magnetic resonance imaging study documenting the influence of the endplate on diffusion in normal and degenerate discs. Spine. 2004;29:2654–67.
19. Nguyen-Minh C, Haughton VM, Papke RA, Censky SC. Measuring diffusion of solutes into intervertebral disks with MR imaging and paramagnetic contrast medium. AJNR Am J Neuroradiol. 1998;19:1781–4.
20. Bydder GM. New approaches to magnetic resonance imaging of intervertebral discs, tendons, ligaments, and menisci. Spine. 2002;27:1264–8.
21. Lama P, Le Maitre CL, Harding IJ, Dolan P, Adams MA. Nerves and blood vessels in degenerated intervertebral discs are confined to physically disrupted tissue. J Anat. 2018;233(1):86–97.
22. Kauppila LI. Ingrowth of blood vessels in disc degeneration. . Angiographic and histological studies of cadaveric spines. JBJS. 1995;77:26–31.
23. Melrose J, Roberts S, Smith S, Menage J, Ghosh P. Increased nerve and blood vessel ingrowth associated with proteoglycan depletion in an ovine anular lesion model of experimental disc degeneration. Spine. 2002;27(12):1278–85.
24. Freemont AJ, Pathab FRC, Peacock TE, Goupille P, Hoyland JA, O'Brien J, Jayson MIV. Nerve ingrowth into diseased intervertebral disc in chronic back pain. Lancet. 1997;350:178–81.
25. Jansen JF, Backes WH, Nicolay K, et al. 1H MR spectroscopy of the brain: absolute quantification of metabolites. Radiology. 2006;240(2):318–32.
26. Preul MC, Caramanos Z, Collins DL, et al. Accurate, noninvasive diagnosis of human brain tumors by using proton magnetic resonance spectroscopy. Nat Med. 1996;2(3):323–5.
27. Mueller-Lisse UG, Scherr M. 1H-MR-spektroskopie der prostata: Ein Überblick [1H magnetic resonance spectroscopy of the prostate]. Radiologe. 2003;43(6):481–8.
28. Tognarelli JM, Dawood M, Shariff MI, et al. Magnetic resonance spectroscopy: principles and techniques: lessons for clinicians. J Clin Exp Hepatol. 2015;5(4):320–8.
29. Gornet MG, Peacock J, Claude J, et al. Magnetic resonance spectroscopy (MRS) can identify painful lumbar discs and may facilitate improved clinical outcomes of lumbar surgeries for discogenic pain. Eur Spine J. 2019;28(4):674–87.
30. Huang T, Tian Z, Li M, Zheng W, Zhang L, Chen J, Zhai J, Li X. Sequestrectomy versus microdiscectomy in the treatment of lumbar disc herniation: a meta-analysis. Int J Clin Exp Med. 2015;8(5):7261–9.
31. https://radiopaedia.org/articles/mr-spectroscopy-1.

# Imaging of the Postoperative Spine

# 6

Mark M. Georgy and Bassem A. Georgy

## 6.1 Introduction

Unsatisfactory results after spinal surgery are often referred to as "failed back surgery syndrome" (FBSS). According to The International Association for the Study of Pain (IASP), FBSS is defined as follows: Lumbar (cervical) pain of unknown origin either persisting despite surgical intervention or appearing after surgical intervention for spinal (original) pain originally in the same topographical distribution [1].The incidence of failure rate of spinal surgery is quoted in the literature between 10–40% [2]. Recently, a European panel has recommended the use of the term persistent pain after spine surgery (PPSS), as the term (FBSS) unilaterally puts the blame on the operation as the cause of the problem, while the etiology is much more complex and often multifactorial [3].

## 6.2 Imaging Techniques

### 6.2.1 Conventional Radiography

Conventional radiography is the most commonly used imaging modality. Radiography during surgery is used to confirm the level of surgery and may be the only imaging technique used in the absence of suspicion of complications. Conventional radiography (X-ray) is particularly useful in surgery involving metal

M. M. Georgy
Ohio State School of Medicine, San Diego, CA, USA
e-mail: mgeorgy@ucsd.edu

B. A. Georgy (✉)
University of California, San Diego, San Diego, CA, USA
e-mail: bgeorgy@ucsd.edu



L. Manfrè, J. Van Goethem (eds.), *The Disc and Degenerative Disc Disease*,
New Procedures in Spinal Interventional Neuroradiology,
https://doi.org/10.1007/978-3-030-03715-4_6

hardware because it is less affected by artifacts produced by other techniques such as computed tomography (CT) and magnetic resonance imaging (MRI).

### 6.2.2 Computed Tomography

CT is the modality of choice for bone and abnormal calcification assessment. CT requires intravenous iodine contrast injection in case of suspected infection. Beam hardening artifacts produced by metallic orthopedic hardware on CT can be reduced during scanning. Image acquisition with the thinnest slice thickness possible using isotropic voxels allows for more accurate z-axis resolution and for multiplanar and volumetric reconstructions with high spatial resolution. Increasing the kilovolts peak increases the mean energy of the X-ray photons, which results in reducing photon starvation and beam hardening. Increasing the milliampere second reduces photon starvation by increasing the total number of photons in the X-ray beam. Lowest pitch possible is used with the highest number of channels. Data should be acquired with a soft tissue reconstruction kernel to reduce artifacts. Using a bone kernel in the postprocessing allows for better assessment of bone structures. Titanium produces less distortion than stainless-steel hardware which in turn produces less distortion than cobalt-chrome [4, 5].

### 6.2.3 Magnetic Resonance Imaging

MRI is the modality of choice in cases where postoperative complications are suspected. The high spatial and contrast resolution of MRI allows for better evaluation of soft tissues, bone marrow, and intraspinal content. Metallic orthopedic hardware produces magnetic susceptibility artifacts. As a general rule, fast spin echo (FSE) sequences are better than conventional spin echo (SE) sequences, and these latter are better than gradient echo (GRE) sequences. The shortest TE possible is recommended for metal artifact reduction in spin echo sequences; however, FSE sequences require longer TR than conventional sequences. A smaller voxel size results in less susceptibility artifacts. The voxel size is determined by the image matrix, the size of the field of view (FOV), and the slice thickness of the image. The use of a larger matrix, a smaller FOV, and thin section images will minimize susceptibility artifacts. The primary drawback of a smaller voxel size is decreased signal-to-noise ratio (SNR). One way to compensate for the loss of SNR is to increase the number of excitations (NEX), which will lead to increased imaging time. Scanning on a lower field strength magnet reduces the degree of susceptibility artifacts by decreasing the magnetization of the implant. Techniques that are relatively insensitive to magnetic field heterogeneity (e.g., STIR and Dixon techniques) produce less artifacts compared with frequency-selective fat-suppression techniques. In addition, the phase encoding direction in both the axial and sagittal planes should be parallel to the long axis of the orthopedic material, since the artifacts produced will be linear and parallel to the metal material, therefore with less interference with image assessment. On MRI, titanium and vitallium hardware produce fewer artifacts than stainless steel.

## 6.3 Clinical Evaluation

For adequate interpretation of postoperative imaging, a good knowledge of the clinical presentation and understanding of the type of surgery is essential for an accurate diagnosis. A patient who is complaining of radicular pain after surgery is most likely to have some type of spinal stenosis that could be due to a recurrent disc herniation, epidural scaring, adjacent level disease, or even a wrong level of surgery. A patient who is presenting with axial low back pain may have a postoperative incisional complication, non-union, facet joint disease, or hardware failure. Understanding the type of surgery and the approach is also essential for accurate diagnosis. As a general rule, spine surgery falls under two big categories, decompression and fusions (Table 6.1).

**Table 6.1** Summary of different surgical techniques

| | |
|---|---|
| *Decompression techniques* | |
| Laminotomy | Resection of a small segment of the inferior margin of the upper lamina and the superior margin of the lower lamina |
| Laminectomy | Resection of the entire width of a lamina |
| Laminectomy and facetectomy | Resection including part or all the facet joint in addition to the laminae |
| Discectomy | Removal of the herniated disc material that is causing compression on neural elements |
| *Fusion techniques* | |
| Rods and plates | Rods can extend to single or multiple spine segments, attached to the spine by pedicle screws. Plates have been developed for anterior or posterior fusion |
| Translaminar or facet screws | They attach the laminae of two adjacent vertebrae |
| Transpedicular screws | The use of pedicle screws in conjunction with plates or rods is generally well accepted as creating a primary stable construct, providing immediate postoperative stabilization without external support |
| Interbody spacers | Inserted into the intervertebral space after removal of the disc material with or without the additional screw and plate/rod fixation. Cages are usually made of titanium, carbon fiber, polyether ether ketone (PEEK), cortical, or cortico-cancellous bone graft. Radiolucent cages contain radiopaque markers to identify their position on radiographs |
| *Surgical approach* | |
| Anterior lumbar interbody fusion (ALIF) | Limited by the potential injury to major vessels and the sympathetic nerve chains |
| Lateral lumbar interbody fusion (XLIF) | Allows for access to the anterior spine through the retroperitoneal space and is less invasive alternative to traditional anterior retroperitoneal approaches |
| Posterior lumbar interbody fusion (PLIF) | Bilateral laminectomies are performed, and bone graft material with a cage or spacer is inserted into the disc space after the disc is removed. Disadvantages include potential injury to the nerve roots and retrograde migration of the graft or cage |
| Transforaminal interbody fusion (TLIF) | Modified posterior lumbar interbody fusion technique that uses a more lateral approach and thus leaves the midline bony structures intact |
| Total disc replacement | Removal of the diseased disc and insertion of a disc prosthesis to alleviate discogenic pain and to restore normal disc height |

## 6.4 Normal Radiological Findings in the Postoperative Spine

A midline approach is the most common approach for lumbar spine surgery, and asymmetry of muscles and fat as well as small seromas and edema of the subcutaneous tissue are not uncommonly observed. During the first 30–60 days, this may cause a posterior mass effect on the thecal sac that will decrease over time.

Edema and enhancement of the vertebral endplates are observed in 19% of patients between 6 and 18 months following surgery [6]. In 20–62% of patients, enhancement of the nerve roots is observed between 3 and 6 weeks following surgery [7]. These enhancements progressively decrease over time, and therefore any enhancement observed after 6 months is considered pathological. Post-discectomy changes may mimic re-herniation. The intraoperative disruption of the annulus fibrosus with resulting edema in the epidural space may efface the thecal sac.

Normal postoperative findings should be distinguished from those associated with early discitis. In these cases, clinical symptoms, laboratory data, and when performed a biopsy of the suspicious lesion should be all correlated. Enhancement associated with bacterial discitis is typically more intense than enhancement seen in the normal postoperative phase. A fluid collection in a paraspinal or anterior epidural location adjacent to the involved disc and enhancement of the psoas muscles are usually indicative of infection. In the laminectomy defect, the dural sac may slightly bulge through the bone defect, which should not be confused with a pseudomeningocele.

## 6.5 Common Radiologic Findings in Postoperative Spine

### 6.5.1 Postoperative Fluid Collections

Hematomas or seromas can be formed in the epidural space or in the postoperative bed posterior to the thecal sac. MR imaging is sensitive in identifying the blood products. Hematomas may be hyperintense on T1-weighted images in the subacute phase because the signal is caused primarily by methemoglobin. Pure seroma should follow cerebrospinal fluid on all pulse sequences. Sterile fluid collections should resolve slowly over time; however, needle aspiration may be necessary to rule out infection (Figs. 6.1 and 6.2).

Pseudomeningocele is a fairly common postoperative finding from dural tears and can get infected. It does not have a true meningeal lining and is usually seen posterior to the thecal sac. They can be complex in signal intensity on MR imaging scans secondary to hemorrhage, and fluid–fluid levels can be present. In chronic cases, the fluid collection should follow cerebrospinal fluid on all sequences;

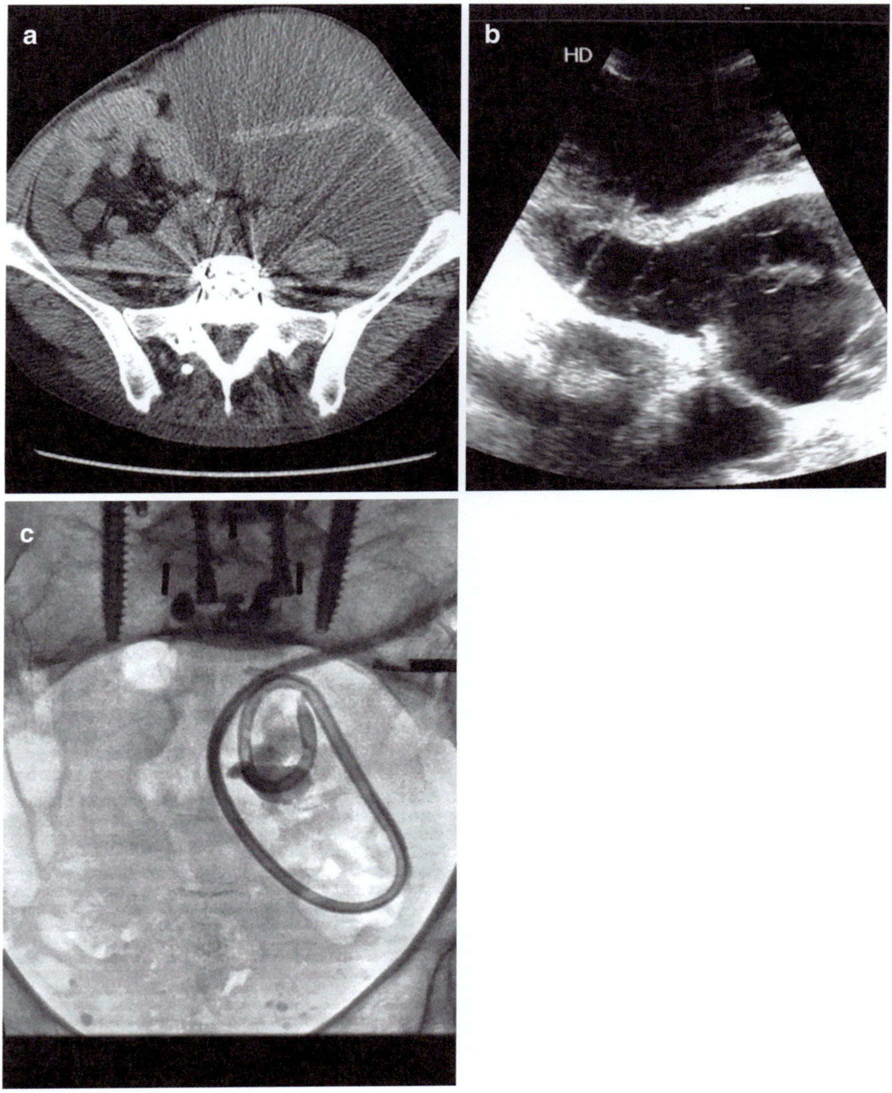


**Fig. 6.1** Postoperative seroma in a 64 year-old woman who underwent anterior fusion at L4–5 and L5–S1 levels presented with back pain and abdominal distension. (**a**) Axial CT examination showing a large cystic lesion extending from the L5–S1 disc space into the left lower quadrant and the anterior abdominal wall. (**b**) Ultrasound examination showing extensive septation of the fluid collection. (**c**) The fluid collection was drained, and a pigtail catheter was placed for continuous drainage

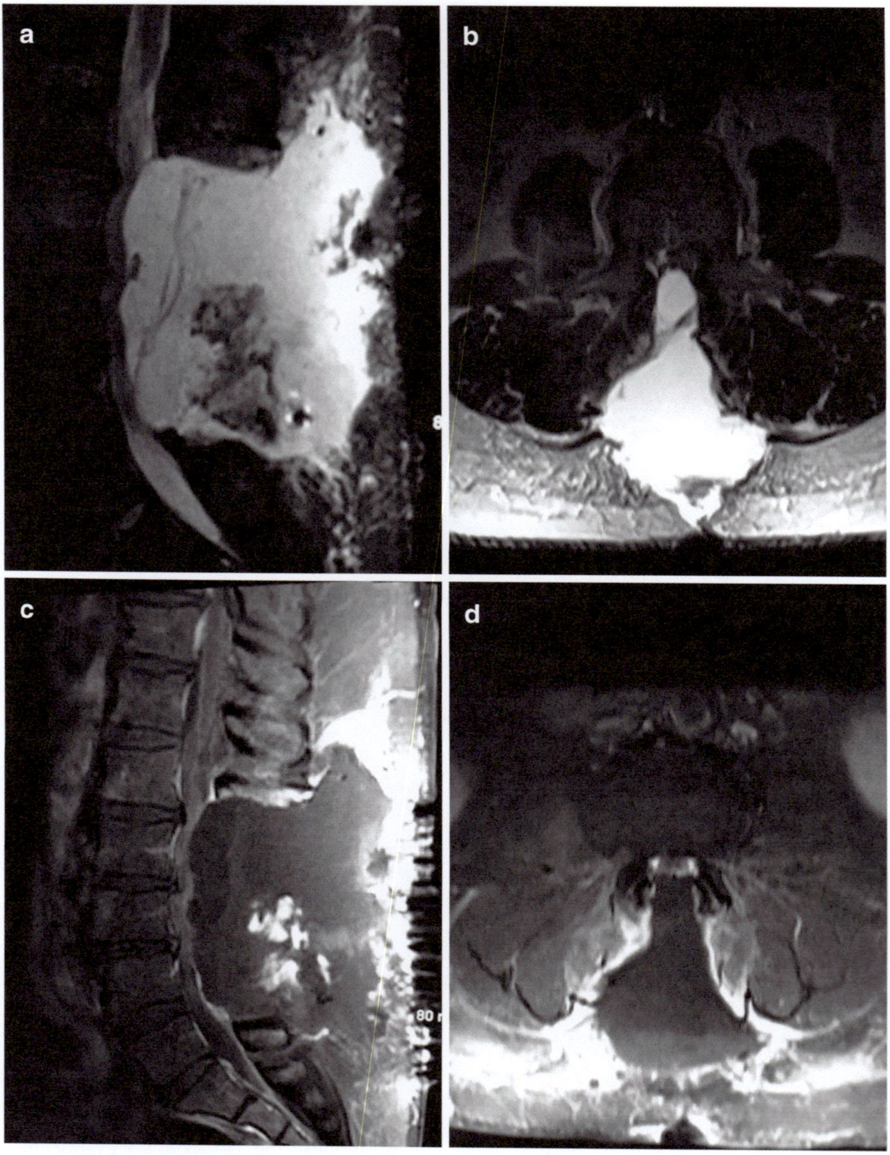

**Fig. 6.2** Postoperative seroma after multilevel laminectomy in the surgery bed in a 66 year-old man. The fluid collection (seroma) is separate from and causing pressure on the thecal sac at the laminectomy defect. (**a**) and (**b**) are sagittal and axial T2-weighted images. (**c**) and (**d**) are sagittal and axial T1-weighted contrast-enhanced fat-suppressed images

**Table 6.2** Abnormal radiological findings in the postoperative spine

| Most common causes of failed back surgery |
|---|
| *Early causes* |
| – Mispositioning of orthopedic hardware |
| – Surgery at a wrong level |
| – Hemorrhage/seroma and postoperative collections |
| – Pseudomeningocele |
| – Infection/discitis, osteomyelitis, and epidural abscess |
| – Canal or foraminal stenosis |
| – Foreign body |
| *Late causes* |
| – Hardware failure including fracture of orthopedic implants |
| – Failed fusion and pseudoarthrosis |
| – Spondylolysis and spondylolisthesis |
| – Accelerated degenerative changes and adjacent level disease |
| – Sterile arachnoiditis |
| – Recurrent disc herniation |
| – Fibrosis |

however, the fluid signal characteristics can differ, depending on the amount of protein or blood. Communication of the cyst with the thecal sac can be observed on T2-weighted sequences as an area of lower signal intensity due to the flow of CSF along this communication. After contrast administration, a fine peripheral enhancement can be visible. More intense irregular enhancement is suggestive of secondary infection (Table 6.2).

### 6.5.2 Postoperative Infections

Postoperative infection initially originates as discitis, less commonly, as facet joint infection and eventually can extend into the epidural space or surgical bed. *Staphylococcus aureus* and *Staphylococcus epidermidis* are the most common causative organisms. At early stages, plain x-rays are usually negative. Later on, erosions and destructive changes are seen in the endplates. Similar findings can be also seen on CT examination. Contrast-enhanced MRI with fat saturation allows for the evaluation of the bone marrow edema and discitis earlier than other imaging techniques7. Diffusion-weighted MRI images show hyperintensity of the central necrotic region of the abscess. Post-contrast images show central hypodense collections with peripheral enhancement. Infections can be also extending or be de-novo into the epidural and paraspinal spaces. (Fig. 6.3).

### 6.5.3 Implant-Related Complications

Implant fractures generally occur secondary to metal fatigue from the repetitive stress of spinal movements. The fractured implant may not be displaced, making its detection difficult. A fractured or dislodged appliance is frequently, but not always,

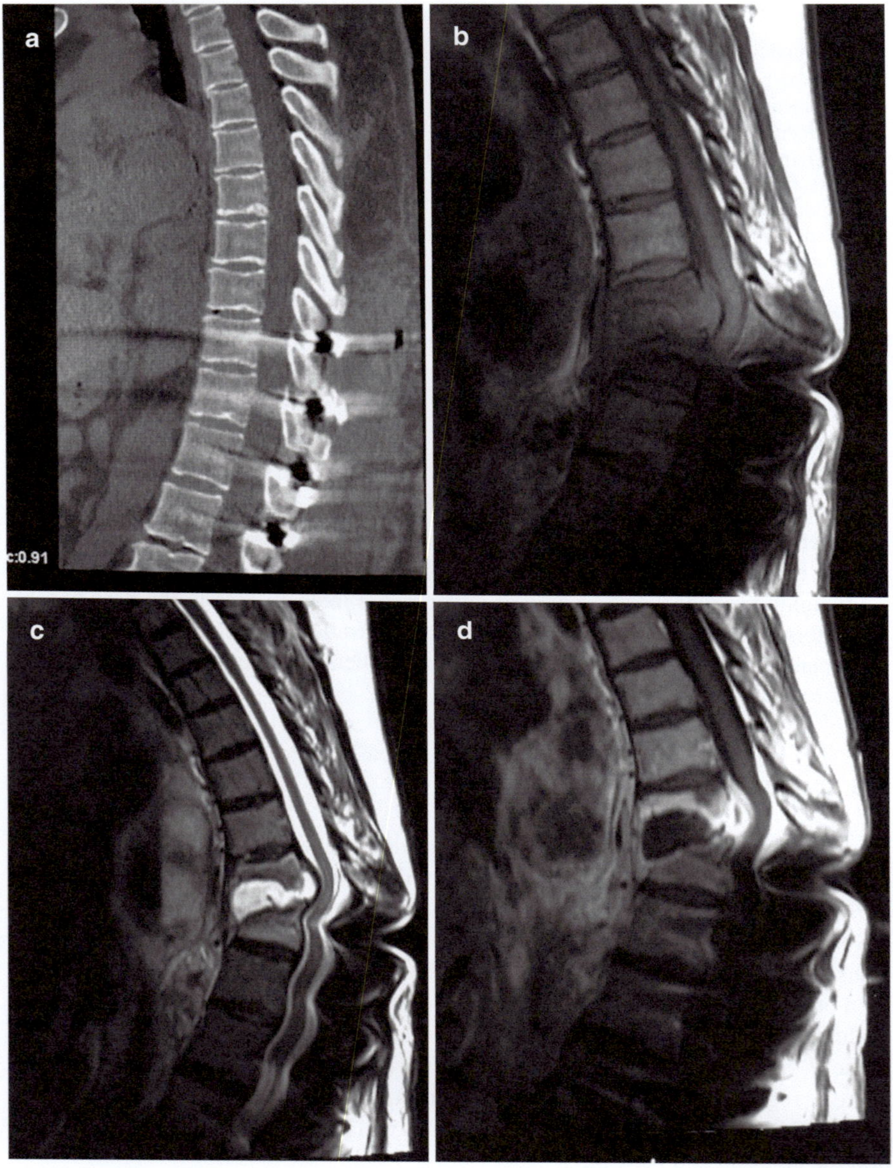


**Fig. 6.3** Adjacent level discitis and epidural infection in a 60-year-old male after thoracolumbar fusion. (**a**) Sagittal CT image showing the pedicle screw fixation. (**b**) Sagittal T1-weighted image showing diffuse decreased signal intensity of the vertebral body above the fusion with epidural soft tissue mass and wide disc space. (**c**) Corresponding sagittal T2-weighted image showing fluid in the widened disc space extending into the epidural collection. Note also the bone marrow edema of the adjacent vertebral bodies. (**d**, **e**) Sagittal (**d**) and axial (**e**) enhanced T1-weighted image with fat suppression showing the enhancing epidural and paraspinal component as well as the vertebral bone marrow. Note that the disc space shows peripheral enhancement of the endplates with central fluid collection

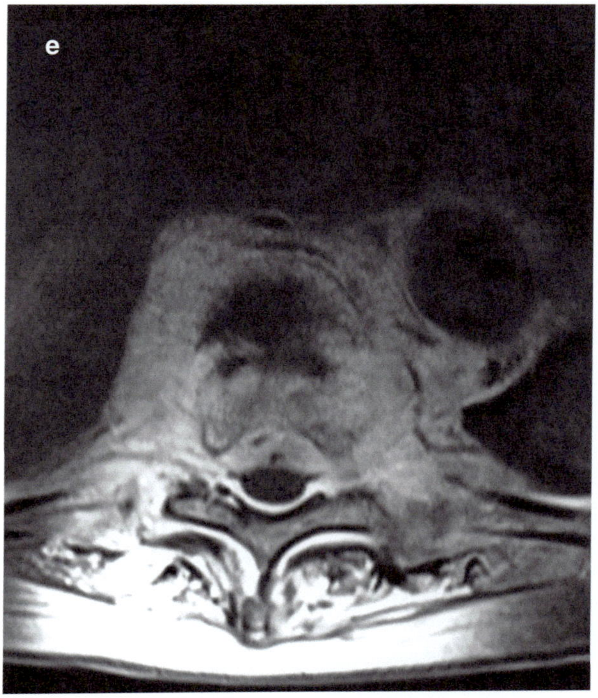


Fig. 6.3 (continued)

associated with regional motion and instability, which may lead to or be the result of pseudarthrosis [8]. Prominence of the instrumentation can cause chronic tissue irritation, leading to pain, bursa formation, and even pressure sores with tissue necrosis, which occasionally can be indications for hardware removal.

The pedicle screw is a commonly used implant that provides stabilization for posterior thoracolumbar fusion procedures. Screw placement is considered optimal when it traverses the central aspect of the pedicle and is aligned parallel to the superior endplate (neutral position) [9]. Careful attention should be paid to pedicle screws because of their close proximity to neurovascular structures. Potential complications are fractures and abnormal screw orientation. The most common clinical complications are nerve root irritation (secondary to excessive medial angulation of the screw) and violation of the medial bony cortex [10] (Fig. 6.4). Lateral position or migration should be carefully evaluated, especially in the cervical spine where the screw can breach the foramen transversarium and potentially damage the vertebral artery. Loosening is defined radiographically as a lucent rim of 2 mm or greater surrounding the hardware, particularly when this lucency enlarges on sequential studies. It is best visualized on CT or plain radiographs [11] (Fig. 6.5).

Restoration of disc height and achievement of anterior fusion are the major goals of interbody spinal surgery, and for this purpose, interbody spacers are used.

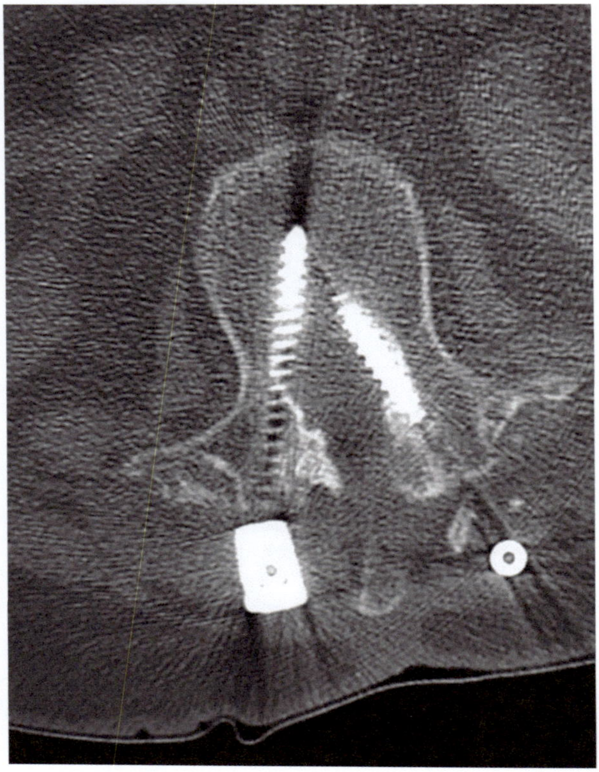

**Fig. 6.4** Sixty-nine-year-old woman with bilateral pedicle screws placed across the lateral recesses bilaterally causing severe bilateral radiculopathy

Radiopaque markers are designed to allow sequential monitoring of cage position in otherwise radiolucent implants. Some degree of subsidence is expected and may facilitate fusion with the bone graft being loaded under compression. However, excessive subsidence leads to loss of disk height and may cause recurrent radicular symptoms secondary to foraminal height loss. Cage subsidence (defined as a migration of >3 mm into the adjacent vertebra) and lateral displacement are disadvantages of mesh and stand-alone cages [12]. Imaging is able to assess for subsidence better in polyether ether ketone and carbon fiber cages since they cause significantly fewer artifacts than older stainless-steel cages.

Other complications of interbody cages include retropulsion (Fig. 6.6). A distance of 2 mm or more between the posterior marker of the cage and the posterior margin of the vertebra should exist to provide reassurance that the cage is not invading the spinal canal. Although bone morphogenetic proteins enhance arthrodesis following spinal fusion, they have been shown to be associated with endplate resorption in 82% of patients following lumbar spinal surgery, resulting in cage subsidence in more than half of the cases [13].

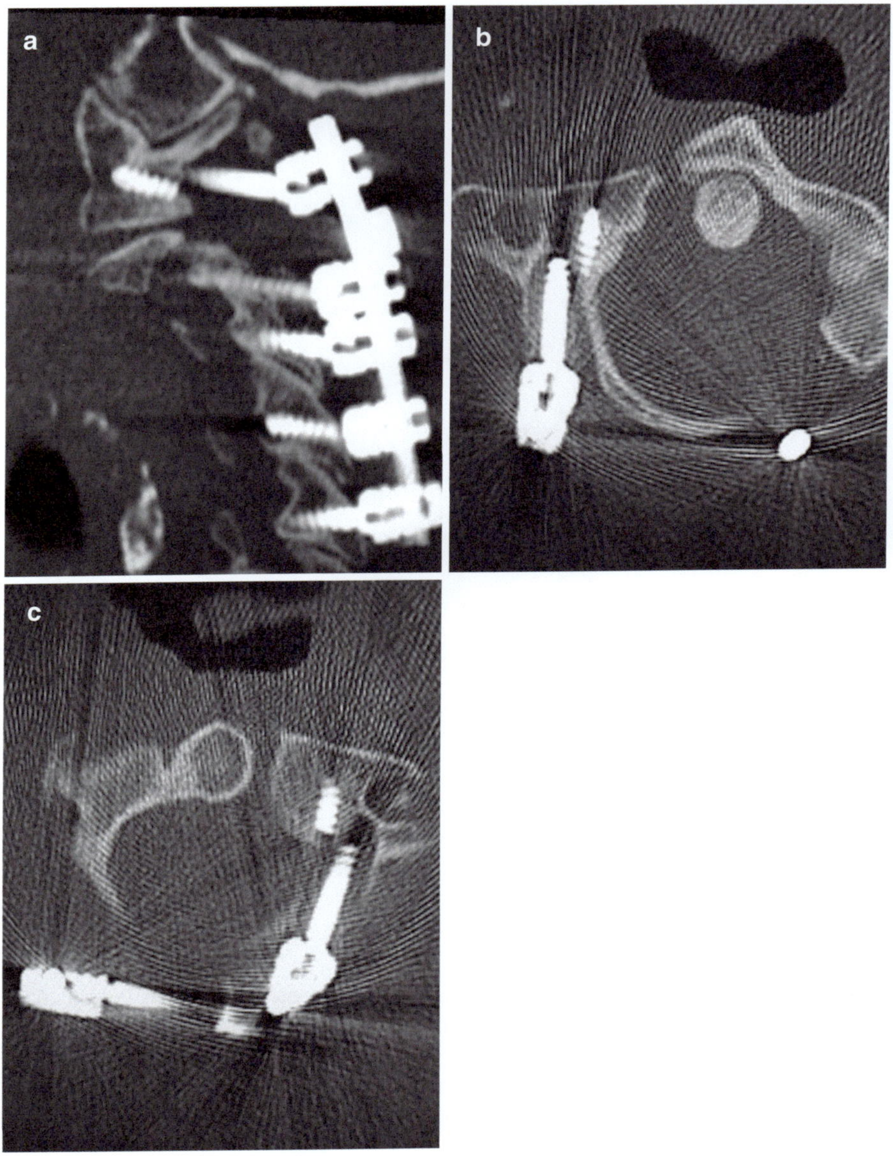


**Fig. 6.5** Sixty-two-year-old-man with hardware failure. (**a**) Sagittal reconstruction images, (**b**, **c**) Axial CT images showing bilateral fractures of the C1 pedicle screws. Note the presence of more than 2 mm lucency around the screws indicating loosening

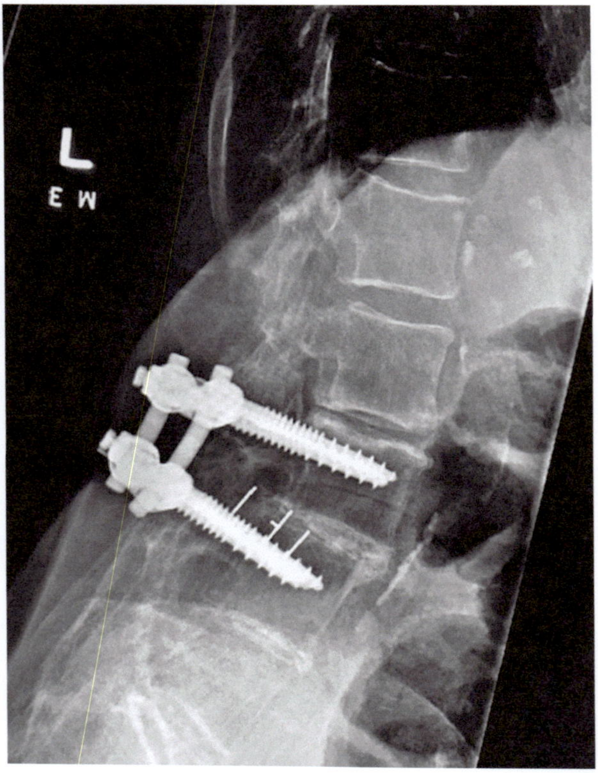


**Fig. 6.6** Postoperative lateral X-ray of the lumbar spine of an 80-year-old female showing posterior pedicle screw fixation at L3–4 level and posterior displacement of the interbody cage behind the posterior border of the vertebrae

## 6.6 Recurrent Disc Herniation and Epidural Fibrosis

### 6.6.1 Recurrent Disc Herniation

Recurrent disc herniation is involved in 7–12% of cases of recurrent lumbar pain following spine surgery [14]. MRI is the modality of choice for assessment of recurrent DH, and the protocol should include T1-weighted and T2-weighted sequences, as well as contrast-enhanced T1-weighted sequences, on the axial and sagittal planes. The herniated disc tissues are isointense with reference to the parent disc, but they may appear hypointense on T1-weighted sequences if calcified or associated with an ex vacuo phenomenon.

Intravenous contrast-enhanced MRI is the modality of choice to differentiate fibrosis from disc herniation with a sensitivity of 96%, which increases with using in T1-weighted fat-saturation sequences [15]. At MRI, fibrosis is isointense on T1-weighted and variable on T2-weighted sequences, with immediate homogeneous enhancement and may be associated with adjacent nerve root thickening (Fig. 6.7). Recurrent disc herniation may show early peripheral and late central enhancement (30 min after contrast agent administration) by diffusion of the contrast material into the center of the disc.

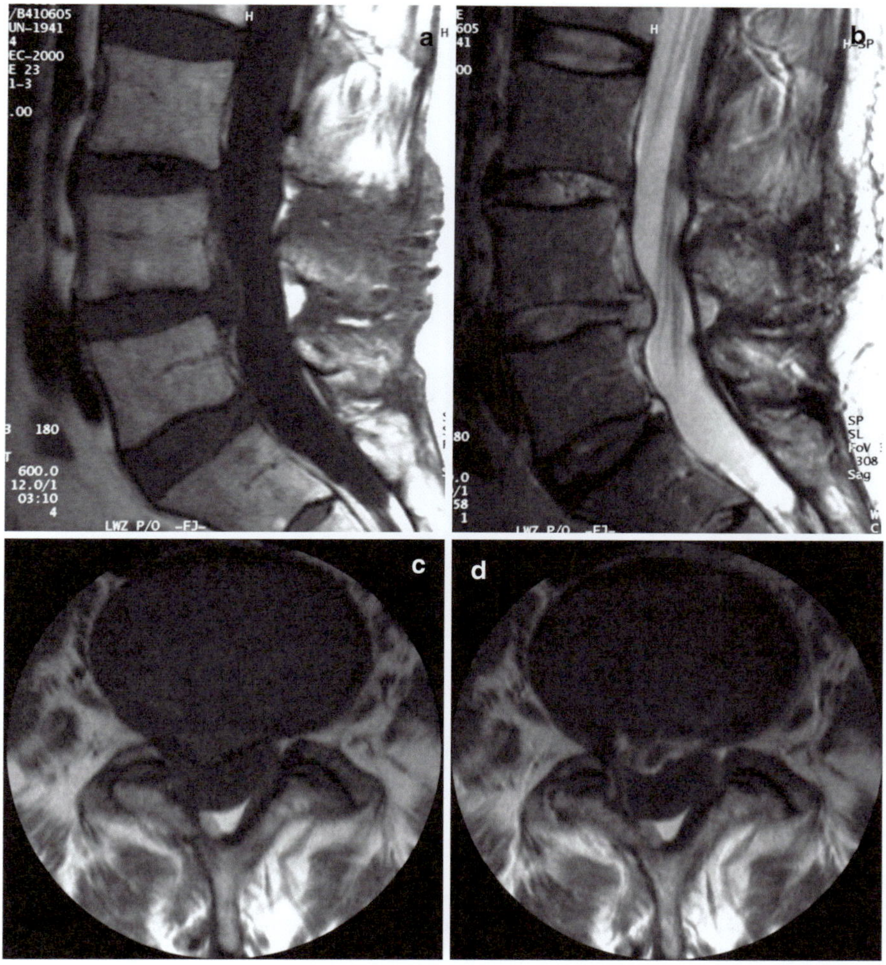

Fig. 6.7 Recurrent disc herniation after previous discectomy and laminectomy (Courtesy of Dr. Johan Van Goethem, Antwerp, Belgium). (**a**, **b**) Sagittal T1-weighted (**a**) and T2-weighted (**b**) images showing recurrent disc herniation at L4–5 level, site of previous discectomy. (**c**, **d**) Axial non-contrast T1-weighted image (**c**) and enhanced T1-weighted image with fat suppression (**d**) showing a peripheral rim of enhancement around the herniated disc material

### 6.6.2 Epidural Fibrosis

This complication is caused by scarring tissue formation in the epidural space after spine surgery. Since epidural scarring is part of the normal reparative mechanism of tissue after surgery, most patients with epidural fibrosis are asymptomatic [16]. However, multicenter studies have demonstrated that extensive epidural fibrosis patients are 3.2 times more likely to experience recurrent radicular pain [17]. Fibrosis-induced pain may be due to irritation, compression, and traction of the fibrotic tissue on adjacent nerve structures (Fig. 6.8). Outcomes after reintervention

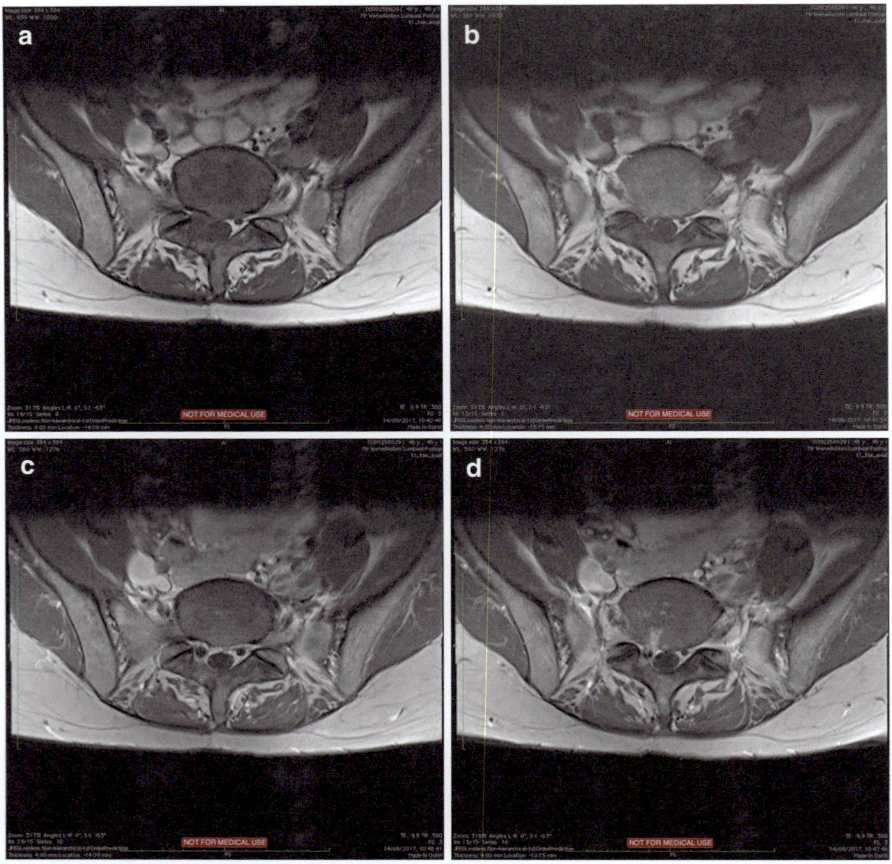


**Fig. 6.8** Epidural fibrosis (Courtesy of Dr. Johan Van Goethem, Antwerp, Belgium). (**a**, **b**) Axial T1-weighted images showing a soft-tissue fullness in the right lateral recess effacing the epidural fat. (**c**, **d**) Corresponding T1-weighted images after contrast enhancement showing the enhancing scar surrounding the swollen nerve root and extending into the disc space in **d**

in patients who only presented with fibrosis are worse than in patients with associated recurrent disc herniation. The main differential diagnosis of epidural fibrosis is recurrent disc herniation.

## 6.7 Sterile Arachnoiditis and Radiculitis

### 6.7.1 Sterile Arachnoiditis

Potential factors leading to arachnoiditis are the surgical procedure itself, the presence of intradural blood after surgery, treated perioperative spinal infection, and the previous use of myelographic contrast media. It occurs in about 3% of the cases of FBSS, excluding lesions caused by a previous myelography [18].

Although not a common finding, calcifications (calcified arachnoiditis) can be observed on CT images. The modality of choice for arachnoiditis evaluation is MR imaging, and axial T2-weighted FSE sequences are the optimal sequences for characterization. There are three patterns of presentation. Type 1 designates a conglomerate of nerve roots and is suggestive of mild involvement. Type 2 refers to peripheral adhesions of the nerve roots to the thecal sac, giving rise to an "empty-sac" appearance. This pattern is associated with moderate involvement. Type 3 refers to an intermediate attenuation mass obliterating the subarachnoid space below the conus medullaris, being the most severe presentation [19] (Fig. 6.9). Contrast enhancement of the thickened meningeal scarring and underlying intrathecal roots may or may not be observed, and the degree of enhancement does not appear to correlate well with the degree of signs and symptoms [20].

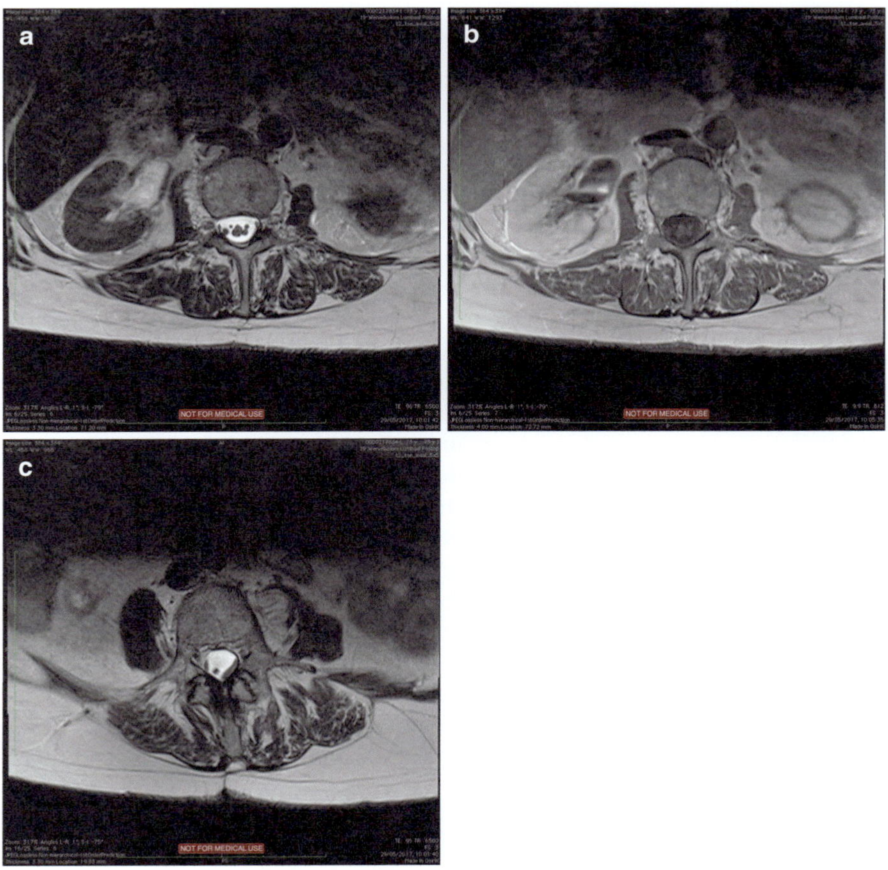


**Fig. 6.9** Arachnoiditis. Type 1 arachnoiditis with clumping of nerve roots seen in T2-weighted image (**a**) and shows no enhancement after contrast enhancement (**b**). Type 2 arachnoiditis, an empty-sac appearance (**c**)

### 6.7.2 Sterile Neuritis

Contrast enhancement of the intrathecal spinal nerve roots of the cauda equina following a conventional dose of gadolinium contrast medium is not a normal finding since spinal nerve roots normally have an intact blood–nerve barrier. On MR imaging, sterile radiculitis is seen as enhancement of the intrathecal spinal nerve roots of the cauda equina because of a breach in the blood–nerve barrier that occurs as a result of chronic neural trauma and/or ischemia. It is believed to be the cause of the abnormal neurophysiologic changes resulting in clinical radiculopathy that may continue long after the disc herniation has been surgically removed. It can extend cranially and caudally away from the surgical site in the chronic postoperative period [21].

Chronic postoperative nerve root enhancement correlates well with a radicular pain pattern in clinical presentation. However, during the first 6–8 months after intervertebral disc surgery, nerve root enhancement can be seen in asymptomatic patients, apparently reflecting transient sterile inflammation within the nerve root undergoing repair. Nevertheless, in the proper clinical setting, that of chronic FBSS, nerve root enhancement may be regarded as a clinically relevant imaging finding in the absence of any other cause of postoperative radiculopathy.

## 6.8 Accelerated Degenerative Changes, Adjacent Segment Disease, and Spinal Stenosis

Adjacent segment disease and junctional stenosis are terms used to designate the development of new clinical symptoms that correlate with radiographic changes adjacent to the level of previous spinal fusion [22]. Premature degenerative changes at the disc levels above or below the fused segments can occur because of the reduced number of mobile segments and by the stress and altered biomechanics following fusion. The reported incidence in the literature is up to 10.2% of patients with posterior fusion and instrumentation [23] and even more frequently at long-term follow-up. It is more common in the lumbosacral spine than in the cervical spine. It is markedly more common in the segment above the fusion because the rostral spine is levered against the fused caudal segment below (Fig. 6.10).

Radiography is the first imaging modality used for the evaluation of these changes. MRI is more accurate in assessing changes in soft tissue and disc contour. The findings are similar to those seen in degenerative changes secondary to other reasons, including intervertebral space narrowing, ex vacuo phenomena, osteophytes, facet arthrosis associated with foraminal stenosis, misalignment, Modic changes in the adjacent vertebral endplates, disc contour abnormalities, and spinal canal stenosis.

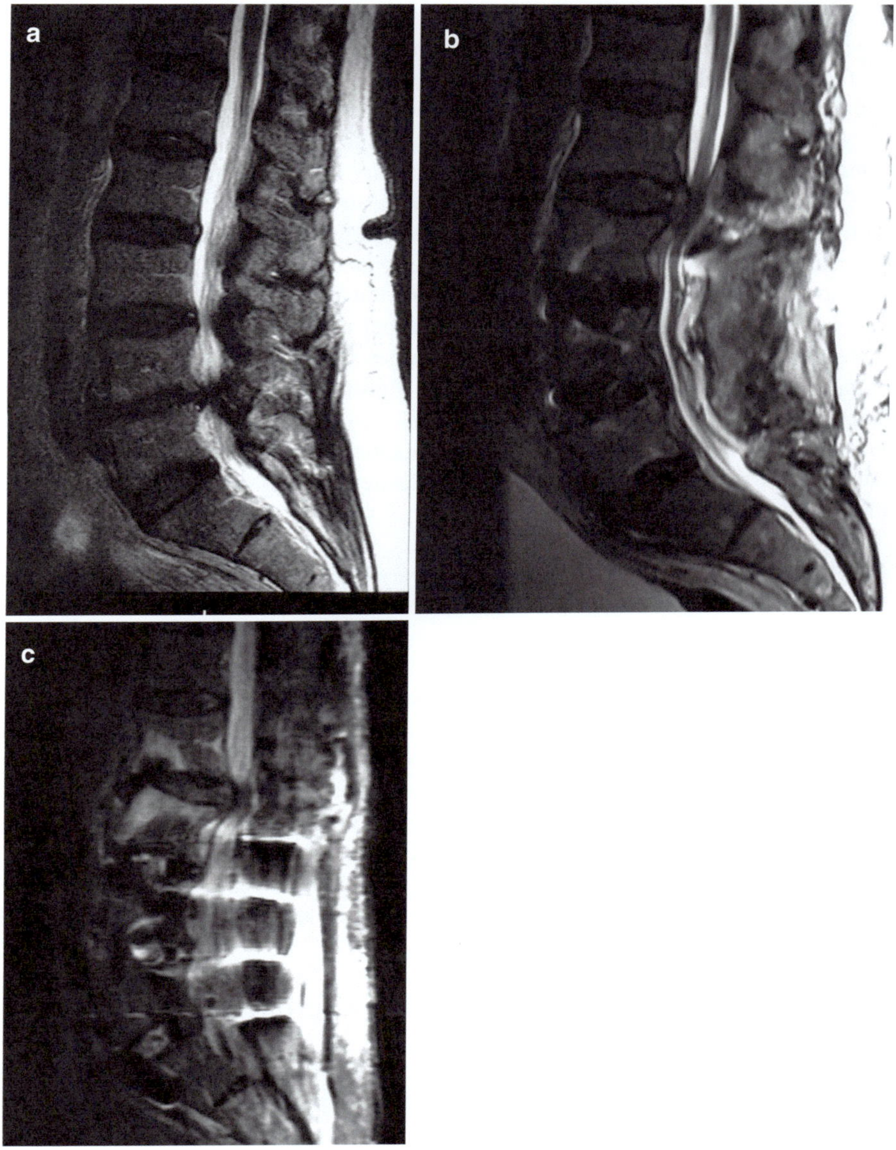


**Fig. 6.10** Seventy-seven-year-old male with adjacent level disease after anterior interbody fusion and posterior laminectomy. (**a**) Preoperative sagittal T2-weighted image showing a posterior disc bulges at L3–4 and L4–5 causing severe central canal stenosis. (**b**, **c**) Postoperative sagittal T2-weighted image 13 months after surgery showing a recurrent disc herniation above the level of the fusion with adjacent degenerative changes

*Stenosis* may present years after a surgical procedure as a result of accelerated degeneration. It is best diagnosed with MR imaging. Bony stenosis may show a variety of changes on MR imaging because of the variability of the marrow content of the vertebral body and bony fusion masses and the degree of bony sclerosis. Parasagittal images are most useful in defining bony foraminal stenosis, whether secondary to osteophyte formation or, more generally, secondary to disc degeneration.

*Spondylolisthesis* can be seen in patients who undergo laminectomy and present with increased instability and deformity. This condition increases with motion and worsens over time. It is more commonly associated with multilevel laminectomy with over 50% resection. A prophylactic fusion is usually performed in these patients. In these cases, dynamic examinations performed with conventional radiography are particularly helpful [24]. These images will show the degree of mobility of various segments in relation to each other. Multiplanar reconstructions with MRI and CT can show anterolisthesis, retrolisthesis, or lateral displacement. These findings should be correlated with previous examinations, preferably including both the latest and earliest ones. This would improve the detection of subtle changes in alignment of vertebral bodies.

## 6.9 Pseudrathrosis

Failure of fusion and the development of *pseudarthrosis* or fibrous union are the sequelae of ongoing low-grade mobility. Pseudarthrosis itself can be a source of pain or it may provide a lead point for ongoing mobility leading to increased stress on hardware and inevitable failure. Radiographic fusion criteria were summarized by Willison et al. [25]: they are presence of at least two visible bone bridges on CT on the level of fusion, absence of any lucency traversing the fusion or graft material, and absence of periprosthetic lucency. Flexion–extension views should show no motion or less that 3-degree motion. There should be no reactive sclerosis in the graft or adjacent vertebrae and no fractures on the device, graft, or vertebrae.

## 6.10 Summary and Problem-Solving Approach to Common Challenges

As seen in the previous discussion, interpretation of postoperative imaging is complex given the patient's underlying preoperative spinal pathology, the altered postsurgical anatomy, and artifacts caused by hardware. In the following discussion, we will focus on common clinically challenging scenarios in the interpretation of postoperative spinal imaging.

### 6.10.1 Infection or Postoperative Change

CT has much greater sensitivity than radiographs for detecting early endplate erosions as well as adjacent paraspinal inflammatory stranding or abscess formation

[26]. Magnetic resonance imaging is the most sensitive modality to identify early findings of postoperative spondylodiscitis. T1-weighted images demonstrate subchondral endplate irregularity and erosions. Adjacent bone marrow edema and purulent collections typically appear as low T1 signal and high T2 signal with enhancement following intravenous gadolinium administration. Infected intervertebral discs demonstrate low T1 signal and high T2 signal with diffuse homogeneous, patchy, or peripheral contrast enhancement [27]. Surrounding mixed T1 and T2 signal, paravertebral inflammatory changes are frequently present.

Similarly, high T2-weighted signal intensities with variable enhancement in an intervertebral disc can be a normal finding for up to 6 months post-discectomy in the absence of infection. Linear disc enhancement is more likely to be postsurgical whereas peripheral enhancement of the residual disc with reactive endplate changes points to infection. Similarly, nerve root enhancement at 3–6 weeks after surgery is a relatively frequent finding, occurring in 20–62% of patients, but persistence of enhancement beyond 6 weeks is abnormal. The presence of enhancing paravertebral or epidural soft tissue greatly increases the likelihood of septic spondylodiscitis. Restricted diffusion within the disc space and endplates is also consistent with spondylodiscitis, but not degenerative change [28]. A recent prospective study reported a sensitivity of 100% for identifying spondylodiscitis using 18FFDG PET/CT in cases of equivocal on MRI [29].

### 6.10.2 Abscess or Sterile Postoperative Fluid Collection

Thin peripheral contrast enhancement may be a normal finding in non-infected hematomas and seromas, but irregularly enhancing walls or adjacent inflammatory change strongly points to infection [30]. Diffusion-weighted imaging can help to identify infected paraspinal collections with developing abscesses demonstrating restricted diffusion [31]. However, it should be noted that chronic hematomas may also demonstrate restricted diffusion due to viscous blood breakdown products. The key finding on MRI to distinguish pseudomeningoceles from other extradural fluid collections is the identification of either direct communication or flow artifact between the thecal sac and the collection.

### 6.10.3 Recurrent Disc Herniation or Fibrosis (Scar)

Imaging too early in the immediate postoperative period is a potential pitfall as annulus fibrosis, epidural space edema, and granulation tissue can mimic a recurrent disc herniation [32]. A disc herniation demonstrates early peripheral enhancement due to granulation tissue or dilated epidural venous plexus, with central non-enhancement area. Conversely, fibrosis enhances rapidly and diffuses over time after contrast injection. It is important that the enhancement pattern be evaluated within the first 5 min after administration of gadolinium as disc herniation may also demonstrate diffuse enhancement on delayed post-gadolinium images [33]. The presence of intermediate signal with irregular margins is more in keeping with fibrosis whereas low signal with smooth margins favors recurrent herniation. In patients who may have both fibrosis and recurrent disc protrusion, it can be difficult to determine the relative contributions of each to the patient's symptoms.

### 6.10.4 Hardware Failure or Acceptable Postoperative Appearance

Hardware-related complications, including implant fracture, loosening, migration, and subsidence, are relatively common and are estimated to occur in 2–40% of spinal fusion patients [34].Persistent motion, pseudoarthrosis, and infection are common predisposing factors to hardware failure. Frank hardware fracture, usually involving fracture of screws or posterior rods, is relatively rare. Screw loosening is suspected when a radiolucent rim is ≥2 mm in width or progressively enlarges over time.

Complications related to interbody cage disc spacer placement involve cage migration, displacement, subsidence, and endplate fracture. Interbody disc cage spacers should lie anterior to the posterior vertebral body margin by at least one-fourth of the endplate length to minimize the potential for spinal canal narrowing and thecal sac impingement. Subsidence is defined as more than 3 mm of migration of the interbody disc spacer into the vertebral endplate, resulting in loss of disc space height. Morselized bone autograft will not be visible on plain radiographs; thus, the appearance of an interbody implant floating in the disc space does not necessarily indicate bone graft failure in the early postoperative period.

Endplate osteolysis and vertebral body bony defects are common in patients undergoing recombinant human bone morphogenetic protein (rhBMP)-assisted spinal fusion, occurring in 100% of cervical spine fusion and 82% of lumbar spine fusions at 6 weeks in a recent case series [35]. This aggressive inflammatory reaction, together with nearly universal endplate osteolysis, can easily be mistaken for either sterile spondylodiscitis or deep surgical site infection.

### 6.10.5 Failed Fusion or Too-Early-to-See Radiographic Fusion?

Greater than 3° of motion between flexion and extension views obtained 8–16 weeks after surgery is suggestive of failed fusion. In adults, posterolateral or facet fusions take longer than interbody fusions (9–12 months vs. 3–9 months) with fusions in the cervical spine occurring faster than thoracic or lumbar spine. With interbody fusion, trabecular bridging begins to develop initially outside the interbody cage spacer by 3 months and should completely bridge the intervertebral disc space by 6 months after cervical and 9 months after lumbar surgery [36]. Radiographic evidence of fusion will appear sooner in patients undergoing rhBMP-assisted procedures and definitely should be evident by 6 months. Central trabecular disruption or misalignment suggests delayed union with ongoing motion, which can lead to development of a pseudoarthrosis. On CT, the absence of mature trabeculations crossing the disc space at 24 months is diagnostic of failed fusion.

## 6.11 Conclusion

Radiological assessment of the postoperative lumbar spine is a common procedure in everyday practice of the radiologist. Despite advances in imaging technology, imaging of the postoperative spine remains a challenging and difficult issue. Knowledge about the different types of surgical procedures and instrumentation, normal postoperative changes, and potential complications are essential for proper evaluation and choice of the radiological technique to use.

## References

1. Merskey H, Bogduk N. Lumbar spinal or radicular pain after failed spinal surgery. Classification of chronic pain IASP second edition. Washington, DC: ISAP; 1994.
2. Thomson S. Failed back surgery syndrome – definition, epidemiology and demographics. Br J Pain. 2013;7(1):56–9.
3. Tronnier VM, Eldabe S, Franke J, Huygen F, Rigoard P, de Andres AJ, Assaker R, Gomez-Rice A, La Grua M, Moens M, Moke L, Perruchoud C, Quraishi NA, Rothenfluh DA, Tabatabaei P, Van Boxem K, Vleggeert-Lankamp C, Zoëga B, Stoevelaar HJ. The appropriate management of persisting pain after spine surgery: a European panel study with recommendations based on the RAND/UCLA method. Eur Spine J. 2019;28(1):31–45.
4. Herrera Herrera I, Moreno de la Presa R, González Gutiérrez R, Bárcena Ruiz E, García Benassi JM. Evaluation of the postoperative lumbar spine. Radiologia. 2013;55(1):12–23.
5. Gupta A, Subhas N, Primak AN, Nittka M, Liu K. Metal artifact reduction standard and advanced magnetic resonance and computed tomography techniques. Radiol Clin N Am. 2015;53:531–47.
6. Grand CM, Bank WO, Balériaux D, Matos C, Levivier M, Brotchi J. Gadolinium enhancement of vertebral endplates following lumbar disc surgery. Neuroradiology. 1993;35:503–5.
7. Van Goethem JW, Van de Kelft E, Biltjes IGGM, van Hasselt BA, van den Hauwel PPM, et al. MRI after successful lumbar discectomy. Neuroradiology. 1996;38(Suppl. 1):S90–6.
8. Venu V, Vertinsky AT, Malfair D, et al. Plain radiograph assessment of spinal hardware. Semin Musculoskelet Radiol. 2011;15:151–62.
9. Rutherford EE, Tarplett LJ, Davies EM, et al. Lumbar spine fusion and stabilization: hardware, techniques, and imaging appearances. Radiographics. 2007;27:1737–49.
10. Young PM, Berquist TH, Bancroft LW, et al. Complications of spinal instrumentation. Radiographics. 2007;27:775–89.
11. Malhotra A, Kalra VB, Wu X, Grant R, Bronen RA, Abbed KM. Imaging of lumbar spinal surgery complications. Insights Imaging. 2015 Dec;6(6):579–90.
12. Gercek E, Arlet V, Delisle J, et al. Subsidence of stand-alone cervical cages in anterior interbody fusion: warning. Eur Spine J. 2003;12:513–6.
13. Sethi A, Craig J, Bartol S, ChenW JM, Coe C, et al. Radiographic and CT evaluation of recombinant human bone morphogenetic protein-2-assisted spinal interbody fusion. AJR Am J Roentgenol. 2011;197(1):W128–33.
14. Suk KS, Lee HM, Moon SH, Kim NH. Recurrent lumbar disc herniation: results of operative management. Spine (Phila Pa 1976). 2001;26:672–6.
15. Georgy BA, Hesselink JR, Middleton MS. Fat-suppression contrast-enhanced MRI in the failed back surgery syndrome: a prospective study. Neuroradiology. 1995;37:51–7.
16. Vogelsang JP, Finkenstaedt M, Vogelsang M, Markakis E. Recurrent pain after lumbar discectomy: the diagnostic value of peridural scar on MRI. Eur Spine J. 1999;8:457–9.
17. Ross JS, Robertson JT, Frederickson RC, Petrie JL, Obuchowski N, Modic MT, et al. Association between peridural scar and recurrent radicular pain after lumbar discectomy: magnetic resonance evaluation. ADCON-L European Study Group. Neurosurgery. 1996;38:855–61.

18. Fitt GJ, Stevens JM. Postoperative arachnoiditis diagnosed by high resolution fast spin-echo MRI of the lumbar spine. Neuroradiology. 1995;37:139–45.
19. Ross JS, Masaryk TJ, Modic MT, Delamater R, Bohlman H, Wilbur G, et al. MR imaging of lumbar arachnoiditis. Am J Roentgenol. 1987;149:1025–32.
20. Jinkins JR. Magnetic resonance imaging of benign nerve root enhancement in the unoperated and postoperative lumbosacral spine. Neuroimag Clin N Am. 1993;3:525–41.
21. Jinkins JR, Roeder MB. MRI of benign lumbosacral nerve root enhancement. Semin Ultrasound CT MR. 1993;14:446–54.
22. Lee CS, Hwang CJ, Lee SW, et al. Risk factors for adjacent segment disease after lumbar fusion. Eur Spine J. 2009;18:1637–43.
23. Cho KJ, Suk SI, Park SR, et al. Complications in posterior fusion and instrumentation for degenerative lumbar scoliosis. Spine (Phila Pa 1976). 2007;32:2232–7.
24. Berquist TH. Imaging of the postoperative spine. Radiol Clin N Am. 2006;44:407–18.
25. Willson MC, Ross JS. Postoperative spine complications. Neuroimaging Clin N Am. 2014;24(2):305–26.
26. Hong SH, Choi JY, Lee JW, et al. MR imaging assessment of the spine: infection or an imitation? Radiographics. 2009;29(2):599–612.
27. Gouliouris T, Aliyu SH, Brown NM. Spondylodiscitis: update on diagnosis and management. J Antimicrob Chemother. 2010;65(Suppl 3):iii11–24.
28. Eguchi Y, Ohtori S, Yamashita M, Yamauchi K, Suzuki M, Orita S, Kamoda H, Arai G, Ishikawa T, Miyagi M, Ochiai N, Kishida S, Masuda Y, Ochi S, Kikawa T, Takaso M, Aoki Y, Inoue G, Toyone T, Takahashi K. Diffusion magnetic resonance imaging to differentiate degenerative from infectious endplate abnormalities in the lumbar spine. Spine (Phila Pa 1976). 2011 Feb 1;36(3):E198–202.
29. Fuster D, Tomás X, Mayoral M, Soriano A, Manchón F, Cardenal C, Monegal A, Granados U, Garcia S, Pons F. Prospective comparison of whole-body (18)F-FDG PET/CT and MRI of the spine in the diagnosis of haematogenous spondylodiscitis. Eur J Nucl Med Mol Imaging. 2015 Feb;42(2):264–71.
30. Jain NK, Dao K, Ortiz AO. Radiologic evaluation and management of postoperative spine paraspinal fluid collections. Neuroimaging Clin N Am. 2014 May;24(2):375–89.
31. Moritani T, Kim J, Capizzano AA, Kirby P, Kademian J, Sato Y. Pyogenic and non-pyogenic spinal infections: emphasis on diffusion-weighted imaging for the detection of abscesses and pus collections. Br J Radiol. 2014;87(1041):20140011.
32. Floris R, Spallone A, Aref TY, Rizzo A, Apruzzese A, Mulas M, Castriota Scanderbeg A, Simonetti G. Early postoperative MRI findings following surgery for herniated lumbar disc. Part II: a gadolinium-enhanced study. Acta Neurochir. 1997;139(12):1101–7.
33. Hueftle MG, Modic MT, Ross JS, Masaryk TJ, Carter JR, Wilber RG, Bohlman HH, Steinberg PM, Delamarter RB. Lumbar spine: postoperative MR imaging with Gd-DTPA. Radiology. 1988 Jun;167(3):817–24.
34. Nasser R, Yadla S, Maltenfort MG, Harrop JS, Anderson DG, Vaccaro AR, Sharan AD, Ratliff JK. Complications in spine surgery. J Neurosurg Spine. 2010 Aug;13(2):144–57.
35. Sethi A, Craig J, Bartol S, Chen W, Jacobson M, Coe C, Vaidya R. Radiographic and CT evaluation of recombinant human bone morphogenetic protein-2-assisted spinal interbody fusion. AJR Am J Roentgenol. 2011;197(1):W128–33. https://doi.org/10.2214/AJR.10.5484. Erratum in: AJR Am J Roentgenol. 2011;197(4):1024.
36. Zampolin R, Erdfarb A, Miller T. Imaging of lumbar spine fusion. Neuroimaging Clin N Am. 2014;24(2):269–86.

# Epidural Steroid Injections: Are They Still Useful?

7

Allan L. Brook, Shafik Boyaji, Christopher J. Gilligan, Joshua A. Hirsch, and R. Jason Yong

## 7.1 Background

Low back pain is one of the leading causes of disability and health care expenditure [1], with escalating prevalence in the United States and globally [2].

Epidural injection with corticosteroids is a common treatment option for patients with lower back pain and sciatica.

Jean Sicard and Fernand Cathelin performed the first epidural injections around 1900 in Paris, injecting small volumes of local anesthetics into the sacral hiatus. The first recorded use of epidural steroid injections dates back to 1952, when Robecchi and Capra reported the relief of lumbar and sciatic pain after a periradicular injection of hydrocortisone onto the first sacral roots through the S1 posterior sacral foramen [3].

Over the past several decades, the technique and indications for epidural injections have changed substantially. A variety of anesthetics as well as a number of glucocorticoids (hydrocortisone, methylprednisolone, triamcinolone, dexamethasone) have been used. The caudal approach, originally described by Sicard and

A. L. Brook (✉)
Department of Radiology, Albert Einstein College of Medicine, Montefiore Medical Center, Bronx, NY, USA
e-mail: abrook@montefiore.org

S. Boyaji · C. J. Gilligan · R. J. Yong
Division of Pain Medicine, Department of Anesthesiology, Perioperative and Pain Medicine, Brigham and Women's Hospital, Harvard Medical School, Boston, MA, USA
e-mail: sboyaji@BWH.Harvard.edu; sboyaji@partners.org; cgilligan@bwh.harvard.edu; ryong@bwh.harvard.edu

J. A. Hirsch
Radiology, Massachusetts General Hospital, Boston, MA, USA
e-mail: jahirsch@mgh.harvard.edu





L. Manfrè, J. Van Goethem (eds.), *The Disc and Degenerative Disc Disease*, New Procedures in Spinal Interventional Neuroradiology,
https://doi.org/10.1007/978-3-030-03715-4_7

Cathelin, has largely been replaced by interlaminar and transforaminal injections that are typically performed with fluoroscopic guidance [4].

Since the 1970s, numerous clinical trials evaluated the effectiveness of epidural corticosteroid injections. Even though, epidural injections are one of the most commonly performed procedures in managing low back and radicular pain, conflicting recommendations have been provided, despite the extensive literature.

## 7.2 Anatomy

The spinal epidural space is located between the fusion of the spinal and periosteal layers of dura mater at the foramen magnum, superiorly and the sacrococcygeal membrane, inferiorly. The posterior longitudinal ligament, vertebral bodies, and discs lie anteriorly and the ligamentum flavum, capsule of facet joints, and laminae lie posteriorly. The pedicles and intervertebral foraminae lie laterally.

The epidural space contains fat, the dural sac, spinal nerves, blood vessels, and connective tissue [5].

## 7.3 Approach

Epidural injections are administered by accessing the lumbar epidural space by multiple routes—caudal, transforaminal, and interlaminar.

*The interlaminar epidural steroid injection (ILESI) approach* is considered to deliver the medication close to the assumed site of pathology, and a parasagittal, paramedian, or midline approach is used through the space between the lamina of the vertebrae. The needle first penetrates the skin, then subcutaneous tissue, paraspinal muscles, (the interspinous ligament—in the case of the midline approach), and then finally the ligamentum flavum. The "loss of resistance" technique is used to verify penetration into the dorsal epidural space and to avoid advancing the needle to far anteriorly and puncturing the dura mater [6].

*The transforaminal epidural steroid injection (TFESI) approach* is considered a target-specific modality requiring the smallest volume to reach the primary site of pathology. The procedure involves administering steroids under fluoroscopic guidance into the intervertebral foramen that lodges the affected spinal nerve. With an oblique needle approach, the most common target area is the posterior surface of the vertebral body, adjacent to the caudal border of the pedicle above the target nerve, commonly described as a subpedicular approach [7]. Two alternative approaches for TFESI include the retroneural approach and the retrodiscal approach.

*The caudal epidural steroid injection (CESI) approach* is considered the safest and perhaps the easiest, with minimal risk of inadvertent dural puncture and, therefore, of inadvertent intrathecal injection. CESIs do require relatively high volumes. The needle is introduced into the epidural space via the sacral hiatus. The needle will pass through the skin, subcutaneous fat, and sacrococcygeal ligament (SCL).

## 7.4 Patients' Selection: Indication

The most common indications for ESI are: radicular pain related to herniated nucleus pulposus, followed by neurogenic claudication or radiculopathy from lumbar spinal stenosis, and to a much lesser extent discogenic pain [8].

## 7.5 Rationale for the Use of ESI

Radicular pain occurs as a result of both mechanical nerve compression and a chemoinflammatory response. Mechanical compression, such as that from herniated disc material or foraminal osteophytes, can cause local structural changes to nerve roots leading to demyelination, axonal transport block, vascular changes, intraneural edema, and stimulation of an inflammatory reaction [9].

One can have classic radicular pain even without neural impingement seen on imaging modalities. This is attributable to the chemoinflammatory response that is best understood as a result of herniated nucleus pulposus. An annular tear exposes the highly antigenic nucleus pulposus, triggering an inflammatory cascade that contributes to localized neural edema, altered nerve function, and sensitization. In essence, the body responds to the herniated disc material as a foreign body [9].

Given the chemoinflammatory contribution to pain, corticosteroids provide a rational treatment approach. Corticosteroids decrease inflammation through inhibition of prostaglandins in the arachidonic acid cascade, which may improve microcirculation through decreasing capillary permeability, nerve root edema, and ischemia [10].

## 7.6 Risk

Complications from LESI are rare and can be classified according to the generic risks of all types of injections in general, those due the pharmacologic effects of steroids and local anesthetic agents, and those pertaining to the epidural site of injection.

Procedural complications include infection, hematoma, intravascular injection, dural puncture, air embolism, vasovagal syncope, intra-arterial injection of particulate steroid, neural puncture, and allergic reaction.

Severe infection is exceedingly rare, with a reported incidence of 0.01–0.1% for all spinal injections. Most often the result of needle introduction of skin flora with inadequate sterile technique during the procedure or the preparation of the injectate, reported infections include meningitis, epidural abscess, vertebral osteomyelitis, and discitis [11]. A large number of devastating fungal infections in the United States were caused by steroid preparations that were produced in a facility with grossly inadequate quality control processes, and the outbreak affected more than 700 patients, some have died, others had major complications, and some suffered chronic sequelae [12]. The primary pathogen was *Exserohilum rostratum*, a plant pathogen that rarely causes human disease. To keep the risk of infection low, ESIs should not be performed when a patient has a concurrent bacterial infection such as a urinary tract infection and cellulitis. In such cases, the injection should be deferred until antibiotics have been completed for several days, and the patient has no signs of ongoing infection.

Epidural hematomas are rare in patients with normal clotting factors, with an overall incidence reported to be 1 in 150,000 epidurals [11], and an unknown proportion developing neurologic injury. Careful screening of patients to identify prescribed anticoagulant medications, clotting disorders, etc., will help to reduce the risk of epidural hematomas.

Vasovagal syncope is a risk with any type of injection, and it occurs in up to 1–2% of LESI patients. Symptoms are usually self-limited with removal of the needle and supportive care.

The incidence of headache is about 1% following lumbar injections. Its mechanism has not been established. It may be due to unrecognized dural puncture with resultant leakage of cerebrospinal fluid or inadvertent injection of air into the subarachnoid space.

The incidence of dural puncture ranges from 0.16% to 1.3% [13]. Inadvertent dural puncture does not constitute a complication in its own right, if it is recognized. The major risk of dural puncture is that, if it goes unrecognized, drugs will be delivered into the intrathecal space. If so injected, local anesthetics may cause spinal anesthesia, and steroid preparations may have neurotoxic effects because of the additives that they contain [14]. The risk of a "high spinal" is far greater during cervical epidural steroid injections, and we recommend using preservative-free corticosteroid and sterile saline with no local anesthetic in the epidural injectate for cervical ESIs.

Intravascular uptake occurs at a rate of 8% for all lumbar injections, and theoretical effects of intravascular anesthetic may include dizziness, tinnitus, nausea, muscle twitching, metallic taste, cardiac arrhythmia, seizures, or coma.

More feared but rare complication is spinal cord injury. There have been very few case reports of this complication in patients who underwent lumbar transforaminal injections [15, 16]. The mechanism of injury has not been explicitly demonstrated, but the prevailing view is that the injection penetrates a radicular artery and that when particulate steroids are injected they act as an embolus and infarct the conus medullaris.

For this reason, investigators have studied the prevalence and size of particles in various steroid preparations. Results have differed with respect to average size of particles and the size of aggregates that they form, but as a general rule, preparations of methylprednisolone and triamcinolone tend to have large particles capable of embolizing a small artery, preparations of betamethasone may or may not have particles, and dexamethasone exhibits no particles [17]. We use non-particulate steroid (dexamethasone) for all transforaminal epidural steroid injections.

Nerve damage also is a theoretical risk with nerve puncture and associated intraneural hematoma formation. Any solution injected into a nerve could potentially be neurotoxic, but this complication is unlikely to occur in an awake patient who will report paresthesias and pain, if the needle tip even grazes the nerve. Advancing the needle very slowly, when it might be in proximity to the nerve, is advisable.

Complications related to the solutions injected are rare. Hypersensitivity or anaphylactic reactions most often occur with contrast, but occasionally to anesthetic or its preservative. Consultation with an allergist may be beneficial when a patient's history of prior reactions raises the concern of a possible reaction during an ESI. In the case of ILESIs, where there is a concern for a possible contrast allergy, we will typically just perform the injection without contrast.

Corticosteroids often cause well-described side effects with systemic therapy, and these can occur to a lesser extent with ESI. Important considerations include elevation of blood sugars in diabetics with an average increase of 106 mg/dl on the evening of the injection and significant increased levels for 3 days [18]. This concern is heightened in patients with a history of brittle diabetes, and consultation with an internist or endocrinologist for recommendations about insulin sliding scales and other measures will reduce the risk of ESIs in such patients. Some fluid retention can occur, and thus caution is taken in patients with congestive heart failure. Case reports also exist of ESI causing Cushingoid syndrome and temporary adrenal suppression, but evidence has not yet linked ESI directly to bone loss or osteonecrosis [11]. Iatrogenic cushing's syndrome has been described in patients who underwent ESIs while taking highly active anti-retroviral therapy [19].

## 7.7 Efficacy

Epidural corticosteroid injections are most commonly performed for radiculopathy due to a herniated disc, but may also be given for spinal stenosis and to a lesser extent axial pain.

Evaluation of the efficacy of ESIs is challenging. Many limitations hinder the comparison of studies: variability in the methods used to select patients for inclusion, the variability of treatment protocols and patient selection, lack of appropriate or uniform outcome measures, and lack of fluoroscopy in many studies.

Given the heterogeneity of primary research, review articles and guidelines understandably arrive at mixed conclusions.

## 7.8 Axial Lower Back Pain

*Sayegh et al.* [20]. Compared blind caudal ESI to caudal injection of lidocaine, in patients with LBP for more than 1 month, with or without sciatica, and MRI evidence of HNP or disc degeneration. They found significant improvement in Oswestry Disability Index in both groups over time up to 1 year, with earlier improvement in disability and straight-leg raise tolerance in the steroid group.

*Southem et al.* [21]. A retrospective study evaluated 84 patients with axial LBP refractory to conservative treatment at 3 months and MRI evidence of disc pathology at L4–5 or L5–S1, without stenosis, who received a fluoroscopically guided caudal ESI. At an average follow-up of 28 months after the injection, only 23% met strict criteria for successful outcome.

## 7.9 Spinal Stenosis

*Botwin et al.* [22]. A prospective cohort study evaluated 34 patients with unilateral radicular pain from degenerative lumbar spinal stenosis who did not respond to conservative management and subsequently underwent fluoroscopically guided lumbar transforaminal epidural injections. Patients were followed up to 12 months after the injection. Seventy five percent of the patient had successful long-term outcome, reporting at least a >50% reduction between preinjection and postinjection pain scores, with an average of 1.9 injections per patient. Sixty-four percentage of patients had improved walking tolerance, and 57% had improved standing tolerance at 12 months. This study had no control group.

*Friedly et al.* [23]. In a multicenter, double-blind trial, 400 patients who had lumbar central spinal stenosis and moderate-to-severe leg pain and disability were randomly assigned to receive epidural injections of glucocorticoids plus lidocaine or lidocaine alone. The patients received one or two injections before the primary outcome evaluation, performed 6 weeks after randomization and the first injection. The primary outcomes were the score on the Roland–Morris Disability Questionnaire (RMDQ) and the rating of the intensity of leg pain. At 6 weeks, there were no significant differences in the RMDQ score or the intensity of leg pain between the two groups. Both groups, lidocaine only and lidocaine with glucocorticoids, improved in the study, raising the possibility that both arms of the trial had a therapeutic effect perhaps by flushing out inflammatory mediators from the epidural space.

## 7.10 Sciatic Pain

### 7.10.1 IESI

*Dilke et al.* [24]. One hundred patients with unilateral sciatic pain due to lumbar disc disease were randomly assigned to the treatment group (epidural injection of 80 mg of methylprednisolone) or the control group (superficial injection of normal saline into the interspinous ligament). Outcome analysis found statistically significant differences only in certain secondary outcome measures, such as return to work at 30 days. With respect to relief of pain, epidural injection of steroids was not demonstrably more effective than injection of normal saline into an interspinous ligament. All the procedures were done by the same physician using non-image-guided technique. One study found that even when the procedure was performed by an experienced anesthesiologist, 25% of the injections were not epidural [25].

*Ridely et al.* [26]. Double-blind study of 39 patients with sciatic pain, who receive either an epidural injection of 80 mg methylprednisolone or an interspinous injection of normal saline. The results showed that epidural injection of steroids achieved greater improvements in pain than did an injection of saline into an interspinous ligament. Baseline data and final outcomes, however, were not reported, and the effects attenuated after 12 weeks.

*Carette et al.* [27]. In a randomized, double-blind trial, comparing the epidural injections of methylprednisolone acetate (80 mg in 8 ml of isotonic saline) or isotonic saline (1 ml) to 158 patients with sciatica due to a herniated nucleus pulposus. Patients were evaluated at 3 weeks, 3 months, and 12 months. The study concluded that epidural injections of methylprednisolone may afford short-term improvement in leg pain and sensory deficits in patients with sciatica due to a herniated nucleus pulposus, but this treatment offers no significant functional benefit nor does it reduce the need for surgery.

*Valat et al.* [28]. In a randomized, double blind, controlled clinical trial, patients with sciatica were assigned to receive three epidural injections (2 day intervals) of either 2 ml prednisolone acetate (50 mg) or 2 ml isotonic saline. Forty two patients were included in the control group and 43 patients in the steroid group. The study found no statistically significant difference in outcome. Although a slightly larger proportion of patients were relieved by steroids at day 20 after treatment, the difference was not significant. By day 35, the proportions relieved were essentially identical.

*Price et al.* [29]. A prospective, multicenter, double blind, randomized, placebo-controlled trial with 12-month follow-up was performed. Total of 228 patients clinically diagnosed unilateral sciatica, aged between 18 and 70 years, who had a duration of symptoms between 4 weeks and 18 months. Patients received up to three injections of epidural steroid and local anesthetic (active), or an injection of normal saline into the interspinous ligament (placebo). ESI led to a transient benefit in Oswestry Disability Questionnaire (ODQ) and pain relief, compared with placebo at 3 weeks There was no benefit over placebo between weeks 6 and 52 (1 year).

### 7.10.2 TFESI

*Weiner et al.* [30]. The only strong evidence that transforaminal injections spare patients from surgery. An observational study that used a novel outcome measure. That study enrolled 30 patients with severe lumbar radiculopathy secondary to foraminal and extraforaminal disc herniation who were on a waiting list for surgery. After being treated with transforaminal injections of steroids, 47% obtained complete relief of pain that was lasting and only 20% required surgery. The efficacy of transforaminal injections was cast in terms of their ability to spare patients from having surgery.

*Lutz et al.* [31]. A prospective observational study reported that 52 out of 69 patients obtained greater than 50% relief of the pain after treatment with transforaminal injections of steroids at follow-up times of between 28 and 144 weeks.

*Riew et al.* [32]. A prospective, randomized, controlled, double-blind study. Used avoidance of surgery as the outcome measure. Fifty five patients who were referred to surgery because of lumbar radicular were prospectively randomized into the study. They then were randomized and referred to a selective nerve root injection with either bupivacaine alone or bupivacaine with betamethasone. It found that only 8 of 28 patients (29%) required surgery after treatment with transforaminal injections of betamethasone, compared with 18 out of 27 patients (67%) treated with transforaminal injections of bupivacaine. The difference in the operative rates between the two groups was highly significant ($p < 0.004$). A later publication [33] reported a 5-year follow-up of these patients, which showed that the majority of patients with lumbar radicular pain who avoid an operation for at least one year after receiving a nerve root injection with bupivacaine alone or in combination with betamethasone will continue to avoid operative intervention for a minimum of five years. In neither publication were pain scores or disability reported.

*Ng et al.* [34]. A randomized, double-blind controlled trial. Eighty-six patients with radicular pain who had unilateral symptoms and who failed conservative management were recruited. The patients were randomized to receive either transforaminal injection of methylprednisolone and bupivacaine with or transforaminal injections of bupivacaine alone. The study found no differences at 1 day, 4 weeks, 6 weeks, or 3 months. In the two groups, pain scores dropped from 73 to 54 and from 77 to 55, respectively.

*Thomas et al.* [35]. Controlled trial compared transforaminal injections of steroids with conventional interlaminar injections. No differences in outcome were evident at 6 days after treatment, but by 30 days and at 6 months after treatment, those patients treated with transforaminal injections showed statistically significant greater improvements in pain and function relating to work and leisure. Small sample of 31 patients.

*Ghahreman et al.* [36]. In a prospective, randomized study, of 150 patients, compared the outcomes of transforaminal injection of steroid and local anesthetic, local anesthetic alone or normal saline, and intramuscular injection of steroid or normal saline. A significantly greater proportion of patients treated with transforaminal injection of steroid (54%) achieved relief of pain than did patients treated with transforaminal injection of local anesthetic (7%) or transforaminal injection of saline (19%), intramuscular steroids (21%), or intramuscular saline (13%). Although the relief of pain was correlated by improvements in function and disability, and reductions in use of other health care, the magnitudes of improvements in desired activities were not significantly different between treatment groups. Over time, the number of patients who maintained relief diminished. Only some maintained relief beyond 12 months.

### 7.10.3 Meta-Analysis

*Pinto et al.* [37]. Epidural Corticosteroid Injections in the Management of Sciatica: A Systematic Review and Meta-analysis.

Twenty three trials were included. The pooled results showed a significant, although small, effect of epidural corticosteroid injections compared with placebo for leg pain in the short term (mean difference, −6.2 [95% CI, −9.4 to −3.0]) and also for disability in the short term (mean difference, −3.1 [CI, −5.0 to −1.2]). The long-term pooled effects were smaller and not statistically significant.

*Cho et al.* [38]. Epidural Corticosteroid Injections for Radiculopathy and Spinal Stenosis. A Systematic Review and Meta-analysis.

Thirty placebo-controlled trials evaluated epidural corticosteroid injections for radiculopathy, and 8 trials were done for spinal stenosis. For radiculopathy, epidural corticosteroids were associated with greater immediate-term reduction in pain (weighted mean difference on a scale of 0 to 100, −7.55 [95% CI, −11.4 to −3.74]), function (standardized mean difference after exclusion of an outlier trial, −0.33 [CI, −0.56 to −0.09]), and short-term surgery risk (relative risk, 0.62 [CI, 0.41–0.92]). Effects were below predefined minimum clinically important difference thresholds, and there were no longer term benefits. Limited evidence showed no clear effects of technical factors, patient characteristics, or comparator interventions on estimates. There were no clear effects of epidural corticosteroid injections for spinal stenosis.

Critique of this study pointed that Cho et al. utilized a novel theory converting active-controlled trials into placebo-controlled trials to prove their hypothesis that epidural steroids do not provide significant benefit.

*Manchikanti et al.* [39]. Epidural Injections for Lumbar Radiculopathy and Spinal Stenosis: A Comparative Systematic Review and Meta-Analysis.

Thirty nine randomized controlled trials met inclusion criteria. There were nine placebo-controlled trials evaluating epidural corticosteroid injections, either with sodium chloride solution or bupivacaine, compared to placebo injections. There were 12 studies comparing local anesthetic alone to local anesthetic with steroid.

A comparison of lidocaine to lidocaine with steroids in seven studies showed significant effectiveness from baseline to long-term follow-up periods.

Meta-analysis showed a similar effectiveness for pain and function without non-inferiority of lidocaine compared to lidocaine with steroid at 3 and 12 months.

## 7.11 Conclusion

Epidural steroid injections have been performed for many decades and are generally considered a very safe and moderately effective treatment for back and leg pain. When performed by an experienced physician using fluoroscopic guidance, the risk of experiencing a serious complication is rare. Overall, ESIs are usually well tolerated and represent a much less invasive option than surgery.

Clinical experience has taught us that ESIs are best used as a part of a multidisciplinary plan; injections are commonly coupled with other treatments (medications, physical therapy, etc.) in an attempt to either maximize the benefit or prolong the effects. Because disc herniations have a favorable history, providing temporary relief to a patient with an ESI may buy time to allow his or her body to resorb the extruded fragment. In some scenarios, this temporary relief may allow a given patient to avoid surgery.

As mentioned earlier, the evaluation of the efficacy of ESI is challenging. Majority of the studies are limited by the small sample size and the inherit difficulty in randomization in interventional procedures. Different studies have different variabilities in patient selection, treatment techniques, outcome measures, and analysis methods. Which make comparison and meta-analysis of these studies difficult to interpret and utilize. Also there is ongoing controversy regarding the choice of steroid.

The current data suggests that ESI is best used for radicular symptoms with the goal of pain management in the acute to subacute setting to help patients be more comfortable as they progress through the generally favorable natural history of spontaneous improvement. The transforaminal route, which has been studied most recently, appears to be the most efficacious approach for monoradicular symptoms, secondary to a disc protrusion. Further placebo-controlled studies are necessary to define more conclusively the role of ESI for the various causes of radicular pain and to define the best technique for each indication.

## References

1. US Burden of Disease Collaborators. The state of US health, 1999–2010: burden of diseases, injuries, and risk factors. JAMA. 2013;310:591–608.
2. Martin BI, Turner JA, Mirza SK, Lee MJ, Comstock BA, Deyo RA. Trends in health care expenditures, utilization, and health status among US adults with spine problems, 1997–2006. Spine (Phila Pa 1976). 2009;34:2077–84.
3. Robechhi A, Capra R. L'idrocortisone (composto F). Prime esperienze cliniche in campo reumatologico. Minerva Med. 1952;98:1259–63.
4. Ter Meulen BC, Weinstein H, Ostelo R, Koehler PJ. The epidural treatment of sciatica: its origin and evolution. Eur Neurol. 2016;75:58–64.
5. Richardson J, Groen GJ. Applied epidural anatomy, continuing education in anaesthesia. Crit Care Pain. 2005;5(3):98–100.
6. Botwin KP, Natalicchio J, Hanna A. Fluoroscopic guided lumbar interlaminar epidural injections: a prospective evaluation of epidurography contrast patterns and anatomical review of the epidural space. Pain Physician. 2004;7:77–80.
7. Bogduk N. Practice guidelines for spinal diagnostic and treatment procedures. 1st ed. San Francisco, CA: International Spine Intervention Society; 2004.
8. Friedrich JM, Harrast MA. Lumbar epidural steroid injections: indications, contraindications, risks, and benefits. Curr Sports Med Rep. 2010;9(1):43–9.
9. Barr KP, Harrast MA. Low back pain. In: Braddom RL, editor. Physical medicine & rehabilitation. 3rd ed. Philadelphia, PA: Elsevier; 2007. p. 888–90.
10. Harrast MA. Epidural steroid injections for lumbar spinal stenosis. Curr Rev Musculoskelet Med. 2008;1(1):32–8.
11. Goodman BS, Posecion LW, Mallempati S, Bayazitoglu M. Complications and pitfalls of lumbar interlaminar and transforaminal epidural injections. Curr Rev Musculoskelet Med. 2008;1(3–4):212–22.
12. Kauffman C, Pappas P, Patterson T. Fungal infections associated with contaminated methylprednisolone injections. N Engl J Med. 2013;368(26):2495–500.
13. Park CH, Lee SH. Lumbar transforaminal epidural blood patch. Pain Med. 2013;14(6):945–7.
14. Bogduk N. Epidural steroids. Spine (Phila Pa 1976). 1995;20(7):845–8.
15. Houten JK, Errico TJ. Paraplegia after lumbosacral nerve root block: report of three cases. Spine J. 2002;2:70–5.
16. Glaser SE, Falco F. Paraplegia following a thoracolumbar transforaminal epidural steroid injection. Pain Physician. 2005;8:309–14.
17. Derby R, Lee SH, Date ES, et al. Size and aggregation of corticosteroids used for epidural injections. Pain Med. 2008;9:227–34.

18. Gonzalaz P, Laker SR, Sullivan W, et al. The effects of epidural betamethasone on blood glucose in patients with diabetes mellitus. PMR. 2009;1:340–5.
19. Maviki M, Cowley P, Marmery H. Injecting epidural and intra-articular triamcinolone in HIV-positive patients on ritonavir: beware of iatrogenic Cushing's syndrome. Skelet Radiol. 2013;42(2):313–5.
20. Sayegh FE, Kenanidis EI, Papavasiliou KA, et al. Efficacy of steroid and non-steroid caudal epidural steroid injections for low back pain and sciatica: a prospective, randomized, double-blind, controlled trial. Spine. 2009;34:1441–7.
21. Southern D, Lutz GE, Cooper G, et al. Are fluoroscopic caudal epidural steroid injections effective for managing chronic low back pain? Pain Phys. 2003;6:167–72.
22. Botwin T, Gruber RD, Bouchlas CG, et al. Fluoroscopically guided lumbar transforaminal epidural steroid injections in degenerative lumbar stenosis: an outcome study. Am J Phys Med Rehabil. 2002;81:898–905.
23. Friedly JL, Comstock BA, Turner JA, et al. A randomized trial of epidural glucocorticoid injections for spinal stenosis. N Engl J Med. 2014;371(1):11–21.
24. Dilke TF, Burry HC, Grahame R. Extradural corticosteroid injection in management of lumbar nerve root compression. BMJ. 1973;2:635–7.
25. White AH, Derby R, Wynne G. Epidural injections for the diagnosis and treatment of low-back pain. Spine. 1980;5(1):78–86.
26. Ridley MG, Kingsley GH, Gibson T, et al. Outpatient lumbar epidural corticosteroid injection in the management of sciatica. Br J Rheumatol. 1988;27:905–9.
27. Carette S, Leclaire R, Marcoux S, et al. Epidural corticosteroid injections for sciatica due to herniated nucleus pulposus. N Engl J Med. 1997;336:1634–40.
28. Valat JP, Giraudeau B, Rozenberg S, et al. Epidural corticosteroid injections for sciatica: a randomized, double-blind, controlled clinical trial. Ann Rheum Dis. 2003;62:639–43.
29. Price C, Arden N, Coglan L, et al. Cost-effectiveness and safety of epidural steroids in the management of sciatica. Health Technol Assess. 2005;9(33):1–74.
30. Weiner BK, Fraser RD. Foraminal injection for lateral lumbar disc herniation. J Bone Joint Surg. 1997;79:804–7.
31. Lutz GE, Vad VB, Wisneski RJ. Fluoroscopic transforaminal lumbar epidural steroids: an outcome study. Arch Phys Med Rehabil. 1998;79:1362–6.
32. Riew KD, Yin Y, Gilula L, et al. The effect of nerve-root injections on the need for operative treatment of lumbar radicular pain: a prospective, randomized, controlled, double-blind study. J Bone Joint Surg Am. 2000;82A:1589–93.
33. Riew KD, Park JB, Cho YS, et al. Nerve root blocks in the treatment of lumbar radicular pain. A minimum five-year follow-up. J Bone Joint Surg. 2006;88:1722–5.
34. Ng L, Chaudhary N, Sell P. The efficacy of corticosteroids in periradicular infiltration for chronic radicular pain. Spine. 2005;30:857–62.
35. Thomas E, Cyteval C, Abiad L, et al. Efficacy of transforaminal versus interspinous corticosteroid injection in discal radiculalgia—a prospective, randomized, double-blind study. Clin Rheumatol. 2003;22:299–304.
36. Ghahreman A, Ferch R, Bogduk N. The efficacy of transforaminal injection of steroids for the treatment of lumbar radicular pain. Pain Med. 2010;11(8):1149–68.
37. Pinto RZ, Maher CG, Ferreira ML, Hancock M, Oliveira VC, McLachlan AJ, et al. Epidural corticosteroid injections in the management of sciatica: a systematic review and meta-analysis. Ann Intern Med. 2012;157:865–77.
38. Chou R, Hashimoto R, Friedly J, Fu R, Bougatsos C, Dana T, et al. Epidural corticosteroid injections for radiculopathy and spinal stenosis: a systematic review and meta-analysis. Ann Intern Med. 2015;163:373–81.
39. Manchikanti L, Knezevic NN, Boswell MV, Kaye AD, Hirsch JA. Epidural injections for lumbar radiculopathy and spinal stenosis: a comparative systematic review and meta-analysis. Pain Physician. 2016;19(3):E365–410.

# 8 Evidentiary Basis of Percutaneous Discectomy

Shafik Boyaji, Christopher J. Gilligan, Joshua A. Hirsch, and R. Jason Yong

## 8.1 Background

The intervertebral disc is part of an anatomic unit that consists of an inner gelatinous nucleus pulposus (NP), an outer annulus fibrosus (AF), and the cartilaginous endplates with their associated capillary beds both cranially and caudally. The central NP is a site of collagen secretion and contains numerous proteoglycans (PG), which facilitate water retention, creating hydrostatic pressure to resist axial compression of the spine. The NP is primarily composed of type II collagen. In contrast, the AF functions to maintain the NP within the center of the disc with low amount of PG and is composed of primarily of type I collagen [1, 2].

The intervertebral disc is one of the largest avascular tissues in the body. Disc tissues derive their nutrition from vessels in the subchondral bone adjacent to the hyaline cartilage of the endplate. Small molecules, such as glucose and oxygen, are carried through the endplate in a passive diffusion process.

The disc matrix is produced by chondrocytes in the nucleus pulposus (NP), and synthesis is promoted by factors such as transforming growth factor (TGF) and insulin-like growth factor (IGF). Under normal conditions, the matrix is in a continuous state of renewal and degradation. The chondrocyte produces enzymes, known matrix metalloproteinases (MMPs), which degrade the matrix. These enzymes are controlled by tissue inhibitors of matrix metalloproteinases (TIMMPs) [3].

S. Boyaji (✉) · C. J. Gilligan · R. J. Yong
Division of Pain Medicine, Department of Anesthesiology, Perioperative and Pain Medicine, Brigham and Women's Hospital, Harvard Medical School, Boston, MA, USA
e-mail: sboyaji@BWH.Harvard.edu

J. A. Hirsch
Radiology, Massachusetts General Hospital, Boston, MA, USA
e-mail: jahirsch@mgh.harvard.edu



L. Manfrè, J. Van Goethem (eds.), *The Disc and Degenerative Disc Disease*, New Procedures in Spinal Interventional Neuroradiology,
https://doi.org/10.1007/978-3-030-03715-4_8

Several changes in the biology of the intervertebral disc may lead to the herniation of the NP through the AF and compression of the thecal sac. These include reduced water retention in the NP, increased percent of type I collagen within the NP and inner AF, degradation of collagen and extracellular matrix (ECM) materials, and upregulation of systems of degradation such as apoptosis, matrix metalloproteinase (MMP) expression, and inflammatory pathways [1, 4, 5]. Axial overloading is another theory for disc herniation that could occur independent of degenerative disease. A subset of patients with LDH lack evidence of severe degenerative disc, thus herniation occurs as a result of spinal overloading [6].

In lumbar disc herniation (LDH), narrowing of the space available for the thecal sac can be due to a protrusion of the disc through an intact AF (contained), an extrusion of the NP through the AF but still maintaining continuity with the disc space (non-contained), or a complete loss of continuity with the disc space and becoming a free fragment (sequestered) [4]. The herniated disc could directly compress the nerves or illicit an inflammatory response in the adjacent neural elements.

The primary signs and symptoms of LDH are radicular pain, sensory abnormalities, and weakness in the distribution of one or more lumbosacral nerve roots. Although the first descriptions of sciatica go back to ancient times, our understanding of LDH as a clinical entity arose in the mid-1700s. Early surgeries for spinal "enchondromas," which very likely were herniated discs, were performed in the first part of the twentieth century [7].

Modern discectomy surgery is usually traced to Mixter and Barr [8] in 1934 when they reported on the open surgical treatment for ruptured intervertebral discs through a laminectomy approach, thereby heralding the beginning of "disc surgery." With the development and advancement in diagnostic and surgical techniques, the surgical approaches became less invasive so that hemilaminectomies were the standard surgical approach for the majority of disc herniations at the beginning of the 1970s [9].

In 1977, Yasargil removed a herniated disc using an operative microscope [10], a technique known as "microsurgical discectomy" or "microdiscectomy," which describes the removal of herniated parts of lumbar intervertebral discs through a posterior approach with the help of a surgical microscope and microsurgical instruments [11].

Despite the significant improvements in surgical treatments of LDH, there were still substantial complications and significant rates of developing "failed back surgery syndrome" (FBSS), otherwise known as "post laminectomy syndrome" [12]. The search for minimally invasive techniques led to the development of percutaneous disc decompression or percutaneous discectomy (PD).

## 8.2 Discussion

The concept behind percutaneous discectomy states that in a contained disc herniation, in which the nucleus pulposus and annulus fibrosis are within a closed hydraulic system, a small reduction in central nucleus pulposus volume causes a large reduction in intradiscal pressure. This allows the nuclear jelly-like material of the herniation to ooze back into the newly created space "Jelly donut theory," decompressing the nerve root responsible for the radicular pain or decreasing inflammatory mediators causing irritation of the nerve root. Thus *a contained disc* is an important prerequisite to the success of PD [9, 13].

The first version of percutaneous discectomy could be attributed to Smith [14], who coined the term chemonucleolysis to describe the enzymatic dissolution of the nucleus pulposus as an alternative and less invasive means of decompressing the herniated disc than surgical discectomy.

In 1975, Hijikata [15] described manual percutaneous lumbar discectomy. And in 1985, Onik et al. [16] described automated percutaneous lumbar discectomy, a minimally invasive method with the aspiration of disc material using a suction cutting device. In 1987, Choy et al. [17] describe the use of laser in percutaneous disc surgery.

With the advancement in biomedical and imaging technologies over the years, new methods and modalities have emerged with variable techniques, advantages, and safety profiles.

There are six major types of PD:

1. Chemonucleolysis.
2. Automated percutaneous lumbar discectomy (APLD).
3. Percutaneous laser disc decompression (PLDD).
4. DeKompressor.
5. Nucleoplasty.
6. Percutaneous endoscopic lumbar discectomy (PELD).

## 8.3 Chemonucleolysis

This is the oldest of the PD techniques, as mentioned earlier, which was described by Smith in 1964 [14]. The two major enzymes used for this purpose are collagenase and chymopapain.

Collagenase is synthesized by *Clostridium histolyticum* consists of varied subenzymes that split the collagen fibers at different locations. The purified collagenase is relatively specific for type 2 collagen, seen mainly in the nucleus pulposus [18]. Collagenase did not gain a significant traction in the clinical treatment of LHD, and there are paucity of literature or evidence for its benefit.

Chymopapain is a proteolytic enzyme derived from the latex of the papaya plant. It catalyzes the hydrolysis of proteins in the nucleus pulposus, decreasing the affinity for water molecules by the proteoglycans, thus causing disc desiccation. The pressure in the disc is lowered, so the disc protrusion decreases, which relieves the tension on the nerve root. Chymopapain is immunoreactive and can be detected in the plasma 30 min after injection, and the half-life is 3 days [18].

Guha et al. [19] published a prospective observational study of 112 patients with magnetic resonance imaging (MRI) proven lumbar disc herniation who underwent treatment with chymopapain chemonuleolysis and were followed up for 5 years. Majority of patients (83%) had excellent/good results, whereas 10% were unchanged and 7% were worse after the procedure. Also noted that the younger patients with single-level discs at L5–S1 had the most successful outcome (Fig. 8.1).

Gibson and Waddell in a Cochrane review [20] found five randomized clinical trials (RCT), which compared the efficacy of chemonucleolysis using chymopapain versus placebo, and the combined results clearly showed that chymopapain was more effective than placebo whether rated by the patients, surgeons, or independent observers. Five trials compared chymopapain to open discectomy of which two trials showed worse results as rated by patients at 1 year. The remaining three trials showed worse results as rated by surgeons at 1 year.

Couto et al. [21] conducted a meta-analysis of 22 clinical trials and concluded that chemonucleolysis with chymopapain was superior to placebo, although comparison to surgery was inconclusive, as the studies were too heterogeneous.

One of the main adverse effects of the treatment with chymopapain was allergic reactions including anaphylaxis with an occurrence of 1.5–2%. More serious and catastrophic adverse events were paraplegia, lumbar subarachnoid hemorrhage, and

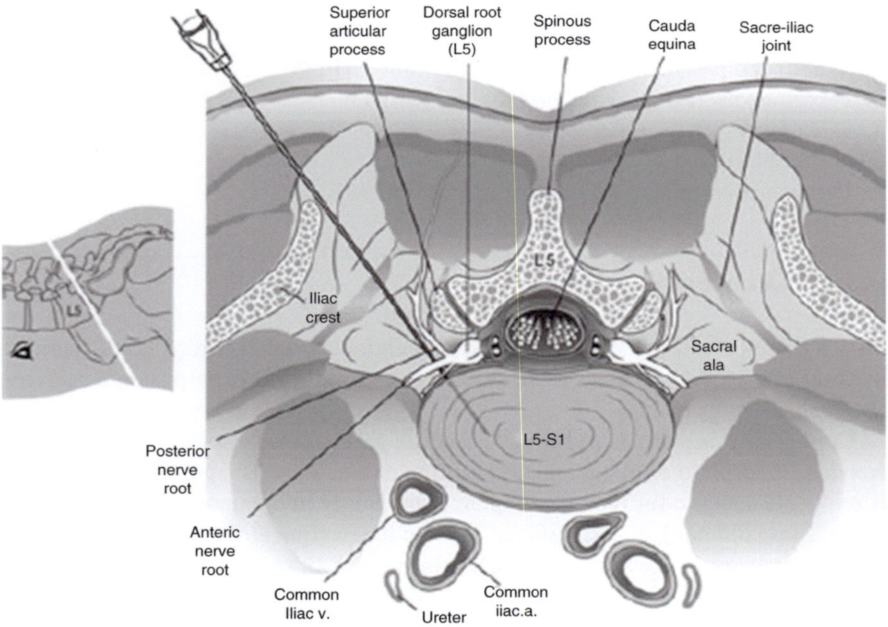


**Fig. 8.1** Axial diagram of L5/S1 discography. The needle enters the posterolateral aspect of the intervertebral disk, just inferomedial to the exiting L5 nerve root. The inset indicates the approximate plane of the L5/S1 disk and needle. All intradiscal treatments share the common element of introducing a hollow needle or introducer cannula percutaneously into the nucleus pulposus of the intervertebral disk (Reproduced with permission from: Rathmell JP. *Atlas of Image-Guided Intervention in Regional Anesthesia and Pain Medicine.* Philadelphia: Lippincott Williams & Wilkins; 2006:107; Fig. 9-7)

death, due to peripheral or intrathecal injections [22]. Nordby et al. [23] evaluated the safety of chymopapain on the basis of 121 "serious" and "unexpected" adverse effects among 135,000 patients in the US reported to the Food and Drug Administration between 1982 and 1991. The incidents ranged from fatal anaphylaxis (seven cases) to infections, hemorrhage, and neurological deficits. The overall mortality rate was 0.019%. This, coupled with the fact that the company that produces chymopapain stopped its production, has made chymopapain administration extremely uncommon.

Ethanol has also been used in the past as a method of chemonucleolysis. Ethanol produces a molecular splitting of proteoglycans that leads to a degradation of these components and a loss of their water-retaining capacity resulting in dehydration and chemical decompression of the disc. Ethanol remained unpopular due to excessive diffusivity and the lack of radiopacity leading to blind injection. But a new preparation that includes ethyl cellulose to make the alcohol solution more viscous and tungsten to facilitate radiological monitoring of the injection (marketed under ethyl alcohol gel or DiscoGel®) is showing promising results. Marcia et al. [24] report on a study of 71 patients who underwent ethyl alcohol gel chemonucleolysis with meaningful improvement in pain and disability and no observed clinical complications. However, further prospective randomized control trials are warranted.

## 8.4 Automated Percutaneous Lumbar Discectomy (APLD)

The introduction of percutaneous chemonucleolysis in 1964 heralded the beginning of new minimally invasive techniques for the treatment of LDH, with the aim to avoid the inherent complications of the traditional laminectomy and discectomy like scar tissue formation, injury to the muscle, the nerve roots and the dural sac, and the development of structural weakness of the lumbar spine due to excessive bone removal.

The initial attempt with percutaneous chymopapin chemonucleolysis was associated with a higher rate of undesired complications and adverse events which made practitioners shy away from its use. As a result, Hijikata [15] pioneered a manual percutaneous lumbar discectomy in 1975 as a method to decompress the disc by mechanical rather than enzymatic action. This method was made popular by Kambin and Gillman [25] in which they used a percutaneous technique with local anesthetic to place an introductory trocar followed by a cannula to pass through to the annulus fibrosis. A cutting instrument is then passed 2 cm beyond the cannula to fragment the herniated disc which is then removed by a specialty designed "punch forceps."

This manual technique required the insertion of relatively large cannulas (> = 6 mm in diameter) in the disc space, which raised the concern about possible nerve injury upon introduction of the cannula. Onik, an interventional radiologist, recognized the similarity between the vitreous material of the eye and the nucleus of the disc and proposed the use of redesigned ophthalmic equipment, known as the "Nucleotome," a mechanical probe with blunted tip, a side shaving port, and a vacuum generator to remove the nucleus pulposus by a "suction and cutting" action while continuous irrigation is applied. The probe was small in size (2 mm in diameter) which minimized the risk of nerve root injury, while its automated action allowed rapid removal of the disc materials. This technique was subsequently named automated percutaneous lumbar discectomy [16, 25].

In a systematic review conducted by Manchikanti et al. [26] to evaluate the effectiveness of APLD, there were no RCTs that met their inclusion criteria. Only 19 observational studies met those criteria, and based on the quality of evidence scale developed by the U.S. Preventive Service Task Force (USPSTF) [27], the indicated evidence for APLD is limited for short- and long-term relief. The authors concluded that APLD may provide appropriate relief in properly selected patients with contained lumbar disc herniation.

Another systematic review by Ong et al. [13] looked into four RCTs [28–31], but all the trials presented with problems in their design, so the results were inconclusive. One observational study [32] showed that APLD was not inferior to microendoscopic discectomy and both techniques show satisfactory long-term efficacy and safety. The author concluded that APLD is efficacious in selected patient group with a low incidence of complication, with evidence score of 2B based on the GRADE guidelines [33] (Table 8.1).

Overall APLD is a safe procedure, with discitis being the main possible complication. Teng et al. [34] in their report of APLD of a prospective multi-institutional study which included 1825 patients, reported a 0.06% incidence of discitis, which was the only complication.

## 8.5 Percutaneous Laser Disc Decompression (PLDD)

In 1987, choy et al. [17] described the use of Nd:YAG laser to perform percutaneous nucleolysis. 18 G needle was inserted into the affected disc under fluoroscopic guidance, with the tip in the nucleus pulposus, then a quartz optical fiber was advanced which through a laser was activated. The absorption of the applied laser energy leads to vaporization of the water content of the nucleus pulposus and a change in its protein structure, causing a decrease in intradiscal pressure. Because the disc is a semi-rigid structure, a small change in volume is associated with a large change in pressure.

There are several types of laser that could be used—Nd:YAG, KTP, CO2, Ho:YAG, and diode laser. The wavelength, pulse interval, and pulse duration can all be adjusted to change the absorption of energy. Low absorption of the energy leads to a low volume of nucleus pulposus removed, while high absorption of energy can cause adjacent tissue damage [13].

There is only one RCT that was recently published, Brouwer et al. [35] conducted a multicenter randomized prospective trial with a non-inferiority design and two-year follow-up to assess the clinical effectiveness of percutaneous laser disc decompression compared to conventional microdiscectomy surgery. Hundred and fifteen patients were enrolled randomly allocated to PLDD ($n = 55$) or conventional surgery ($n = 57$). The main outcome measures for this trial were the Roland-Morris

**Table 8.1** Grading recommendations

| Grade of recommendation/ description | Benefit vs. risk and burdens | Methodological quality of supporting evidence | Implications |
|---|---|---|---|
| 1A/strong recommendation, high-quality evidence | Benefits clearly outweigh risk and burdens, or vice versa | RCTs without important limitations or overwhelming evidence from observational studies | Strong recommendation, can apply to most patients in most circumstances without reservation |
| 1B/strong recommendation, moderate quality evidence | Benefits clearly outweigh risk and burdens, or vice vena | RCTs with important limitations (inconsistent results, methodological flaws, indirect, or imprecise) or exceptionally strong evidence from observational studies | Strong recommendation, can apply to most patients in most circumstances without reservation |
| 1C/strong recommendation, low-quality or very low-quality evidence | Benefits clearly outweigh risk and burdens, or vice versa | Observational studies or case series | Strong recommendation but may change when higher quality evidence becomes available |
| 2A/weak recommendation. High-quality evidence | Benefits closely balanced with risks and burden | RCIs without important limitations or overwhelming evidence from observational studies | Weak recommendation, best action may differ depending on circumstances or patients or societal values |
| 2B/weak recommendation, moderate-quality evidence | Benefits closely balanced with risks and burden | RCTs with important limitations (inconsistent results, methodological flaws, indirect, or imprecise) or exceptionally strong evidence from observational studies | Weak recommendation, best action may differ depending on circumstances or patients or societal values |
| 2C/weak recommendation, low-quality or very low-quality evidence | Uncertainty in the estimates of benefits. Risks, and burden; benefits, risk, and burden may be closely balanced | Observational studies or ease series | Very weak recommendations; other alternatives may be equally reasonable |

Disability Questionnaire for sciatica, visual analogue scores (VAS) for back and leg pain, and the patient's report of perceived recovery. Three patients were excluded after randomization and seven patients lost to follow-up. The primary outcome measures showed no significant difference or clinically relevant difference between the two groups at two-year follow-up. The reoperation rate was 21% in the surgery group, which is relatively high, and with an even higher 52% in the percutaneous laser disc decompression group. The authors concluded that despite a small sample size of the study, a strategy of percutaneous laser disc decompression, followed by surgery if needed, resulted in non-inferior outcomes compared to a strategy of microdiscectomy. Although the rate of reoperation in the percutaneous laser disc decompression group was higher than expected, surgery could be avoided in 48% of those patients that were originally candidates for surgery.

Schenk et al. [37] conducted a systematic review in 2006. There were no randomized controlled trials identified at that time, but 16 clinical trials were included in this review, representing a total of 1579 patients. Success rates varied from 75% to 87% with broad 95% CIs that made interpretation of success rates difficult. The authors concluded that scientific proof of PLDD's efficacy still remains relatively poor, though the potential medical and economic benefits of PLDD are too high to justify discarding it as experimental or ineffective on the sole basis of insufficient scientific proof.

Sing et al. [36] performed a systematic review in 2013; while no RCT was identified at that time, and there were 15 observational studies of moderate-to-high quality. All studies showed positive outcome regarding pain relief at >12 months. However, overall level of evidence (based on USPSTF quality of evidence scale) for percutaneous lumbar laser disc decompression is limited for short- and long-term relief.

The most common complication of PLDD is discitis, both aseptic and septic, between 0% and 1.2% [36]. Aseptic discitis is likely secondary to thermal damage to either the disc itself or the vertebral endplates. In a case series in which CO2 laser was used, they reported an 8% incidence of thermal nerve root damage. As the CO2 laser needed a fixed metal cannula to be introduced to the disc, it is postulated that it is the heating of the metal cannula that caused such a high incidence of nerve root damage. As such, this complication should not be taken to represent all PLDD techniques [37].

## 8.6 DeKompressor

The Dekompressor® system (from Stryker) is a single-use probe intended for percutaneous discectomies under fluoroscopic imaging. The probe (a titanium auger) is introduced through a 1.5-mm-diameter cannula after the insertion of a hollow 17 G cannula into the disc, and the auger is connected to a disposable rotational motor, which mechanically aspirates nucleus material along the proximal chamber. The device removes a predetermined amount of disc material from the herniated disc, reducing pressure in the disc and the surrounding area. Advantages purported by proponents are that Dekompressor does not accelerate disc degeneration, allows collection of disc material for histology, and has minimal damage to adjacent tissues [38].

Manchikanti et al. [39] performed a systematic review in 2013, no RCT met their inclusion criteria and only three non-randomized prospective studies were evaluated [38, 40, 41]. Although these studies showed positive short- and long-term results with follow-up over 6 and 12 months. The level of evidence for percutaneous discectomy with Dekompressor® is limited.

Erginousakis et al. [42] presented RCT in 2011 comparing Dekompressor against conservative treatment (analgesics, anti-inflammatory drugs, muscle relaxants, and physiotherapy) with a follow-up of 2 years. There was an 86% decrease in pain scores in the Dekompressor group versus 36% in the conservative group.

An observational study by Lemcke et al. [43] compared results of Dekompressor against nucleoplasty. Both groups had reductions in VAS scores and improvement in ability to work and to participate in activities of daily living, demonstrating that both Dekompressor and nucleoplasty are efficacious.

Recent long-term outcome study by McCormick et al. [44] investigated the long-term efficacy of percutaneous disc decompression with Dekompressor for discogenic radicular pain that has failed conservative management. Seventy patients underwent the procedure, and 40 and 25 patients were successfully contacted at 1- and 8-year follow-up, respectively. Using intention to treat analysis, at 1 and 8 years, numerical rating scale (NRS) pain scores were reduced >50% in both groups 47% and 29%, respectively; Oswestry Disability Index (ODI) score were improved >30% in 43% and 26% of patients, respectively. Of the patients who followed up at 8 years, 36% had undergone surgery.

Overall, this procedure has a low reported complication rate, and only one serious complication related to critical failure of the Dekompressor probe was reported. When the probe was removed after operating, the instrument tip broke off and remained embedded in the patient. The tip was needed to be removed surgically, and the patient recovered without any major complications [45].

## 8.7 Nucleoplasty

Nucleoplasty is an innovative percutaneous disc decompression procedure developed by ArthroCare. Nucleoplasty uses coblation technology, which is a controlled, non-heat driven process of tissue ablation.

Nucleoplasty involves removing a portion of the nucleus tissue using a 1 mm diameter bipolar instrument with radiofrequency energy that excites the electrolytes in the disc material creating a highly focused plasma field around the electrodes. The energized particles have a sufficient force to break down molecular bonds, which dissolves the soft-tissue material of the nucleus pulposus, producing a zone of thermal coagulation. Thus, nucleoplasty combines coagulation and tissue ablation (patented Coblation technology). Removal of tissue at relatively low temperatures (typically 40–70 °C) preserves the integrity of surrounding healthy tissue, therefore reducing the risk of damage to remaining disc tissue and the endplate cartilage [46, 47].

Nucleoplasty, sometimes also referred to as plasma disc decompression (PDD), is one of the most published technique among the PD procedures in recent years. There is one RCT published by Gerstzen et al. [48] in 2010, this was a multicenter randomized controlled clinical study and 90 patients who had sciatica associated with a single-level lumbar contained disc herniation were enrolled. These patients were refractory to initial conservative care and one epidural steroid injection. Participants were randomly assigned to receive either nucleoplasty (46 patients) or transforaminal epidural steroid injection (TFESI) (44 patients, up to two injections).

Patients in the plasma disc decompression group had significantly greater reduction in leg pain scores, ODI, and 36-Item Short Form Health Survey (SF-36). During the two-year follow-up, 56% of the patients in the PDD group and 28% of those in the TFESI group remained free from having a second procedure, following the study procedure. Adverse events, including injection site pain, increased leg or back pain, weakness, and lightheadedness, were observed in five patients in the PDD Group and seven in the TFESI Group.

A prospective comparative study by Adam et al. [49] compared patients with disc herniations <6 mm who underwent nucleoplasty (80 patients) to patients with herniations >6 mm that underwent open microdiscectomy (80 patients). Although the initial drop in VAS scores in the microdiscectomy group was more pronounced, the VAS scores between the two groups were similar by the end of 1 year. Compared to microdiscectomy, significantly more patients who underwent nucleoplasty returned to work.

Gerges et al. [50] published a systematic review on the effectiveness of nucleoplasty in 2010. The review included one RCT and 13 observational studies. The quality of evidence for improvement in pain or function after a nucleoplasty procedure is Level II-3, based on the quality of evidence developed by USPSTF for therapeutic interventions. The recommendation is level 1C based on the Grading Recommendation, strongly supporting the therapeutic efficacy of this procedure. However, the authors enforce the need for prospective randomized controlled trials with higher quality of evidence to confirm efficacy and risks and to determine ideal patient selection for this procedure.

In 2013, Manchikanti et al. [47] published and updated a systematic review including one RCT and 14 observational studies. The review concluded that there is limited to fair evidence for nucleoplasty in managing radicular pain secondary to contained disc herniations.

The majority of reviewed studies reported no significant complications related to nucleoplasty. However, Gerszten et al. [48] reported that 11% of patients in the nucleoplasty group had procedure-related adverse events such as increased radicular pain, pain at the injection site, increased back pain, increased weakness, and increased muscle spasms. One study by Azzazi et al. [51] had a 10% discitis rate, but it resolved in all five patients by 2 months. Rathmell et al. [52] described that even though the introducer cannula used for nucleoplasty is larger in diameter than the typical 22-G spinal needle used to perform discography, there is no evidence to suggest that there is a higher complication rate associated with the use of this large-bore introducer.

## 8.8 Percutaneous Endoscopic Lumbar Discectomy

Percutaneous endoscopic lumbar discectomy is a relatively new technique for the decompression of the lumbar disc space and removal of nucleus pulposus via a posterolateral approach. This was originally described by Mayer et al. [53] in 1987 but received more attention in the early 1990s.

In this technique, a working cannula is placed at the dorsal lateral border of the disc, then the disc space is visualized with an endoscope. The disc space is opened with anulus trephines and the nucleus pulposus is removed with forceps and an automated shaver system under intermittent endoscopic control [54]. PELD can be subclassified into the percutaneous endoscopic transforaminal discectomy (PETD) and percutaneous endoscopic interlaminar discectomy (PEID) according to the approach to the herniated disc material.

In 1993, Mayer et al. [54] published a study of 30 patients who underwent this procedure. The results were graded by the percentage of symptom relief and their own assessment of the results according to four categories (excellent/good/fair/bad). Patients were followed-up for 6 months, and 22 patients reported excellent or good relief, six patients reported fair relief, and two patients reported bad relief. Of these 30 patients, seven ultimately underwent open lumbar microdiscectomy, but the author indicated that three of them were operations on the same level or site of the procedure (true failures) and four were on a different level or site (false failures). There was only one complication in the study with one patient developing acute spondylodiscitis 36-h after the procedure. The patient was then immobilized and treated with antibiotics which led to the relief of the symptoms within 5 days.

In 2008, Ruetten et al. [55] published a prospective randomized controlled trial comparing the results of endoscopic interlaminar and transforaminal lumbar discectomies with the conventional microsurgical technique. In this study, 200 patients were enrolled but only 178 patients followed up for the full 24 months of the study. The results showed significant improvement in VAS pain scores, ODI scores, and North American Spine Society Instrument scores in both groups. After 2 years, 82% of the patients no longer had leg pain, 14% of patients reported pain occasionally or the pain was greatly reduced, and 4% of the patients experienced essentially no improvement. The differences in results between the groups were not significant. The recurrence rate was 6.2% with no difference between the groups. There were no serious complications in either group, such as dural/nerve injury or cauda equine syndrome. However, in the surgery group, two patients had postoperative bleeding, one patient suffered from delayed wound-healing, one patient developed a soft tissue infection, and three patients developed transient urinary retention. The complication rates were significantly elevated in the surgery group ($P < 0.05$). Another significant difference was in the mean postoperative work disability days which were 25 days in the PELD group versus 49 days in the surgery group ($P < 0.01$). Although the clinical results of the percutaneous endoscopic technique are equal to those of the microsurgical technique, the study pointed that there are advantages of the endoscopic technique in rehabilitation, complications, and reduced traumatization. With endoscopic surgery is a sufficient and safe supplementation and alternative to microsurgical procedures.

Most recent meta-analysis by Li et al. [56] compared PELD and standard discectomy (SD). The meta-analysis compiled 1301 cases from four randomized controlled trials and three retrospective studies. Compared with SD, PELD showed shorter operative times, less blood loss, shorter hospital stays, and shorter mean disability periods. However, there were no significant differences in the visual analogue scale (VAS) scores at the final follow-up, Macnab criteria at the final follow-up, complications, recurrence rates, or reoperation rates. The authors concluded that PELD can be a feasible alternative to the conventional surgical approach in the treatment of the LDH, but high-quality RCTs with sufficiently large sample sizes are necessary to further confirm these results.

An important point was mentioned in this study that could apply not only to PELD but also to all of the minimally invasive PD technique, is the steep learning curve that could be the main reason contributing to complication and the heterogeneity of results. Referring to the studies by Wang [57] and Lee [58] which have shown that the complication rate remarkably decreased after the first-twenty patients. To overcome the problem of the steep learning curve, Gibson [59] recommend that surgeons should start performing the procedure under experienced guidance, after attending cadaveric workshops. Additionally, the surgeon should have enough patience to learn PELD, especially for those who are unfamiliar with percutaneous techniques.

## 8.9 Conclusion

With the growing popularity of minimally invasive techniques in almost all fields of surgery, spine interventions have received significant attention and development over the last two decades. Percutaneous discectomy presents as a safe and less invasive technique than microdiscectomy, which has been considered the "gold standard" for the treatment of herniated discs.

Nucleoplasty is an attractive treatment option because of its minimally invasive nature and the corresponding decreased risk of structural damage to the muscles, bone, ligaments, and nerves. This may result in a lower prevalence rate of failed back surgery syndrome. In addition, the patients are expected to have less back pain, shorter hospitalization stays, and shorter recovery periods than conventional surgery. Furthermore, the procedure can be done under local anesthesia which adds a significant economic advantage, especially in the current environment with increased emphasis on cost and efficiency.

In general, there is a paucity of high-quality literature around percutaneous discectomy which is multifactorial: small sample sizes, short durations of follow up, and large losses of patients' data on subsequent follow ups. It is difficult to compare the results of different studies due to wide variations in inclusion criteria, interventional protocols, and outcome measures. And it is extremely hard to conduct double-blinded, placebo-controlled studies with interventional procedures, and there are additional ethical concerns about exposing patients to the risk of the procedure without any added benefit in the placebo arms.

With any intradiscal technique, discitis is an inherent risk that can be difficult to diagnose and treat. Rathmell et al. [52] recommend the regular use of prophylactic antibiotics, a comprehensive knowledge of the anatomy of the intervertebral space and the meticulous use of radiographic guidance in multiple planes. Additionally, an adequate level of sedation that still allows the patient to communicate verbally is warranted to notify the proceduralist of potential nerve damage before permanent injury.

While open surgical discectomy is the best option for sequestered, non-contained or large herniations, PDD has been demonstrated to be the best option to treat small contained disc herniations [60–62].

## References

1. Kadow T, Sowa G, Vo N, Kang JD. Molecular basis of intervertebral disc degeneration and herniations: what are the important translational questions? Clin Orthop Relat Res. 2015;473(6):1903–12.
2. Kalb S, Martirosyan NL, Kalani MYS, Broc GG, Theodore N. Genetics of the degenerated intervertebral disc. World Neurosurg. 2012;77(3–4):491–501.
3. Hadjipavlou AG, Tzermiadianos MN, Bogduk N, et al. The pathophysiology of disc degeneration: a critical review. J Bone Joint Surg. 2008;90-B(10):1261–70.
4. Amin RM, Andrade NS, Neuman BJ. Lumbar disc herniation. Curr Rev Musculoskelet Med. 2017;10(4):507–16. https://doi.org/10.1007/s12178-017-9441-4.
5. Kepler CK, Ponnappan RK, Tannoury CA, Risbud MV, Anderson DG. The molecular basis of intervertebral disc degeneration. Spine J. 2013;13(3):318–30.
6. Lotz JC, Chin JR. Intervertebral disc cell death is dependent on the magnitude and duration of spinal loading. Spine (Phila Pa 1976). 2000;25(12):1477–83.
7. ruumees E. A history of lumbar disc herniation from Hippocrates to the 1990s. Clin Orthop Relat Res 2014;473(6):1885–1895. doi:https://doi.org/10.1007/s11999-014-3633-7.
8. Mixter W, Barr J. Rupture of the intervertebral disc with involvement of the spinal canal. N Engl J Med. 1934;211:210–5.
9. Mayer H. Minimally invasive spine surgery: a surgical manual (2nd [completely rev. and expanded] ed.). Berlin: Springer; 2006.
10. Yasargil MG. Microsurgical operation for herniated disc. Adv Neurosurg. 1977;81:9.
11. Caspar W. A new surgical procedure for lumbar disc herniation causing less tissue damage through a microsurgical approach. Adv Neurosurg. 1977;4:74–7.
12. Baber Z, Erdek MA. Failed back surgery syndrome: current perspectives. J Pain Res. 2016;9:979–87.
13. Ong D, Chua NH, Vissers K. Percutaneous disc decompression for lumbar radicular pain: a review article. Pain Pract. 2016;16(1):111–26.
14. Smith L. Enzyme dissolution of the nucleus pulposus in humans. JAMA. 1964;187:137–40.
15. Hijikata S. Percutaneous nucleotomy: a method of percutaneous nuclear extraction. J Toden Hosp. 1975;5:39–44.
16. Onik G, Helms C, Ginsburg L, Hoaglund FT, Morris J. Percutaneous lumbar discectomy using a new aspiration probe. AJNR. 1985;6:290–3.
17. Choy DS, Case RB, Fielding W, Hughes J, Liebler W, Ascher P. Percutaneous laser nucleolysis of lumbar discs. N Engl J Med. 1987;317:771–2.
18. Wittenberg RH, Oppel S, Rubenthaler FA, et al. Five year results from chemonucleolysis with chymopapain or collagenase: a prospective randomized study. Spine. 2001;26:1835–41.
19. Guha AR, Debnath UK, D'Souza S. Chemonucleolysis revisited: a prospective outcome study in symptomatic lumbar disc prolapse. J Spinal Disord Tech. 2006;19:167–70.
20. Gibson JN, Waddell G. Surgical interventions for lumbar disc prolapse: updated cochrane review. Spine. 2007;32:1735–47.
21. Couto JM, Castilho EA, Menezes PR. Chemonucleolysis in lumbar disc herniation: a meta-analysis. Clinics (Sao Paulo). 2007;62:175–80.
22. Simmons JW, Nordby EJ, Hadjipavlou AG. Chemonucleolysis: the state of the art. Eur Spine J. 2001;10:192–202.

23. Nordby EJ, Wright PH, Schofield SR. Safety of chemonucleolysis. Adverse effects reported in the United States, 1982–1991. Clin Orthop. 1993;293:122–34.
24. Marcia S, Bellin M, Hirsch J, Chandra R, Piras E, Marras M, et al. Efficacy of an ethyl alcohol gel in symptomatic disc herniation. Eur J Radiol. 2018;109:101–7.
25. Kambin P, Gellman H. Percutaneous lateral discectomy of the lumbar spine a preliminary report. Clin Orthop Relat Res. 1983;174:127–32.
26. Manchikanti L, Singh V, Falco F, Calodney A, Onyewu O, Helm S, et al. An updated review of automated percutaneous mechanical lumbar discectomy for the contained herniated lumbar disc. Pain Physician. 2013;16(2 Suppl):SE151–84.
27. Harris RP, Helfand M, Woolf SH, Lohr KN, Mulrow CD, Teutsch SM, Atkins D, Methods Work Group, Third US Preventive Services Task Force. Current methods of the US Preventive Services Task Force. Am J Prevent Med. 2001;20:21–35.
28. Revel M, Payan C, Vallee C, et al. Automated percutaneous lumbar discectomy versus chemonucleolysis in the treatment of sciatica. A randomized multicenter trial. Spine. 1993;18:1–7.
29. Chatterjee S, Foy PM, Findlay GF. Report of a controlled clinical trial comparing automated percutaneous lumbar discectomy and microdiscectomy in the treatment of contained lumbar disc herniation. Spine. 1995;20:734–8.
30. Krugluger J, Knahr K. Chemonucleolysis and automated percutaneous discectomy—a prospective randomized comparison. Int Orthop. 2000;24:167–9.
31. Haines SJ, Jordan N, Boen JR, et al. Discectomy strategies for lumbar disc herniation: results of the LAPDOG trial. J Clin Neurosci. 2002;9:411–7.
32. Liu WG, Wu XT, Guo JH, et al. Long-term outcomes of patients with lumbar disc herniation treated with percutaneous discectomy: comparative study with microendoscopic discectomy. Cardiovasc Intervent Radiol. 2010;33:780–6.
33. Guyatt G, Gutterman D, Baumann MH, et al. Grading strength of recommendations and quality of evidence in clinical guidelines: report from an American College of Chest Physicians Task Force. Chest. 2006;129:174–81.
34. Teng GJ, Jeffery RF, Guo JH, He SC, Zhu HZ, Wang XH, et al. Automated percutaneous lumbar discectomy: a prospective multi-institutional study. J Vasc Interv Radiol. 1997;8:457–63.
35. Brouwer PA, Brand R, van den Akker-van Marle ME, et al. Percutaneous laser disc decompression versus conventional microdiscectomy for patients with sciatica: two-year results of a randomised controlled trial. Interv Neuroradiol. 2017;23(3):313–24.
36. Singh V, Manchikanti L, Calodney AK, Staats PS, Falco FJ, Caraway DL, Hirsch JA, Cohen SP. Percutaneous lumbar laser disc decompression: an update of current evidence. Pain Physician. 2013;16(2 Suppl):SE229–60.
37. Schenk B, Brouwer PA, Peul WC, van Buchem MA. Percutaneous laser disc decompression: a review of the literature. AJNR Am J Neuroradiol. 2006;27:232–5.
38. Alò K, Wright R, Sutcliffe J, Brandt S. Percutaneous lumbar discectomy: one-year follow-up in an initial cohort of fifty consecutive patients with chronic radicular pain. Pain Pract. 2005;5(2):116–24.
39. Manchikanti L, Singh V, Calodney AK, Helm S 2nd, Deer TR, Benyamin RM, Falco FJ, Hirsch JA. Percutaneous lumbar mechanical disc decompression utilizing Dekompressor®: an update of current evidence. Pain Physician. 2013;16(2 Suppl):SE1–24.
40. Lierz P, Alo KM, Felleiter P. Percutaneous lumbar discectomy using the Dekompressor® system under CT-control. Pain Pract. 2009;9:216–20.
41. Amoretti N, David P, Grimaud A, Flory P, Hovorka I, Roux C, Chevallier P, Bruneton JN. Clinical follow up of 50 patients treated by percutaneous lumbar discectomy. Clin Imaging. 2006;30:242–4.
42. Erginousakis D, Filippiadis DK, Malagari A, et al. Comparative prospective randomized study comparing conservative treatment and percutaneous disc decompression for treatment of intervertebral disc herniation. Radiology. 2011;260:487–93.
43. Lemcke J, Al-Zain F, Mutze S, et al. Minimally invasive spinal surgery using nucleoplasty and the Dekompressor tool: a comparison of two methods in a one year follow-up. Minim Invasive Neurosurg. 2010;53:236–42.

44. McCormick ZL, Slipman C, Kotcharian A, Chhatre A, Bender FJ 3rd, Salam A, Menkin S, Kennedy DJ, Plastaras C. Percutaneous lumbar disc decompression using the Dekompressor: a prospective long-term outcome study. Pain Med. 2016; https://doi.org/10.1093/pm/pnv122.
45. Domsky R, Goldberg ME, Hirsh RA, et al. Critical failure of a percutaneous discectomy probe requiring surgical removal during disc decompression. Reg Anesth Pain Med. 2006;31:177–9.
46. Chen YC, Lee SH, Saenz Y, Lehman NL. Histologic findings of disc, end plate and neural elements after coblation of nucleus pulposus: an experimental nucleoplasty study. Spine J. 2003;3:466–70.
47. Manchikanti L, Falco FJ, Benyamin RM, Caraway DL, Deer TR, Singh V, Hameed H, Hirsch JA. An update of the systematic assessment of mechanical lumbar disc decompression with nucleoplasty. Pain Physician. 2013;16(2 Suppl):SE25–54.
48. Gerszten PC, Smuck M, Rathmell JP, Simopoulos TT, Bhagia SM, Mocek CK, Crabtree T, Bloch DA, SPINE Study Group. Plasma disc decompression compared with fluoroscopy-guided transforaminal epidural steroid injections for symptomatic contained lumbar disc herniation: a prospective, randomized, controlled trial. J Neurosurg Spine. 2010;12:357–71.
49. Adam D, Pevzner E, Gepstein R. Comparison of percutaneous nucleoplasty and open discectomy in patients with lumbar disc protrusions. Chirurgia (Bucur). 2013;108:94–8.
50. Gerges FJ, Lipsitz SR, Nedeljkovic SS. A systematic review on the effectiveness of the nucleoplasty procedure for discogenic pain. Pain Physician. 2010;13:117–32.
51. Azzazi A, AlMekawi S, Zein M. Lumbar disc nucleoplasty using coblation technology: clinical outcome. J Neurointerv Surg. 2011;3:288–92.
52. Rathmell JP, Saal JS, Saal J. Discography, IDET, percutaneous discectomy, and nucleoplasty: complications and their prevention. Pain Med. 2008;9:S73–81.
53. Mayer HM, Brock M. Behandlung des lumbalen Bandscheibenvorfalls: Die perkutane Discektomie. Deutsches Arzteblatt. 1988;85:853–8.
54. Mayer HM, Brock M. Percutaneous endoscopic lumbar discectomy (PELD). Neurosurg Rev. 1993;16(2):115–20.
55. Ruetten S, Komp M, Merk H, Godolias G. Full-endoscopic interlaminar and transforaminal lumbar discectomy versus conventional microsurgical technique: a prospective, randomized, controlled study. Spine (Phila Pa 1976). 2008;33(9):931–9.
56. Li X, Han Y, Di Z, Cui J, Pan J, Yang M, Sun G, Tan J, Li L. Percutaneous endoscopic lumbar discectomy for lumbar disc herniation. J Clin Neurosci. 2016;33:19–27. https://doi.org/10.1016/j.jocn.2016.01.043.
57. Wang H, Huang B, Li C. Learning curve for percutaneous endoscopic lumbar discectomy depending on the surgeon's training level of minimally invasive spine surgery. Clin Neurol Neurosurg. 2013;115:1987–91.
58. Lee DY, Lee SH. Learning curve for percutaneous endoscopic lumbar discectomy. Neurol Med Chir (Tokyo). 2008;48:383–8.
59. Gibson JN, Cowie JG, Iprenburg M. Transforaminal endoscopic spinal surgery: the future 'gold standard' for discectomy? A review. Surgeon. 2012;10(5):290–6.
60. Zhang B, Liu S, Liu J, et al. Transforaminal endoscopic discectomy versus conventional microdiscectomy for lumbar discherniation: a systematic review and meta-analysis. J Orthop Surg Res. 2018;13(1):169.
61. Dewing CB, Provencher MT, Riffenburgh RH, et al. The outcomes of lumbar microdiscectomy in a young, active population: correlation by herniation type and level. Spine. 2008;33:33–8.
62. Carragee EJ, Han MY, Suen PW, et al. Clinical outcomes after lumbar discectomy for sciatica: the effects of fragment type and anular competence. J Bone Joint Surg Am. 2003;85-A:102–8.

# 9 Minimally Invasive Treatment of Herniated Disc: How to Remove the Disc with Chemical Tools

Giuseppe Leone, Massimo Muto, Gianluigi Guarnieri, Luigi Della Gatta, Matteo Bonetti, and Mario Muto

## 9.1 Introduction

Lumbar disc herniation is the most common cause of low back pain and sciatica in Western country with classical irradiation along the nerve root course. Around 80% of adults suffer from low back pain during a lifetime, and 55% are suffering from back pain associated with radicular syndrome [1].

The natural history of herniated disc at cervical and lumbar level is well-described by several epidemiological study and with MRI correlation [2–5]. Normally, it is characterized by a disappearance of clinical symptoms in up to 70% with conservative treatment through simple rest for about 6 weeks of patients and shrinkage of the disc herniation revealed by CT or MR scans within 8–9 months after the onset of back pain [6–8]. It has also been demonstrated that the mean space-occupying ratio of herniation significantly decrease during 2-year MR follow-up with a progression of degeneration of the intervertebral disc and morphologic changes of lumbar disc herniation [9]. About 88% of patients affected by herniated disc show >50% reduction of the hernia during 3–12 months at MR follow-up after onset, with morphologic changes of the herniated mass well correlated with the clinical outcome [10, 11].

Nowadays, surgery is confined for treatment of patients with progressive neurological deficit, cauda equina syndrome, and severe intolerable pain, which makes it the treatment of choice quite often for extruded, migrated, and free fragment herniated disc.

G. Leone · M. Muto · G. Guarnieri · L. D. Gatta · M. Muto (✉)
Department of Neuroradiology, Antonio Cardarelli Azienda Ospedaliera di Rilievo Nazionale, Naples, Italy

M. Bonetti
Department of Neuroradiology, Istituto Clinico Città di Brescia, Brescia, Italy



L. Manfrè, J. Van Goethem (eds.), *The Disc and Degenerative Disc Disease*, New Procedures in Spinal Interventional Neuroradiology,
https://doi.org/10.1007/978-3-030-03715-4_9

Therefore, different minimally invasive, well-tolerated, and low-cost procedures have been developed to provide good clinical results without the associated drawbacks of surgery.

Chemiodiscolysis can be realized by two main chemical agents: O2–O3 mixture and radiopaque gelled ethanol (DiscoGel®) [12, 13].

Chemiodiscolysis with O2–O3 mixture with periradicular and periganglionic infiltration is a recent percutaneous technique widespread in Europe; it was first proposed in Italy in the 1980s as a treatment for herniated disc.

Ozone (O3), the triatomic form of oxygen, is a strong oxidant, capable of inducing several useful biological responses and, eventually, reversing chronic oxidative stresses such as those derived from degenerative processes. Ozone (O3) is a strongly oxidant gas with antiseptic, immunomodulating, analgesic, and anti-inflammatory properties.

O3 is administered in the form of O2–O3 at nontoxic concentrations ranging from 1 to 40 mg of O3 per mL of oxygen, using various percutaneous methods.

A mixture of ozone and oxygen (O2–O3) can be injected directly in the disc aiming to reduce herniation, relieving nerve root compression, with potential analgesic and anti-inflammatory effects [12].

On the other hand, DiscoGel® has indication in patients with poor therapeutic outcome following O2–O3 therapy [13, 14].

## 9.2 Ozone Mechanism of Action

The ozone and oxygen mechanisms of action are currently being investigated and include inhibition of inflammatory inducers and pain-producing mediators in the disease site [15].

Oxygen–ozone inhibits the synthesis and release of prostaglandins, bradykinin, and various algogenic molecules and increases the release of antagonists of proinflammatory cytokines. The effect of ozone on solving or decreasing chemical radiculitis can also explain the clinical effectiveness of intraforaminal O2–O3 injection without intradiscal therapy. Moreover, the direct effect of ozone on the mucopolysaccharides can release the mechanical pressure and compression on the nerves. The effect was confirmed by histologic disc specimens removed during surgical microdiscectomy, previously treated with intradiscal O2–O3 mixture injection, with features of nucleus pulposus fibrillary matrix dehydration and signs of regression [15–22].

On the other side, oxygen–ozone plays significant role in hyper-oxygenation of the area of interest; disc herniation impinges on the venous and arterial flow, causing phlebostasis and arteriolo-stenosis, which lead to hypoxemia of the tissues; by applying O2–O3 mixture in the herniated site and oxygen concentration increases.

O2–O3 mechanism of action has been investigated using three approaches: mathematical models of intervertebral disc space to explore the relationship between disc pressure and volume; ozonolysis experiments using glycosaminoglycans (GAGs) from a Chinese hamster ovary cell line that were similar in composition to GAGs found in human nucleus pulposus; and experiments in which live Yucatan miniature pigs received various concentrations of percutaneous, image-guided intradiscal oxygen–ozone treatment and were examined (after sacrifice) with histology and semiquantitative analysis of disc cytokine concentrations [23].

Porcine disc histology and Chinese hamster ovary GAG ozonolysis results showed that administered ozone reacted with fragmented disc proteoglycans, reducing disc volume through disc dehydration. Cytokine analysis of porcine discs found that each of four cytokines measured (interleukin [IL]-1β, IL-6, IL-8, and tumor necrosis factor α) increased in concentration after 2-week ozone treatment [23].

Finally, ozone stimulates the repair process, promoting the fibroblastic activity and inducing collagen deposition. Experimental studies have demonstrated that a mixture of O2–O3 at concentration used by intradiscal injection produced the same results of steroid on cytokine production and so it reduces pain.

It was evidenced that the mixture of O3–O2 has dose-related effects. At "high" concentrations (40–70 μg O3/O2 mL), it enhances alterations and destruction of tissue structures, at medium concentrations (20–30 μg O3/O2 mL), it appears to affect the regulation of the immune system, and at lower concentrations (<20 μg O3/O2 mL), it improves microcirculation [15, 24].

The administrated dose for treating the disc is 30–40 μm/mL, and it is resulted to be the best concentration to dehydrate the nucleus and to reduce the inflammation, according to experimental studies [23]. A recent study has evaluated the quality of pain alleviation using two different doses of intradiscal injections of O3–O2 mixture of 40 and 30 μg/mL [25]. There were no significant differences between the two groups regarding the clinical outcomes; however, both the ODI and VAS evaluations showed highly significant improvement (decreased) ($P < 0.01$) after injection and during the entire follow-up period [25].

## 9.3 The Selection of Patients: Indication and Contraindications

The selection of patients undergoing minimally invasive treatments is the most important factor for the technique's success and most of all because it is an alternative treatment to classical surgery, already standardized by world guidelines. The following selection criteria are usually adopted for enrolment.

General exclusion criteria are:

- Extruded herniated disc.
- Free herniated fragment.
- Spine infection.
- High arm and foot progressive motor deficit.
- Cono-cauda syndrome.
- Hyperalgesic sciatica.

Last three conditions are absolute indication to surgery.

Among all the techniques illustrated, the oxygen–ozone therapy has the advantage of no absolute contraindications.

The best results are reported for small and medium size herniations with a normal spinal canal, without calcifications. Prognostic factors for an unsuccessful outcome are the presence of a calcified herniated disc, a high grade of spinal stenosis, presence of a small descending herniated disc in the lateral spinal recess, or recurred herniation.

Inclusion criteria are:

1. Clinical criteria: low back pain and sciatica resistant to conservative medical therapy, physical therapy, and others manipulations for a time not shorter than 2–3 months.
2. Neurological criteria: paresthesia or hypoesthesia over the dermatome involved, mild muscle weakness and signs of root-ganglion irritation.
3. Psychological criteria: a firm resolve on the part of the patient to recover with a commitment to cooperate and undergo subsequent physiotherapy with postural and motor rehabilitation.
4. Neuroradiological (CT, MR).
   (a) Evidence of small- and medium-sized herniated discs correlating with the patient's symptoms with or without degenerative disc vertebral disease complicated by intervertebral disc changes (protrusion, herniation).
   (b) Residual of surgical (micro)-discectomy with herniation recurrence and/or hypertrophic fibrous scarring.

## 9.4 Neuroradiological Technique

The choice among any different techniques depends on the confidence of the operator about the technique itself and availability of a good quality machine on the territory. All techniques need a radiological specific support: CT or fluoroscopic guide.

A standard technical protocol has not yet been provided, and every operator develops his own technique on the basis of experience and resources availability. Working in sterile conditions is essential. Fluoro- (Fig. 9.1) or computed tomography (CT) guidance are both feasible depending on the operator choice. The patient lies in a prone position and a pillow can be placed under the abdomen to increase the lumbosacral angle. The approach with the patient lying laterally on the healthy site has been also described.

CT guide allows the operator to avoid the intradiscal administration of contrast that even if with low dose reduces the ozone absorption and causes obstruction to the intraforaminal injection of the mixture O2–O3.

Disc access is gained with a posterolateral extra-pedicular approach on the symptomatic side at the level of the disc herniation (Fig. 9.2), even if the puncture site is 6–10 cm away from the vertebral midline, using a 15 cm needle 19–22 G, depending on the patient build, with an angle of about 40–45°. When the needle enters the disc, a soft resistance is felt. The needle position in the centre of the disc

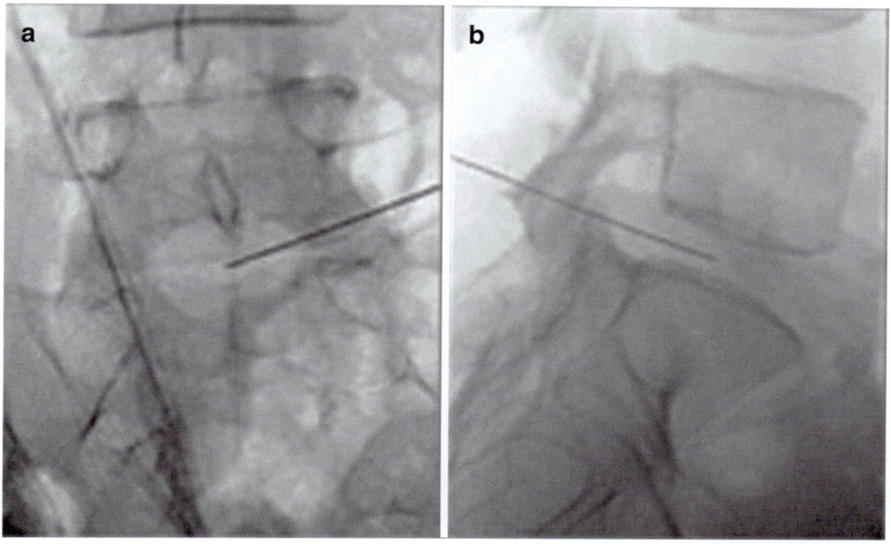


**Fig. 9.1** Patient affected by herniated disc at L5–S1 level: (**a**, **b**) under fluoroscopy guidance, the LL and PA X-ray control show the right position of the needle into disc in patient in prone position

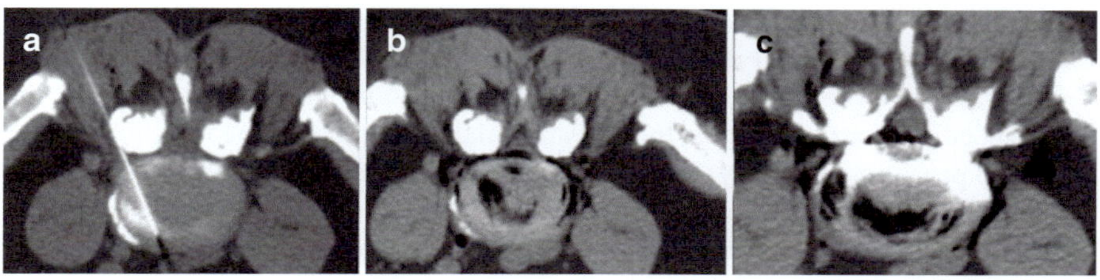


**Fig. 9.2** Patient affected by herniated disc at L4–L5 level: (**a**) CT control shows the right position of the needle in the disc at L4–L5 level by posterolateral approach in patient in prone position; (**b**, **c**) CT control shows the right distribution of O2–O3 in the herniated disc

must be confirmed by fluoroscopy or CT imaging; the ideal needle position is considered to be at the junction between the posterior and the middle third of the disc. Gas mixture (1–3 mL: 2% O3 (30–40 mg/mL) in 98% O2) is injected into the disc. Then the needle tip is withdrawn into the intervertebral foramen (where the operator feels minor resistance) where another 10 mL of O2–O3 and 2 mL of corticosteroid/local anesthetic (1/1) are injected; indeed the rationale to puncture the symptomatic and not the healthy side when adopting this technique is based on the concept that the effects of the O2–O3 and corticosteroid/local anesthetic mixture are not limited to the disc but affect the intraforaminal nerve root tract as well.

Under CT guidance, the distribution of the O2–O3 in the disc, foraminal-perigangliar, and epidural spaces can be observed. Finally, the needle is removed, and the patient is required to lie in the bed (in a supine position) for 1 h before being dismissed to home. Heavy activity must be avoided for the following two weeks.

If the posterolateral approach at L5–S1 level is unfeasible due to the high position of the iliac crests, a curved steerable needle can be adopted: these devices are able to deflect from a straight rigid direction and the tip can be bent in order to bypass a bone structure. If these devices are not available, a translaminar approach can be considered (Fig. 9.3). In this case, CT guidance is advised because it allows the visualization of the dural sac. The puncture site is 2 cm away from the diseased spinal process in the intervertebral space, and the needle is advanced stepwise into the hernia through the space between the medial border of the articular process and the lateral border of the dural sac; the ideal position of the needle tip is inside the herniated portion of the disc. Before injecting slowly O2–O3 (5–6 mL), an aspiration test is mandatory to make sure that the needle tip is not located in a blood vessel or in the subarachnoidal space, containing cerebrospinal fluid.

Differently from other percutaneous techniques, the infiltration of mixture of O2–O3 can be performed safely at the cervical level with some differences compared to the lumbar level.

The indications are very restricted and selective.

Only the soft herniated disc without calcified element or central spinal stenosis or lateral foraminal stenosis associated can be treated. Symptomatic herniated disc with important motor deficit at upper limb is contraindicated and it is a surgery indication. A pretreatment imaging with CT, MR, and EMG are recommended.

Then for the treatment at cervical level, there are same technical differences: the needle used for cervical level is thinner and smaller than other one used for lumbar level; the procedure is always performed in patient in supine position and it can be done under CT guidance or fluoroscopy; the technique is always performed by right anterolateral approach with carotid-axis manual dislocation; the amount of mixture of O2–O3 is less than lumbar level: only 1–2 cc must be injected into cervical disc; the procedure is never associated with anesthetic drug injection to avoid breathing disturbances; as for lumbar level, a peri-foraminal steroid injection can be associated.

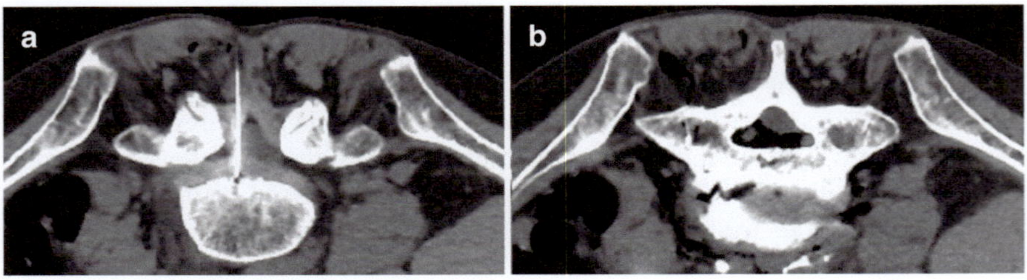


**Fig. 9.3** Patient affected by herniated disc at L5–S1 (**a**) CT control shows the right position of the needle in the disc at L4–L5 level by translaminar approach in patient in prone position; (**b**) CT control shows the right distribution of O2–O3 in the herniated disc

## 9.5 Complication and Results

The O2–O3 chemonucleolysis is as effective as other percutaneous disc decompression techniques, which has a high therapeutic success rate (70–80%) with the lowest cost (best cost/benefit ratio) and lowest complication rate (<0.1%) [16–22, 26]. No early or late neurological or infectious complications have been reported following O2–O3 injection [16–22].

In the literature, there have been reported: bilateral vitreoretinal haemorrhages; thunderclap headache after O2–O3 therapy related to pneumoencephalus as a consequence of inadvertent intrathecal puncture; paresthesias on the anterolateral portion of the left leg and foot, suggesting nerve injury; a few temporary episodes of impaired sensitivity; one case of vertebrobasilar stroke and a subcutaneous haematoma at the puncture site [27].

Regarding infections, a case of L5–S1 discitis and a case of fatal septicaemia have been described. As O2–O3 has disinfecting properties, it is not likely for the gas mixture to be infected; probably these complications were due to inadequate asepsis and iatrogenic inoculation of the bacteria during the injection [27].

In the study of Dall'Olio et al. [24], the pain relief and motor improvement were noted early after 2 weeks. Some researchers studied local ozone injection for low back pain in one group of patients and in one definite dose.

In 2013, Magalhães et al. [28] investigated the epidural injection of ozone upon a single group of 13 sequential adult patients with chronic low lumbar pain after failed back surgery syndrome. The patients had a reduction of low back pain by 43.7% in 6 months followed by 44.0% of improvement in the ODI. Another single group of 30 adult patients with LBP with DH underwent intradiscal injection of O3–O2 mixture (4 mL, 40 μg/mL).

Some studies compared O3–O2 mixtures alone and with additives upon a series of cases of herniated disc. In 2013, some Authors [29] compared the epidural usage of O3–O2 mixture and with steroids added to the same mixture in two groups of 172 patients with disc herniation who failed to respond to conventional therapy and found excellent pain alleviation by nucleolysis in both the groups with insignificant difference. They recommended that the use of O3–O2 could only be sufficient to reduce the disc size and alleviate the pain. They also recommended the use of ozone before recourse to surgical intervention or when surgery is not possible.

A comparison was done by Apuzzo et al. [30] between O3–O2 therapy and global postural reeducation in complicated chronic LBP reeducation or a combination of the two therapeutic options. Follow-up showed that pain severity was lower in the O3–O2 group than in the global postural reeducation alone group. This study denoted that ozone alone can produce a sharp decrease of pain in short term, and the use of global postural education could increase the duration of pain alleviation.

In the appropriate clinical/imaging context, intra-discal injection of O2–O3 has a reported success rate that reaches 90% at short-term follow-up (6 months) and a 75–82% success rate at long-term follow-up (12 months) with no major or minor side effects. Around 73% of the patients who went through O2–O3 therapy are still better at 5 and 10 years [12].

An average reduction in pain intensity in VAS from 7.58 before treatment to 2.64 two years after treatment has been reported, with similar results in ODI classification [12].

Muto et al. [17, 20, 24] reported their experience in three studies published in the course of 10 years enrolling more than 3500 patients and they found an 80% success rate; they used CT guidance and excluded subjects with extruded hernia and free disc fragments; furthermore, they reassessed patient status after 1 month, and those showing only partial success were scheduled for a second treatment session.

Andreula et al. [18] treated 600 patients and compared intradiscal O2–O3 and intradiscal O2–O3 associated with periganglionic injection of corticosteroid and anesthetic: they found success in 70% with intradiscal O2–O3 alone and in 78% with intradiscal O2–O3 and periganglionic injection, concluding that combined intradiscal and periganglionic injection have a cumulative effect enhancing the overall outcome of treatment. Oder et al. [31] reported successful treatment in 620 subjects with reduction of pain measured by means of a VAS score with excellent results in one-third of the patients (reduction from 8 to <3); the better results were encountered in those patients with a single disc herniation <50 years of age.

The study group of Lehnert et al. [32] focused on the physical effects of O2–O3 on the disc volume: they analysed data from 283 treated lumbar disc herniations and concluded that intradiscal administration of medical ozone is associated in 96% of the cases with a statistically significant volume reduction of the herniated lumbar disc. This value correlates negatively with the patient's age and positively with the initial disc volume; on the other hand, patient's sex does not affect the volume change after therapy.

Xu et al. [33] treated 187 patients and they followed their cohort up to 4 years with an effective rate of 82%; interestingly they divided this sample into three groups according to the number of O2–O3 sessions (1, 2, or 3), and they did not describe any significant correlation between the injections number and success rate.

Alexandre et al. [34] published a multicentre study reporting follow-up at 5 years on 6665 patients treated in Italy, Spain, and Argentina treated with intradiscal ozone followed by four paravertebral injections, and they reported complete elimination of pain in 80%, improvement in 12% and no improvement in 7%.

Buric et al. [35] reported on 108 patients treated with a single intradiscal injection of O2–O3. They followed up with 107 patients at 5 years and 60 patients at 10 years; They acquired MR imaging at 6 months after the ozone injection that demonstrated a reduction of the disc herniation volume in 79%. During the long-term follow-up, only 19 of 107 patients underwent to surgery while among those that avoided surgery 82% were improved at 5 years and 88% were improved at 10 years. Critically on long-term follow-up, on MR imaging the treated discs stayed hydrated and did not become a low signal. At 6 months MR follow-up, approximately 75–96% of patients had a significant herniation volume reduction, with the higher reduction observed in larger discs. It has been recently reported that the T2 shine-through effect increases already 2 months after O2–O3 nucleolysis, which, in the future, may be used to predict shrinkage of lumbar disc herniation. Furthermore, the high negative predictive value of DWI-ADC analysis could be useful to select those patients who will require further treatment with ozone. Moreover, starting a physical rehabilitation programme is strongly recommended.

Recently, Ezeldin et al. [26] have analyzed 52 patients, with symptomatic herniated lumbar discs, who underwent fluoroscopic-guided intradiscal oxygen–ozone mixture injection (5 mL) at a concentration of 27–30 μg/mL and periradicular injection of the same O2–O3 mixture (10 mL), steroid (1 mL), and local anesthetic (1 mL). Clinical outcomes were evaluated, based on the Oswestry Disability Index (ODI) and pain intensity (0–5) scale results, which were obtained initially and at 2- and 6-month controls. They proved a significant decrease in pain disability and intensity, with a significant reduction in ODI. Negative results were related to long symptoms duration of more than 1 year. No complications were recorded.

## 9.6 Radiopaque Gelled Ethanol (DiscoGel®)

Radiopaque gelled ethanol (DiscoGel®) is a sterile viscous solution containing ethyl alcohol, cellulose derivative product, added to a radiopaque element, the tungsten, that, injected into the vertebral disc, relieves low back pain, radicular, or lumbar-radicular pain. The 96% pure ethyl alcohol produces a local necrosis of the nucleus pulposus. Its action is mechanical via a dehydration of the turgescent and protruding disc, which is compressing the peripheral nerves of the rachis and causing extreme pain. The product is injected into the nucleus pulposus under radiological control (CT or fluoroscopy guide) with posterolateral approach for thoracic or lumbar level and anterolateral approach for the cervical level [13].

Generally, a small 18-G needle is used for thoracic and lumbar level, while for cervical level it is recommended to use a 20-G needle [13, 14, 36].

*Inclusion criteria* for DiscoGel® chemonucleolysis are:

- Lumbago, cruralgia, and sciatica lasting at least 3 months and resistant to conservative management, medication, and physical therapies; sometimes in association with paresthesia.
- Poor therapeutic outcome following O2–O3 therapy performed at least 6 months before DiscoGel® treatment.

  *Neuroradiological criteria (CT and/or MR)*:
- Imaging findings of one or more small or medium uncalcified disc herniations in a location congruent with symptoms, complicated or not by degenerative disc disease.

  *Exclusion criteria* for treatment with O2–O3 and DiscoGel® were:
- Neuroradiological evidence of calcified herniation or free disc fragments.
- Major neurological deficit with impaired lower limber motility congruent with observed disc disease (this criterion is an indication for surgery).

The quantity of jellified ethyl alcohol injected varies between 0.2 and 0.8 mL, according to the dimension of the disc and extent of the hernia.

It is recommended to use:

- 0.2 mL of jellified ethyl alcohol for cervical discs.
- 0.3–0.5 mL of jellified ethyl alcohol for thoracic discs.
- 0.6–0.8 mL of jellified ethyl alcohol for lumbar discs.

At the beginning of the injection, the patient may experience a transitional scalding sensation in the region of injection which disappears in the course of injection. To minimize this risk, the product must be injected very slowly. Once the product has been injected, the needle is left 2 min before being withdrawn.

The viscosity of jellified ethyl alcohol depends on the temperature. Avoid an administration of the product warmed up above room temperature because gel becomes more liquid and is below optimum viscosity. To increase its viscosity, jellified ethyl alcohol can be refrigerated just prior to injection.

It is not indicated for pregnant woman and for patients known to be allergic to one of the components, patients in severe depression, or any other condition making the interpretation of pain difficult.

Experimental study on pigs performed by injecting DiscoGel intradiscal, intraforaminal, epidural and, intramuscular elements demonstrated that the DiscoGel® does not produce any morpho-structural changes in contact with nervous structures or muscular tissue. In fact, no tissue alteration was found but only some inflammatory elements like lympho-monocyte cells and venous stasis with same granular material colored black by hematoxylin and eosin method (the tungsten) in paravertebral tissue in the muscular and connective tissue. The nucleus pulposus, disc, chondro-myxoid, and root ganglion were normal, without morpho-structural changes in nuclear tissue and annulus at contact with DiscoGel [36].

The success rate is achieved between 89% and 91% of cases without any minor or major complications [13, 14, 36].

## 9.7 Conclusion

Percutaneous techniques, in particular chemodiscolysis, can be a good alternative to surgery treatment for herniated disc for patients affected by low back pain and sciatica.

They have a low rate of complications and easy feasibility. They do not need a long hospitalization period, and they do not exclude the possibility, in case of failed treatment, to undergo surgery afterwards.

Literature data have demonstrated that they play relevant role in the treatment of low back pain resistant to conservative therapy without motoric deficits.

In our experience, among all techniques, chemodiscolysis with O2–O3 mixture with periradicular and periganglionic infiltration is the best and most competitive technique with good therapeutic results and lower costs, also related to cost-benefit ratio and absence of complications.

Surgery is really indicated in emergency cases of cono-cauda syndrome, progressive neurologic deficit and hyperalgesic sciatica.

## References


1. Long MD. Decision making in lumbar disc disease. Clinical Neurosurg. 2001;39:36–51.
2. Bozzao A, Gallucci M, Masciocchi C, Aprile I, Barile A, Passariello R. Lumbar disk herniation: MR imaging assessment of natural history in patients treated without surgery. Radiology. 1992;185(1):135–41.
3. Splendiani A, Puglielli E, De Amicis R, Barile A, Masciocchi C, Gallucci M. Spontaneous resolution of lumbar disk herniation: predictive signs for prognostic evaluation. Neuroradiology. 2004;46(11):916–22.
4. Casey E. Natural history of radiculopathy. Phys Med Rehabil Clin N Am. 2011;22(1):1–5.
5. Awad JN, Moskovich R. Lumbar disc herniations: surgical versus nonsurgical treatment. Clin Orthop Relat Res. 2006;443:183–97.
6. Muto M, De Maria G, Izzo R, Fucci G. Non-discal lumbar radiculopathy: combined approach by CT and MR. Riv Neuroradiol. 1997;10:165–73.
7. Bush K, Cowan N, Katz DE, Gishen P. The natural history of sciatica associated with disc pathology. A prospective study with clinical and independent radiologic follow-up. Spine. 1992;17(10):1205–12.
8. Van de Velden J, de Bakker DH. Basis rapport: morbiditeit in de huisartsenpraktijk. Utrecht: Nivel; 1990.
9. Masui T, Yukawa Y, Nakamura S, Kajino G, Matsubara Y, Kato F, Ishiguro N. Natural history of patients with lumbar disc herniation observed by magnetic resonance imaging for minimum 7 years. J Spinal Disord Tech. 2005;18(2):121–6.
10. Takada E, Takahashi M, Shimada K. Natural history of lumbar disc hernia with radicular leg pain: spontaneous MRI changes of the herniated mass and correlation with clinical outcome. J Orthop Surg. 2001;9(1):1–7.
11. Singh V, Piryani C, Liao K. Percutaneous disc decompression using coblation in the treatment of chronic discogenic pain. Pain Phys. 2002;5:250–9.
12. Giurazza F, Guarnieri G, Murphy KJ, Muto M. Intradiscal O2O3: rationale, injection technique, short- and long-term outcomes for the treatment of low back pain due to disc herniation. Can Assoc Radiol J. 2017;68(2):171–7.
13. Guarnieri G, De Dominicis G, Muto M. Intradiscal and intramuscular injection of Discogel(®)—radiopaque gelified ethanol: pathological evaluation. Neuroradiol J. 2010;23(2):249–52.
14. Stagni S, Simonetti L, Stafa A, Leonardi M, et al. A minimally invasive treatment for lumbar disc herniation: DiscoGel® chemonucleolysis in patients unresponsive to chemonucleolysis with oxygen-ozone. Interv Neuroradiol. 2012;18(1):97–104.
15. Chang JD, Lu HS, Chang YF, Wang D. Ameliorative effect on ozone on cytokine production in mice injected with human rheumatoid arthritis synovial fibroblast cells. Rheumatol Int. 2005;26:141–51.
16. Andreula C, Muto M, Leonardi M. Interventional spinal procedures. Eur J Radiol. 2004;50:112–9.
17. Muto M, Andreula C, Leonardi M. Treatment of herniated lumbar disc by intradiscal and intraforaminal oxygen-ozone injection. J Neuroradiol. 2004;31(3):183–9.
18. Andreula CF, Simonetti L, Leonardi M. Minimally invasive oxygen-ozone therapy for lumbar disk herniation. AJNR. 2003;24:996–1000.
19. Tian JL, et al. Changes of CSF and spinal path-morphology after hight concentration ozone injection into the subarachnoid space:an experimental study in pigs. AJNR. 2007;28:1051–4.
20. Muto M, Avella F. Percutaneous treatment of herniated lumbar disc by intradiscal oxygen-ozone injection. Interv Neuroradiol. 1998;4(4):279–86.

21. Muto M, Guarnieri G, et al. Low back pain and sciatica: treatment with intradiscal-intraforaminal O(2)-O (3) injection. Our experience. Radiol Med. 2008;113(5):695–706.
22. Bonetti M, Cotticelli B, et al. Oxygen-ozone therapy versus epidural steroid injection. Riv Neuroradiol. 2000;13:203–6.
23. Murphy K, Elias G, Steppan J, Boxley C, Balagurunathan K, Victor X, Meaders T, Muto M. Percutaneous treatment of herniated lumbar discs with ozone: investigation of the mechanisms of action. J Vasc Interv Radiol. 2016;27(8):1242–1250.e3.
24. Dall'Olio M, Princiotta C, Cirillo L, Budai C, de Santis F, Bartolini S, Serchi E, Leonardi M. Oxygen-ozone therapy for herniated lumbar disc in patients with subacute partial motor weakness due to nerve root compression. Interv Neuroradiol. 2014;20:547–54.
25. Elawamy A, Kamel EZ, Hassanien M, Wahba OM, Amin SE. Implication of two different doses of intradiscal ozone-oxygen injection upon the pain alleviation in patients with low back pain: a randomized, single-blind study. Pain Physician. 2018;21(1):E25–31.
26. Ezeldin M, Leonardi M, Princiotta C, Dall'olio M, Tharwat M, Zaki M, Abdel-Wanis ME, Cirillo L. Percutaneous ozone nucleolysis for lumbar disc herniation. Neuroradiology. 2018;60(11):1231–41. https://doi.org/10.1007/s0O234-018-2083-4.
27. De Oliveira MF, Dotta L, Sasse A, et al. Ozone therapy as a treatment for low back pain secondary to herniated disc: a systematic review and meta-analysis of randomized controlled trials. Pain Physician. 2012;15:E115–29.
28. Magalhães FN, Soares SC, Torres JM, Ungaretti A, Cacciacarro MF, Teixeira MJ, Fonoff ET. Effects of ozone applied by spinal endoscopy in patients with chronic pain related to failed back surgery syndrome: a pilot study. Neuropsychiatr Dis Treat. 2013;9:1759–66.
29. Zhang Y, Ma Y, Jiang J, Ding T, Wang J. Treatment of the lumbar disc herniation with intradiscal and intraforaminal injection of oxygen-ozone. J Back Musculoskelet Rehabil. 2013;26:317–22.
30. Apuzzo D, Giotti C, Pasqualetti P, Ferrazza P, Soldati P, Zucco GM. An observational retrospective/horizontal study to compare oxygen-ozone therapy and/ or global postural re-education in complicated chronic low back pain. Funct Neurol. 2014;29:31–9.
31. Oder B, Loewe M, Reisegger M, Lang W, Ilias W, Thurnher SA. CT-guided ozone/steroid therapy for the treatment of degenerative spinal disease: effect of age, gender, disc pathology and multi-segmental changes. Neuroradiology. 2008;50:777e85.
32. Lehnert T, Naguib N, Wutzler S, et al. Analysis of disk volume before and after CT-guided intradiscal and periganglionic ozoneeoxygen injection for the treatment of lumbar disk herniation. J Vasc Interv Radiol. 2012;23:1430e6.
33. Xu L, Li ZL, He XF, et al. Evaluation of the clinical curative effect of an O2-O3 mixture to treat lumbar disc herniation with different treat- ment sessions. Interv Neuroradiol. 2009;15:159e63.
34. Alexandre A, Buric J, Paradiso R, et al. Intradiscal injection of O2-O3 to treat lumbar disc herniations. Results at five years. Riv Ital Ossigeno Ozonoterapia. 2002;1:165e9.
35. Buric J, Rigobello L, Hooper D. Five and ten year follow-up on intradiscal ozone injection for disc herniation. Int J Spine Surg. 2014;8:17.
36. Theron J, Guimaraens L, Casasco A, Sola T, Cuellar H, Courtheoux P. Percutaneous treatment of lumbar intervertebral disk hernias with radiopaque gelified ethanol: a preliminary study. J Spinal Disord Tech. 2007;20:526–32.

# Minimally Invasive Treatment of Herniated Discs: How to Remove the Disc with Physical Tools

# 10

Giuseppe Bonaldi and Alessandro Cianfoni

## 10.1 Introduction

Radicular pain, which is usually caused by herniation of an intervertebral disc, is a common problem with an annual incidence of 5 per 1000 [1, 2]. Radiculopathy arises from direct neural compression by disc herniations and associated inflammatory and ischemic phenomena. Symptoms can also arise from a disc protrusion because of the effect on heavily innervated surrounding structures such as the outer annulus and posterior longitudinal ligament. The severity of symptoms does not always correlate with the extent of the herniation [3]. Sensitization of the central nervous system has also been suggested to be a possible causative factor of chronicity in some spinal pain conditions.

Patients suffering from radicular pain, in which spinal imaging shows a herniated disc compressing the nerve root involved in the radiculopathy, have historically been considered as possible candidates for open surgical discectomy, with the intent of providing decompression of the nerve root by removing the herniated disc. With surgical approaches, there is direct visualization of the herniated disc and removal of the portion of the disc compressing the adjacent nerve root. Numerous surgical

G. Bonaldi (✉)
Giuseppe Bonaldi, Neurosurgery Department, Casa di Cura Igea, Milan, Italy

Neurosurgery Department, Casa di Cura Igea, Milan, Italy

A. Cianfoni
Department of Neuroradiology, Neurocenter of Southern Switzerland, Ospedale Regionale di Lugano, Lugano, Switzerland

Department of Interventional and Diagnostic Neuroradiology, Inselspital University Hospital of Bern, Bern, Switzerland
e-mail: alessandro.cianfoni@eoc.ch



L. Manfrè, J. Van Goethem (eds.), *The Disc and Degenerative Disc Disease*, New Procedures in Spinal Interventional Neuroradiology,
https://doi.org/10.1007/978-3-030-03715-4_10

treatments for discogenic pain have been developed, ranging from disc excision with laminectomy, microdiscectomy, spinal fusion to artificial disc replacement. Although open surgery is effective, it has well-known disadvantages, including epidural scarring, damage to bone, denervation of paraspinal muscles with consequent lumbar instability, long postoperative inactivity, and the not infrequent "failed back surgery syndrome." Patients with the latter are in fact often untreatable and severely disabled. Because of the considerable morbidity and convalescence period inherent to conventional lumbar disc surgery, there has been an ongoing search for less invasive methods of treatment. Lyman Smith opened the path in 1963, describing a minimally invasive attempt to treat sciatica through a percutaneous injection of chymopapain into the disc, with the intent of achieving enzymatic chemolysis of the nucleus pulposus and of its protruding fragments compressing the nerve root [4–6]. Since then, and from the 1970s onwards, multiple percutaneous minimally invasive interventional techniques to achieve disc decompression have been described, entailing both chemical and physical tools [7–13]. The latter will be discussed in this chapter.

Percutaneous discectomy techniques attempt nerve root decompression indirectly by decreasing the central disc pressure. The treatment principle of percutaneous disc decompression is based on the concept of the intervertebral disc being a closed hydraulic system. This system consists of the nucleus pulposus, containing a large amount of water, surrounded by the inelastic annulus fibrosus. An increase in water content of the nucleus pulposus leads to a disproportional increase of intradiscal pressure. On the other hand, a decrease of intradiscal volume causes a disproportionally large decrease in intradiscal pressure [14, 15]. Central decompression is achieved by the removal of material from the nucleus pulposus. The most often stated goal of central nuclear decompression is to lower the pressure in the nucleus and to allow room for the herniated fragment to recede inward. The theory postulates that intact outer annular fibers will be able to contract enough to reduce the tension on both the nerve root and annulus. Additional suggested effects of central decompression include denaturation and fibrotic changes in the nucleus pulposus, which should in turn limit the ability of the nuclear matrix to attract water, thereby causing a long-lasting pressure reduction [16], and reinforce the inner annular fibers, reducing the tendency of the central components of the disc to herniate toward the spinal canal [17]. The goal is to allow sufficient tissue removal while minimizing collateral tissue damage and avoiding destabilization of the disco-vertebral unit. The benefits of percutaneous discectomy are greater than just avoidance of open surgery. Small contained disc protrusions have been shown to be less likely than larger disc extrusions to undergo spontaneous resorption [18] and are associated with worse surgical outcomes following discectomy [19]. Fortunately, this is the subtype of herniation most responsive to percutaneous techniques. Finally, percutaneous disc procedures have the advantage of a high patient psychological acceptance, tolerance, and satisfaction.

## 10.2 Indications

Percutaneous decompression has been shown effective in relieving radicular pain and to a lesser extent axial pain from contained disc protrusions. Patient selection criteria include the presence of a contained disc herniation documented by spinal imaging, causing radicular pain greater than axial pain, for 6 months or longer, and the patient having failed conservative measures, including anti-inflammatory and analgesic medications and physical therapy. Imaging and clinical correlation is of utmost importance. In doubtful cases, diagnostic selective nerve root blocks, facet blocks, and provocative discography might help target the correct pain generator. The success of the procedure depends greatly on selecting the lesions to treat (Fig. 10.1); the protruding nucleus pulposus must be at least partially contained by the external fibers of the disc, without a large extrusion or migrated fragments [20, 21]. The herniation should not be pinched off by the endplates and should be without significant prolapse above or below the disc level. The disc should have maintained at least 50% of its height on imaging studies. The discs with more advanced degrees of degeneration are more difficult to access and are less likely to achieve much further pressure reduction [22]. Contained disc herniations are often circumferential bulges or protrusions, which appear broad on axial MRI or computed tomography (CT) [21–24]. Because MRI and CT do not usually enable distinction of a contained from an uncontained prolapse, in doubtful cases, discography or CT discography may help in assessing annular tears and extruded lesions, revealed by epidural spread of contrast injected in the nucleus pulposus (Fig. 10.1). CT discography may also show the size of the "neck" connecting the protruded part of the disc with the central nucleus pulposus: the wider the connection, the more likely efficient transmission of pressure toward the center of the disc, and the more likely the clinical success of the procedure [24–26].

Purely, clinical criteria are also very important. Patients with a contained herniation, a good indication for percutaneous treatment, typically have a relatively long history (6 months or more) of back and/or leg pain of variable intensity, more intense under loading of the lumbar spine and particularly in a sitting position (typically, driving a car). The pain is not disabling, but becomes more and more incompatible with a good quality of life, in part because of a progressive reduction in the psychological threshold of pain tolerance. It is probable that these features correlate with a contained disc lesion, and root compression becomes evident only when a static or dynamic load on the spine provokes outward transmission of pressure from the center of the disc through rents in the inner fibers of the annulus, with secondary increase in the external diameter of the disc. The pressure within the disc and its volume decrease with rest, owing to integrity of the outer annular fibers and ligaments. Uncontained extrusions of the nucleus pulposus or sequestrated fragments, which are not a good indication for disc decompression, cause sustained, firmer compression of the nerve root (probably along with inflammatory phenomena

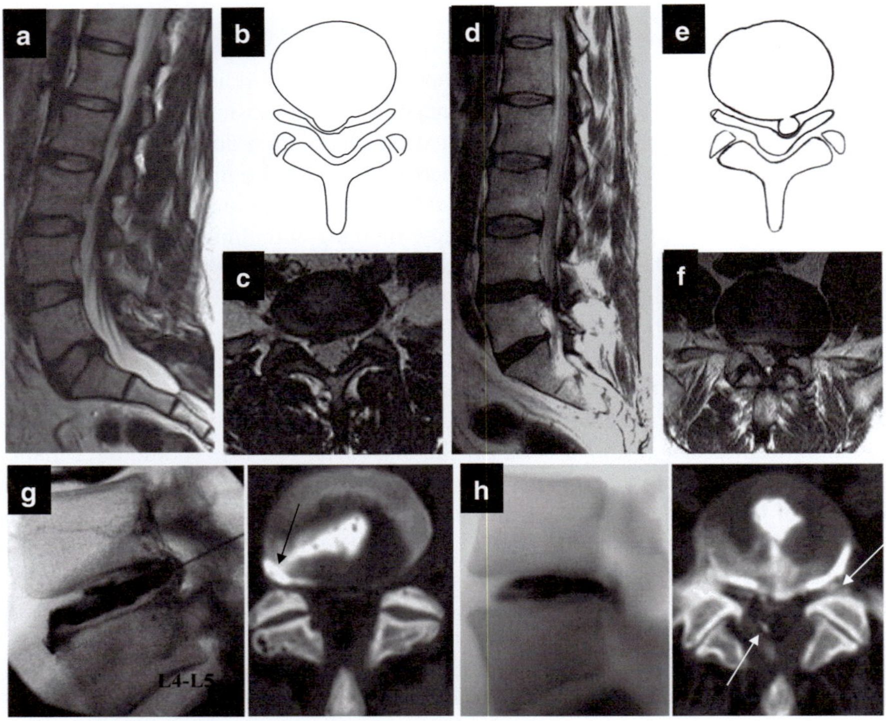


**Fig. 10.1** Contained and extruded disc herniations. (**a–c**) Show the MR appearance and the schematic drawing of a contained disc herniation; note the broad base on axial and sagittal plane, the disc-endplates do not "pinch off" the herniation, and the disc height is preserved; in the appropriate clinical setting this might represent a good indication for disc decompression. (**d–f**) Show the non-contained counterpart of disc herniation, with long sagittal dimension, and "pinched-off" aspect, that, based on morphological characteristics, is not likely to respond to a procedure of disc decompression. (**g**) Shows the discography and CT discography features of a contained disc herniation (arrow), with contrast contained by the external fibers of the annulus, while (**h**) shows a non-contained disc herniation, as revealed by epidural spread of contrast injected in the nucleus pulposus (arrows). CT discography is the most accurate imaging technique to differentiate between contained and non-contained disc herniations

primed by the presence of nucleus pulposus, recognized as a foreign body, in the epidural space) and therefore more constant, intense, and often disabling pain. These clinical landmarks, when they last for at least 6–8 weeks, justify open surgery as the treatment of choice.

Contraindications include sequestered herniation, herniation greater than one-third of the sagittal diameter of the spinal canal, progressive neurologic deficit, infection, bony deformity not allowing a safe percutaneous image-guided disc access, or other bone lesions which could compress a root and cause radicular symptoms [27]. Applying strict selection criteria, Onik estimated that only 5–10% of the patients with disc herniation who eventually undergo surgery would be eligible for percutaneous disc decompression [28]. Given its low morbidity, however, disclosing the lesser likelihood of clinical success of the procedure, the minimally invasive therapeutic option can be ethically offered to a wider range of patients, such as the ones with partially uncontained prolapses, as an attempt to avoid surgery, or when the risks of open surgery are higher because of age, general medical conditions, or other contraindications [28]. This typically applies to patients who have already undergone open surgery at the same level because of the possibility of symptomatic epidural scar and to elderly people. In fact, an observational study on a large cohort of patients reports these subgroups of patients as good responders to automated disc decompression (APLD) [17]. Although the satisfactory outcome can be attributed to several factors, the one that supersedes all is that in these patients, with a nerve root confined and compressed in a small space, either due to epidural fibrosis or arthropathic degenerative bone changes, even a small reduction in the volume of the disc by disc decompression might result in radicular decompression and clinical improvement.

## 10.3 Techniques of Percutaneous Disc Access

The procedure can be performed with the patient in either the prone or lateral decubitus position. When the prone position is used, bolsters are placed underneath the patient's abdomen to flatten the lordosis and open the disc spaces posteriorly (Fig. 10.2). This will allow easier disc access and better transmission of the pressure drop caused in the center of the disc by the decompression procedure to the

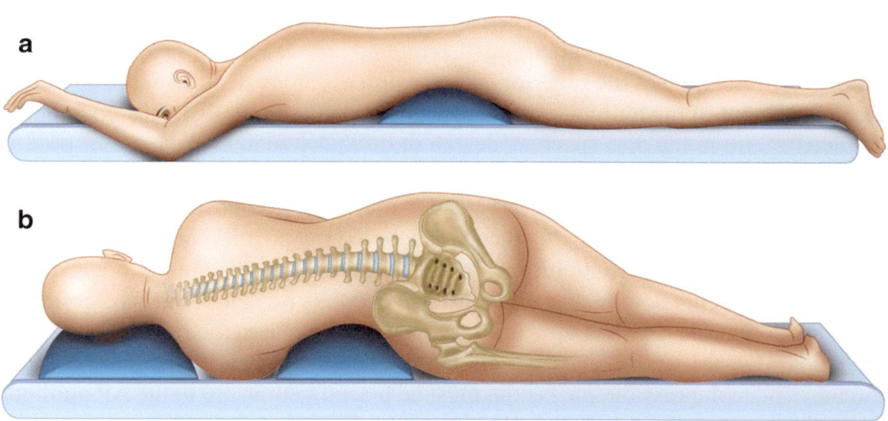


**Fig. 10.2** Patient positioning for lumbar discectomy. (**a**) Shows the use of a bolster to be placed under the lower abdomen when the patient is in prone decubitus, to flatten the lumbar lordosis, and to open the disc space posteriorly for an easier access and better transmission of the pressure drop to the herniated disc component. Similarly, the patient is flexed when in the lateral decubitus position, by positioning a bolster under the recumbent side (**b**), approximately at the level of the disc to be treated, with the intent of opening the disc space on the entry side, and of tilting away the iliac crest for access to the L5–S1 disc

herniated disc component. For the same reason, the patient is flexed when in the lateral decubitus position, by positioning a bolster under the recumbent side, approximately at the level of the disc to be treated (Fig. 10.2). The entry route is posterolateral. Correct positioning of the guiding needle in the disc is the most delicate part of the procedure and is crucial to the result. The procedure is monitored fluoroscopically. If, while approaching the disc, a radicular paresthesia or a true radicular pain is elicited, the needle needs to be retracted and redirected. If the nerve root is touched, the patient experiences radicular symptoms, usually a sensation described as a sudden "electrical shock" which may radiate as distal as the foot, depending on the root that has been abutted. In contrast, the pain originating directly from the nociceptive fibers of the external annulus is less intense and does not typically refers below the knee.

### 10.3.1 Oblique View for Disc Access

The most reliable, standardized, and safe technique to perform percutaneous fluoroscopy guided lumbar disc access implies the use of the so-called tunnel vision view. According to this technique, the fluoroscopy tube is angled along the projected path of the needle from the skin to the desired final position of the needle tip within the disc, with an oblique posterolateral paravertebral approach. To identify the correct angle and obliquity of the access, from a true AP view of the disc space of interest, the tube is angled obliquely, toward the side of the preferred approach, under continuous fluoroscopic view, until the anatomical landmark of the "Scottie dog" appears, with its ear (the superior articular process of the vertebra below) superimposed on the disc space. The target point is in the middle of the disc space, as seen on this oblique projection, just lateral and anterior to the superior articular process. The position of the superior articular process along the disc endplate line is the determinant of the obliquity of the disc access and eventually of the position of the needle's tip in the disc space. A degree of obliquity such as the anterior profile of the ear of the Scottie dog bisects the endplate line ensures a final position of the needle's tip in the exact center of the disc. A more external position of the Scottie dog's ear predicts a more peripheral and ipsilateral final position of the needle's tip, along with a higher chance to hit the exiting nerve root, while a more medial position of the ear of the Scottie dog along the disc endplate line allows a more posterior final position of the needle's tip within the disc, but increases the risk of straying in the epidural space and potentially entering the dural sac (Fig. 10.3). For a routine intradiscal decompression, the needle must be placed with its tip in the AP midline, at the junction of the middle and posterior thirds of the disc, where the normal nucleus pulposus lies. In cases of large, posterior protrusions indenting the spinal canal, it is preferable to aim for a more posterior position of the needle; therefore, a more oblique view, with the ear of the Scottie dog located toward the medial end of the disc endplate line, is chosen. Eventually, the degree of obliquity and the

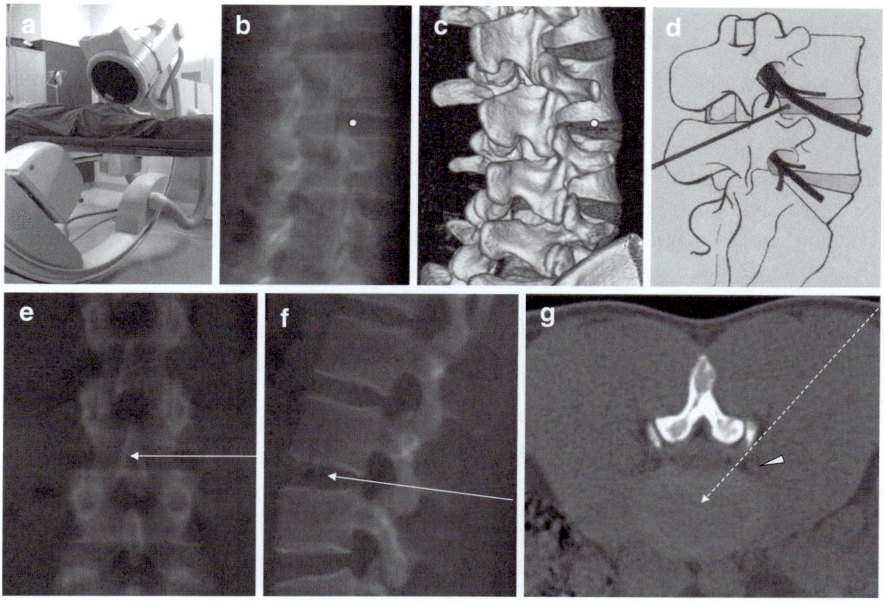


**Fig. 10.3** Fluoroscopy and CT correlates of disc access anatomy. (**a**) shows the fluoroscopic tube angle to obtain a correct "tunnel vision" for a right posterolateral percutaneous access to the disc L3–L4 (**b**), as also shown on the correspondent 3D volume rendering CT model (**c**). The cranio-caudal angle of the tube is such that the disc space is well profiled at the level of interest, and the right-to-left (RL) obliquity is such that the superior articular process (ear of the Scottie dog) of L4 is superimposed on the midpoint of the disc-endplate line. This ensures an access window for the needle (white dot on **b** and **c**) posterior, inferior, and medial to the exiting nerve root (**d**). (**e, f**) show the final location of the needle (arrow) in the center of the nucleus pulposus on the AP and LL views. (**g**) shows the axial CT section through the disc space and the ideal needle path (dashed arrow); note that steep obliquity, tangent to the superior articular process of the facet, is necessary to have a correct access to the disc and to avoid the exiting nerve root (arrowhead)

trajectory of the needle as tangent as possible to the ear of the Scottie dog determine the safety of this trajectory in avoiding the exiting nerve root, usually located superior and anterior to the needle's entry point in the annulus. Once the specific oblique projection has been identified, the entry point of the needle in the skin projects over the target, and the needle is inserted accordingly to the tube angle, and along its whole path, from the skin to the target and it will appear as a single radiopaque dot superimposed to the target. Of course, as always in radiology, the position of an object must be confirmed in two orthogonal projections; in this case, the depth of the needle tip and its final correct position on the target must be controlled intermittently, and finally confirmed, by the two strict AP and LL views. Adherence to this, methodology guarantees the safest and most reproducible needle approach to the disc.

### 10.3.2 L5–S1 Disc Access: Special Considerations

The anatomy, and consequently the fluoroscopic views, is different at the L5–S1 level because of the prominent lordosis and the presence of the iliac crest. The presence of the iliac crests often obstructs the desired posteriolateral oblique trajectory of the needle into the disc space. Performing the procedure with the patient lying in the lateral decubitus position increases the probability of correctly entering the L5–S1 disc. A soft silicone gel cushion or other similar prop wedged just superior to the iliac crest will laterally flex and lower the iliac crest on the entry side, thus opening a trajectory to access the L5–S1 disc (Fig. 10.2). When moving the C-arm to the oblique orientation, as mentioned above, the L5–S1 facet joint moves across the disc space and the iliac crest starts to overlap the disc. When the beam is at approximately a 45° angle, the superior articular process of S1 is seen bisecting the S1 endplate, and a triangular window at the center of the disc space is seen (Fig. 10.4). This triangle is bounded laterally by the iliac crest, medially by the anterior surface of the superior articular process of S1, and superiorly by the inferior endplate of the L5 vertebra. The center of the triangle, superimposed on the disc space, is our target.

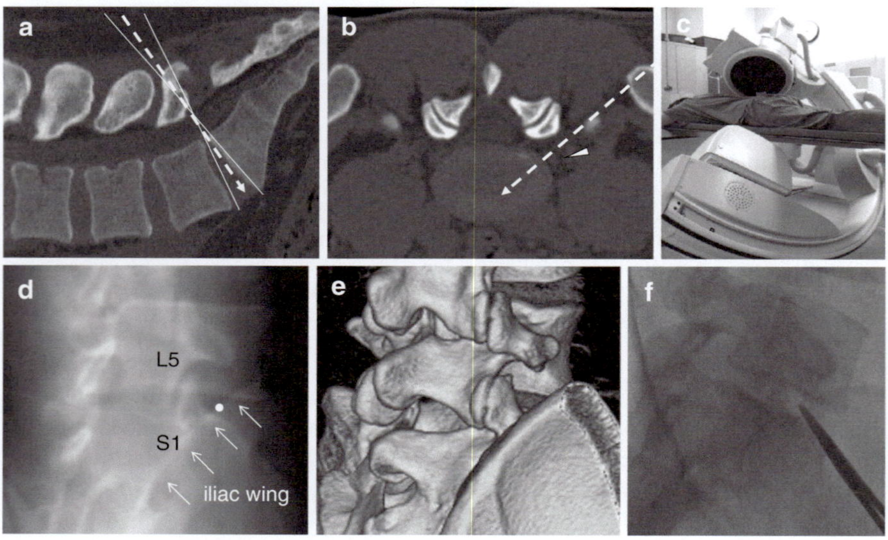


**Fig. 10.4** L5–S1 disc access. (**a**) Shows how the lordotic curvature causes the disc-endplates not to be parallel mainly at L5–S1, and in some patients also at L4–L5. The most appropriate cranio-caudal obliquity of the fluoroscopy tube to access these discs (dashed arrow) is, therefore, in between the angles necessary to profile the superior and the inferior disc-endplates (dotted lines). (**b**) shows the CT axial section through the L5–S1 disc; note that the RL obliquity of the disc access (dashed arrow) is limited by the iliac crest and by the superior articular facet, whereas the needle trajectory needs to avoid the nerve root (arrowhead). (**c–f**) show the fluoroscopic access to the L5–S1 disc, with the 3D-CT correlate. The angle of the tube can be extreme, in the CC and RL direction. The target (dot on **d**) is the center of the clear triangle formed by the superior margin of iliac wing, the lateral margin of the S1 articular process, and the L5 inferior endplate

Not uncommonly, high iliac crests cover the lateral oblique approach to the disc space, and the triangular window is visible only when the superior articular process of S1 is projected on the lateral third of the S1 endplate; any further obliquity of the X-ray beam brings the iliac crest to obstruct the path from the desired skin entry point to the disc space. Consequently, the entry route has to be less oblique (which means that the entry point in the skin is closer to the midline of the spine, for the needle to pass medially to the iliac crest) or must originate from a more cephalad starting point. With both approaches (more medial and more cephalad), there are instances in which straight instrumentation will not enter the disc correctly. If the trajectory of the needle is not obliquely angled enough, as discussed previously, it might be impossible to position the needle's tip in the desired position in the center of the nucleus pulposus, as it will tend to be too lateral and anterior in the disc. If the trajectory comes from a more cephalad entry point, the needle might still enter the disc, but will not be parallel to the disc endplates, and therefore, it will not advance in the disc space to the center of the nucleus pulposus. If the correct intradiscal position cannot be achieved with a straight cannula, a curved needle can be used. Although some operators might use a curved cannula as the introducing needle alone, this technique is very dependent on personal skills and expertise and might require several attempts to achieve the proper trajectory (Fig. 10.5).

### 10.3.3 Transdural Posterior Approach

If desired, using an appropriately small caliber needle (21–22 G) and CT guidance, the disc space can be accessed from a posterior transdural approach at the lower lumbar levels, below the position of the conus medullaris. This access is feasible with straight needles when local anatomy permits an axial oblique plane parallel to the disc space passing through the interlaminar space. At certain levels, and in

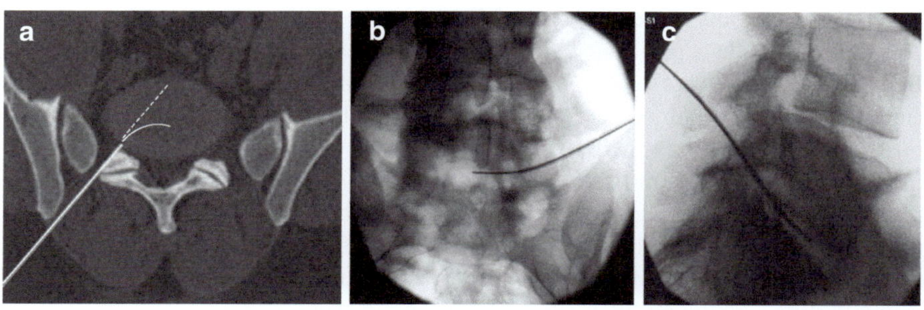

**Fig. 10.5** Coaxial curved needle access to the L5–S1 disc. In certain patients, the degree of lateral obliquity of the access to the L5–S1 disc is limited by the iliac crest, as shown by an oblique axial CT view through the disc space (**a**). In such cases, it is possible to reach the center of the nucleus pulposus using a coaxial system; a straight cannula is brought to the annulus, and exchanged with a K-wire; then a curved tip cannula is brought to the annulus along the K-wire; the K-wire is retracted, and the curved tip of the cannula is deployed, advanced, and directed to the center of the nucleus pulposus, as shown on **b**, **c**

certain patients, the oblique plane passing through the disc space corresponds posteriorly to the bony laminae, which would clearly obstruct the needle path. The path of the needle is just lateral to midline where the spinous process is, entering the central canal through the ligamentum flavum, piercing the dura along the posterior and anterior aspect of the dural sac, and thereby entering the disc from the posterior longitudinal ligament. The nerve roots of the cauda equina easily allow this needle access, when performed gently. Although this is a potentially easy and effective access to the center of the nucleus pulposus in selected instances, it carries additional risks of cerebrospinal fluid leak and headache, cerebrospinal fluid infection, and epidural hematoma.

### 10.3.4 Approach to Cervical Discs

The procedure is performed under fluoroscopy using a C-arm unit, with the patient placed in supine position, and using an anterior approach. The procedure is usually conducted under general anesthesia, although it is also doable under local anesthesia with sedation as necessary, particularly in fragile patients. The head and neck are slightly hyperextended to facilitate access to the cervical discs. For better visualization of the lower cervical discs, it is beneficial to stabilize the shoulders. In these cases, traction is achieved by tying a belt to the patient's wrists, and the belt is fixed to the foot of the table and pulled, if necessary, during the procedure to uncover the lower discs from the shoulders. The entry point for the port cannula is placed off-midline toward the patient's right side in order to make an anterolateral approach. Local anesthetic is administered using a 22-G needle and inserted as deep as the annulus fibrosus; the anesthesia needle is positioned using an extended holder to reduce x-ray exposure to the surgeon's hands (Fig. 10.6). While palpating vital structures away from the surgical pathway (the trachea is pushed across the midline, while the neurovascular bundle, the carotid artery in particular, and sternocleidomastoid muscle are maneuvered laterally and protected manually) (Fig. 10.7), a 18- or 19-G needle is positioned against the anterior surface of the annulus fibrosus. Because the esophagus resides to the left of the midline, a relatively more right-sided approach is deemed safer at the more caudal cervical levels. The C-arm is positioned to gain a lateral view of the surgical field and the needle advanced under fluoroscopic guidance into the disc. The mandrel is withdrawn and the needle is replaced, by means of a guide wire of proper size, by the cannula needed to introduce into the nucleus pulposus the desired device for disc decompression. At the end of the procedure, the cannula is removed and manual compression is applied for a few minutes on the surgical site to favor hemostasis. Alternatively, the surgeon could choose to position the cannula under CT guidance and switch to direct fluoroscopy for the remainder of the procedure. The use of CT allows a better control of the position of the decompressive device, particularly when it must be positioned inside the spinal canal or foramen for treatment of larger herniations (Figs. 10.8 and 10.9).

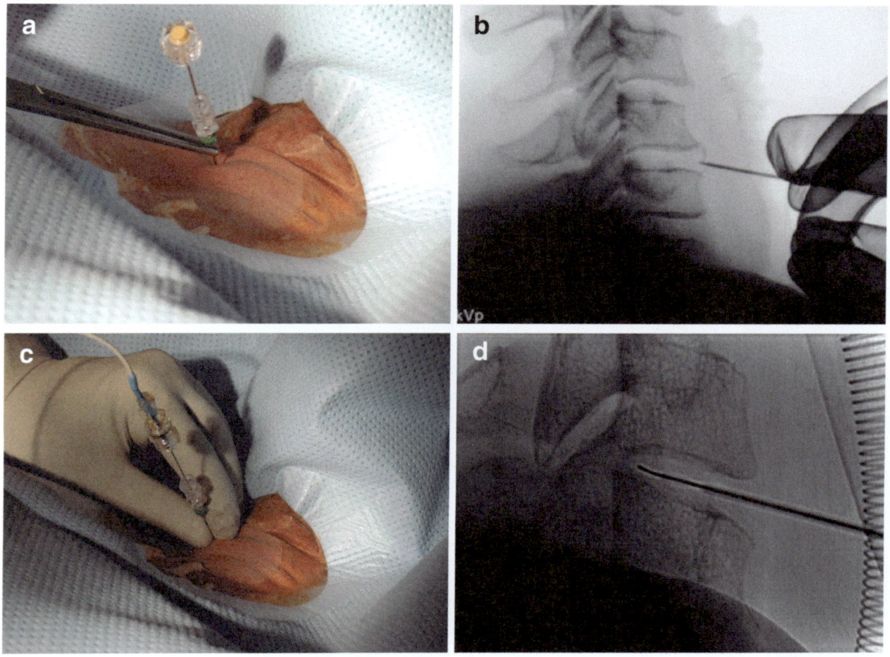


**Fig. 10.6** (**a**) The 19-G cannula with an internal mandrel is positioned against the anterior surface of the annulus fibrosus. The cannula is held by surgical forceps to minimize X-ray exposure of the surgeon's hand. (**b**) Cannula placement as observed under fluoroscopy. (**c**, **d**) The cannula is advanced into the disk, and the coblation probe is introduced into the nucleus pulposus via the cannula

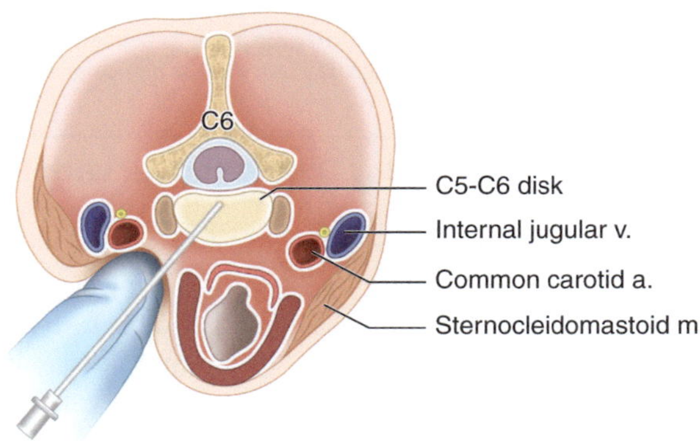


**Fig. 10.7** A schematic drawing shows the entry route, with the clinician's fingers pushing the trachea across the midline while protecting the neurovascular bundle

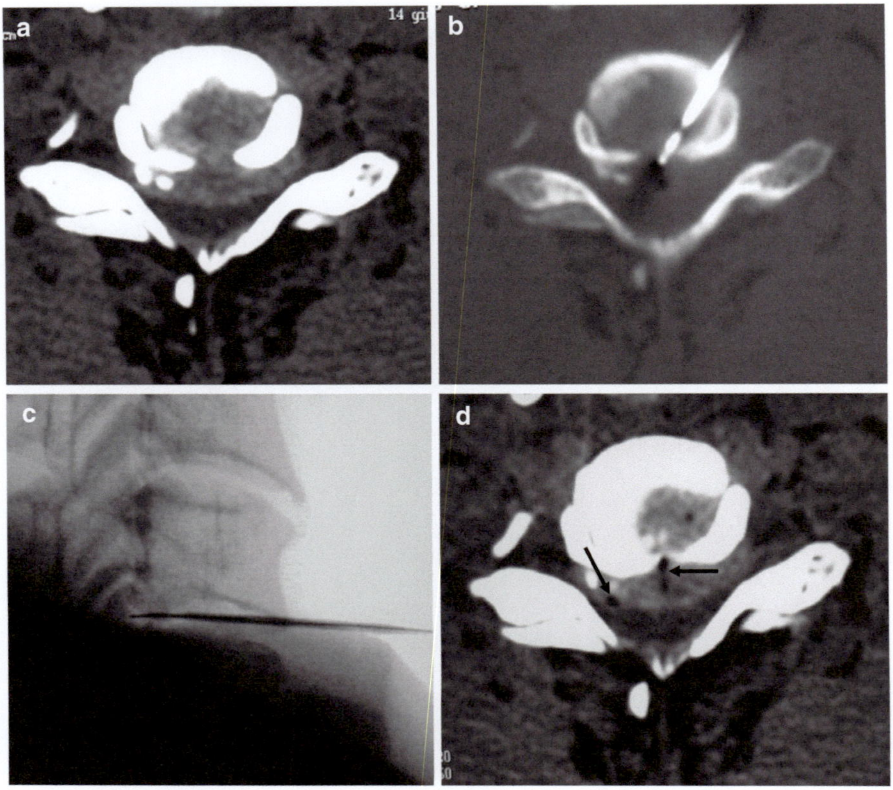

**Fig. 10.8** (**a**) Bilateral disk herniation at C6–C7 encroaching the spinal canal. The intervention was conducted under CT guidance for positioning the coblation bipolar probe, switching to direct fluoroscopy during the ablation procedure. This allows activation of the plasma-field energy directly inside the herniation. (**b**, **c**) The active electrode is beyond the posterior limit of the vertebral body, inside the spinal canal. In (**d**) the trajectory of the device and gas from tissue excision (arrows)

## 10.4 Techniques for Disc Removal with Physical Tools

### 10.4.1 Mechanical

In 1975, Hijikata [29], in Japan, published his results with a series of patients who underwent lumbar discectomy performed percutaneously. He used specially designed instruments placed through a 5-mm cannula inserted through the lateral annulus. A circular incision was made in the annulus, and the herniated disc material was grasped with modified pituitary-type rongeurs. In his initial published findings, Hijikata reported that approximately 80% of his patients experienced improvement after this procedure. Variations on this method have been subsequently popularized by Kambin [30, 31] in Philadelphia and Suezawa [32] in Switzerland. Using Craig-type biopsy instruments under fluoroscopic control, Kambin inserted a large trocar through the lateral annulus fibrosus, grasped the herniated disc, and removed it. He reported excellent results with no significant complications in 85%

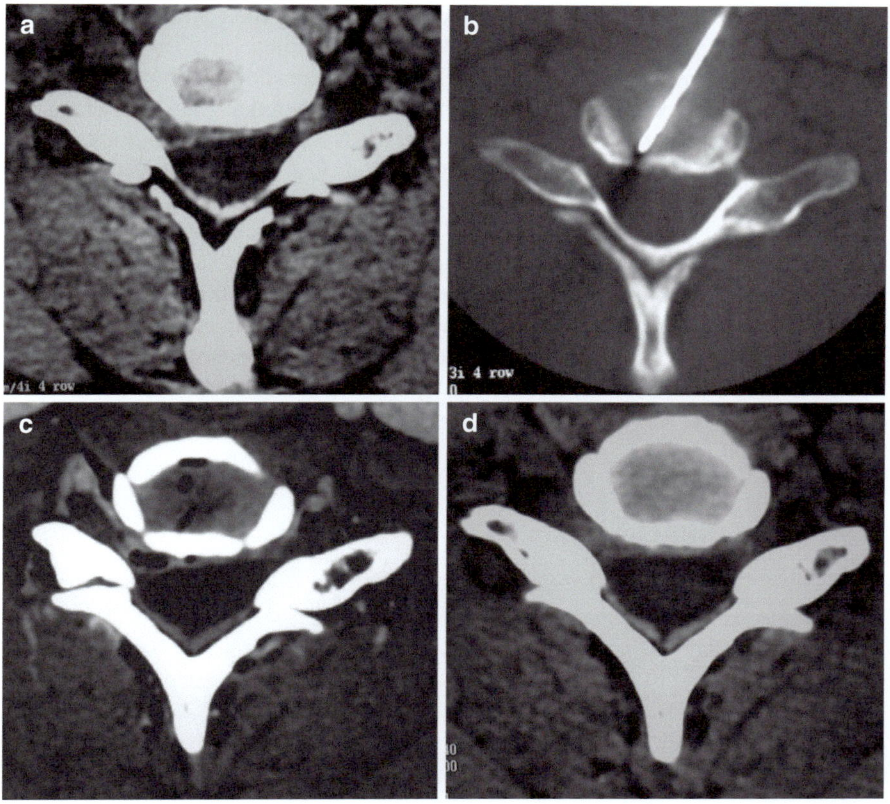


**Fig. 10.9** (**a**) Lateral disk herniation compressing the nerve root. (**b**) The cannula and coblation probe are positioned under CT guidance and then safely and precisely directed toward the herniation. (**c**) Note gas from tissue ablation diffusing inside the herniation itself. (**d**) A 4-month CT follow-up shows partial regression of the lesion; the patient reports a definite clinical improvement

of 50 patients. Suezawa used the instruments designed by Hijikata and in addition he inserted a discoscope through a contralateral approach. This was essentially a fiberoptic system used to visualize the disc material being removed. Excellent results were reported in 67% of 47 patients, although the majority of these patients showed complicating factors, such as spinal stenosis.

In another development, Jacobson [33], a neurosurgeon in Miami, designed his own instruments and used a direct lateral approach to remove herniated discs percutaneously in more than 300 patients. With the patient under general anesthesia, a 10- to 11-mm cannula was introduced through the lateral annulus. Using his own patented instruments, Jacobson grasped and removed disc material with overall good results in terms of pain relief. Unfortunately, unacceptable injury of bowel and peripheral nerves occurred. Friedman [8] studied Jacobson's technique in cadavers and demonstrated that the anatomical variations were such, that an unacceptably high rate of morbidity and potential mortality could be expected with this technique. Friedman therefore recommended against its use.

After surveying the previous techniques and assessing their potential problems, Gary Onik working with engineers from Surgical Dynamics, Inc., designed his own instruments for lumbar discectomy in 1984 and introduced it in clinical practice in 1985 [34–37]. The technique was called "automated" percutaneous lumbar discectomy because it involves a mechanical probe, the Nucleotome, which removes the nucleus pulposus by a "suction and cutting" action (Fig. 10.10). The device is now manufactured by Clarus Medical, LLC. The probe tip, excluding the handle, is 20.2 cm long and has an outer diameter of 2.2 mm. The negative pressure for aspiration is generated by the vacuum-generating console. A vacuum is created that draws nuclear material into the side port, which is located a few millimeters proximal to the distal tip of the probe. The cutting blade for fragmentation of nucleus pulposus aspirated through the port works with a reciprocal, not rotatory motion. This type of movement is a safety feature because the "guillotine" blade is contained within the

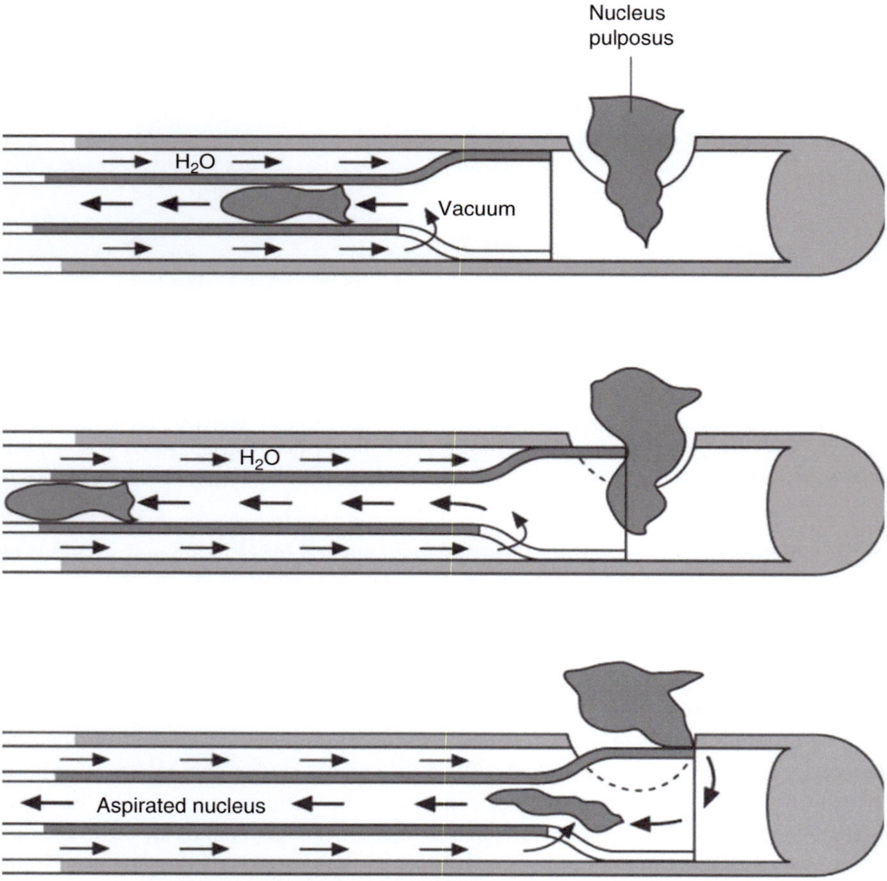




**Fig. 10.10** Onik's nucleotome mechanical aspiration probe, with its blunt, rounded tip. Internal irrigation and cutting functions are incorporated. The aspirated nucleus pulposus enters the side port and is resected by a pneumatically driven "guillotine blade," which has a reciprocal not rotary movement

probe. Consequently, only the nuclear material that is drawn into the port can be cut. The material aspirated from the inner disc and exiting through the metallic probe is ultimately deposited into a filter in a disposable collection bottle. The extracted nucleus pulposus is thus available for quantitative and macroscopic qualitative evaluation, or even for histology examination. A sequence of devices is used for introduction of the probe inside the disc, the last one being a cannula, straight with an outer diameter of 2.8 mm, or a curved one, with an outer diameter of 3.8 mm, better suited for access to the L5–S1 disc space, when the direct path from the skin is covered by the iliac crest. The reason for a larger diameter in the latter is that it is internally coated by a Teflon layer, which reduces friction and favors the sliding of the flexible but straight probe. APLD as proposed by Onik has lost the favor of most operators and discussion of the reasons of that falls beyond the limits of this chapter. One of the authors (GB) of this chapter has developed a large experience with very good results, depending on a strict and wise selection of patients, and still uses it in few, very selected cases [17]. In any case, Onik's remains the percutaneous procedure that removes the largest amounts of nuclear material from within the intervertebral disc. Another advantage, when comparing APLD with physical techniques that blindly destroy the disc (such as laser, RF or coblation), is that the surgeon can verify directly and visually the quantity of disc material removed, as well as its "quality." The extracted nucleus pulposus can be observed as it passes through the transparent tubing that connects to the filter. How much nucleus is taken out and how degenerated it is, are important procedural and prognostic pieces of information. For example, viewing the quantity of removed nuclear tissue and comparing it with the amount that was anticipated to be extracted from interpreting the preoperative imaging provide critical information to determine whether the probe worked in the correct intranuclear location. Observing blood coming from the disc could suggest the presence of unexpected degeneration, or of painful granulation tissue inside the disc, or prompt arrest of the procedure so as not to damage the endplate cartilage. Another important safety feature is that, once the Nucleotome is safely within the disc, it is unable, unlike other devices, to cut its way out of the disc space to cause injury to vital structures.

The notion that Onik's proposal was meritorious is suggested by the recent resurgence of new devices designed to mechanically remove the nucleus pulposus in an "automated" mode by aspiration. Observational studies are available, together with four RCTs [38–41]. In a review published in 2009, the level of evidence for clinical effectiveness of APLD, as determined based on the US Preventive Services Task Force (USPSTF) criteria [42], using five levels, ranging from I to III with three subcategories in level II, is level II-2 for short- and long-term relief [43]. This review was updated in 2013 [44], and the indicated evidence was considered limited for short- and long-term relief. However, APLD does not appear to compare favorably against chymopapain injection and open discectomy [39, 41].

A similar hydraulic aspiration principle is utilized by the SpineJet probe, produced by HydroCision. The disposable SpineJet probe simultaneously cuts and aspirates nucleus; a round atraumatic tip design reduces risks of annular puncture and endplate damage. The SpineJet HydroSurgery system utilizes a reusable power console with foot pedal activation (Fig. 10.11). Both the Nucleotome and the

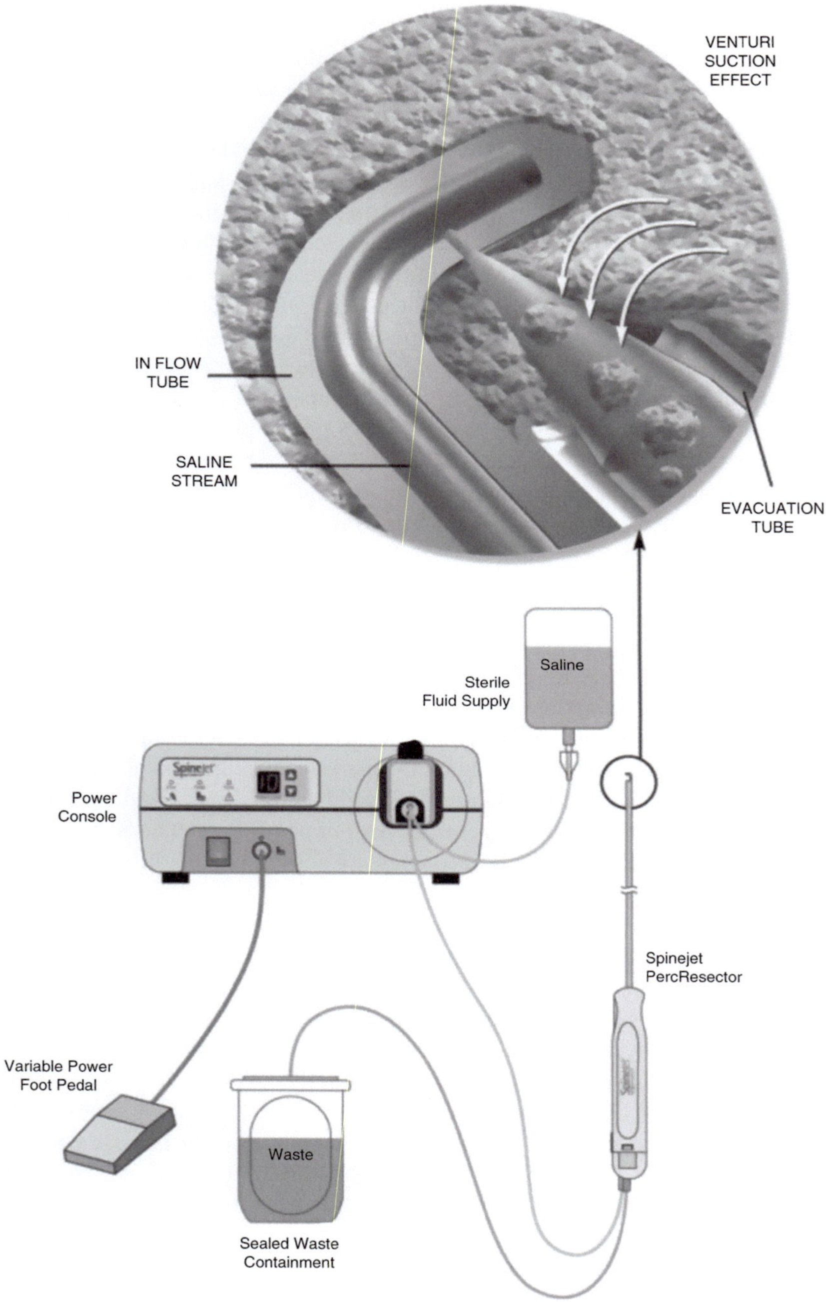


**Fig. 10.11** The SpineJet HydroDiscectomy mechanical aspiration system; the nucleus pulposus is fragmented by the high-speed water jet, while a Venturi suction effect aspirates and removes the fragments through the evacuation port and tube

SpineJet are fluid-based systems, that is, the inner disc material is hydrated while the probe's aspiration action is active for tissue removal: consequently, they can, unlike every other system (purely mechanical, thermal, laser, etc.), efficiently ablate tissue regardless of patient's age and disc hydration. Moreover, internal irrigation with sterile saline is a vehicle for easy aspiration, to prevent accumulation of nuclear material and consequent clogging inside the probe.

The Dekompressor, proposed by the Stryker Company in 2003 and now provided by other companies after patent expiration, is a single-use probe, introduced through a 15-mm cannula, intended for percutaneous discectomy in the lumbar, thoracic, and cervical spine. Under fluoroscopic imaging, the Dekompressor utilizes an Archimedes pump principle to remove nucleus material from the disc. The rotating screw blade is spun by a disposable rotational motor (Fig. 10.12). The single-use probe is smaller than Onik's Nucleotome or the SpineJet, with no need for a console or other external control to make it operate properly. It is also cheaper. Unlike the Nucleotome and the SpineJet, the Dekompressor does not entail a hydration of the inner disc to favor tissue removal (purely mechanical extraction), and the quantity of extracted nucleus material is significantly lower. Case series are available [45–49], although no controlled studies have to date been performed. The level of evidence for clinical effectiveness, based on USPSTF criteria [42], is level III for short- and long-term relief [50]. In a new review of 2013 [51], only five studies were considered for inclusion; of those, only three met inclusion criteria. Based on USPSTF criteria, the level of evidence for PDD with Dekompressor is considered limited. Recently Amoretti et al. published a favorable series in patients treated under CT guidance [52].

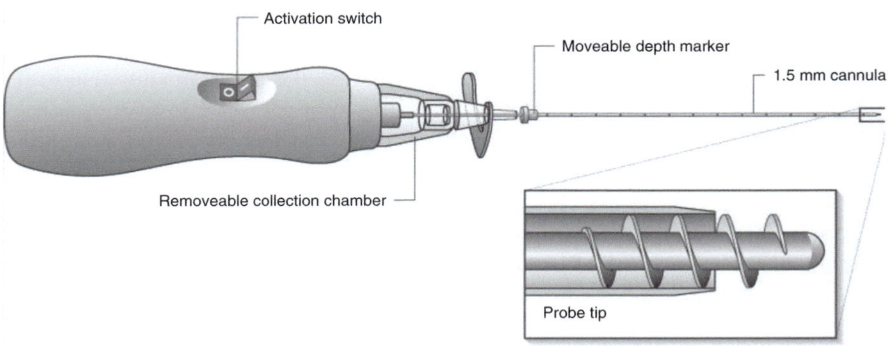




**Fig. 10.12** The Stryker Lumbar Dekompressor single-use aspiration probe; the rotating, helical screw blade carves the nucleus pulposus and pushes it inside the cannula and through it up to the clear collection chamber for visual monitoring of the extracted material. Approximately 1 cc of tissue has been removed once the tissue becomes visible at the collection chamber entrance. This material can then be collected and sent for examination

### 10.4.2 RF Thermal Ablation

The use of thermal energy to modulate and ablate tissue is not new. Electrical current, in one form or another, has been applied to human tissues as a surgical modality for more than 100 years. RF energy occupies a range upon the electromagnetic radiation spectrum. The frequency at which the device operates determines the absorption characteristics and tissue effects. Electrosurgical units based on standard monopolar or bipolar devices generally operate from 200 to 500 kHz, and they are limitedly applied or avoided to prevent unwanted tissue destruction. Devices operating in this frequency range cause the electrode that comes in contact with the tissue to become hot, therefore acting like true heat cautery. RF in the radio wave range (between 1.7 and 4.0 MHz) of the radiation spectrum emits energy that is nonthermal with optimal controlled absorption characteristics of water-rich tissues, with minimal tissue alteration. High-frequency radiosurgery, above 1500 kHz (1.5 MHz), transmits pure radio waves to the tissue without heating the electrode. The heat for this ablation is generated by a natural resistance of the tissue, which comes in the path of the waves released through the electrode tip of the device. The cellular water in the soft tissues gets heated and when the temperature reaches 100 °C, it starts boiling, and produces steam, which results in cellular molecular dissolution of individual tissue cells. The cells exposed to these waves are destroyed whereas the surrounding tissues remain unaffected. This property of radiofrequencies eliminates the possibility of undesired damage to the normal tissues, while improving the surgical precision.

The Disc-FX discectomy system is proposed by elliquence, LLC, formerly Ellman Innovations, LLC, New York. It works in bipolar mode at 1.7 MHz. In particular, the Bipolar Trigger-Flex probe is used to obtain a radio wave energy application both for removal of nucleus material and a modulation of weak collagen fibrils and sealing of annular tears (shrinking or eliminating defects in the annulus) and contributing to depopulating nerve fibers sensitizing the outer annulus due to its smooth thermal effect.

The two different effects in the nucleus (ablation for decompression) and in the annulus (annulus modulation) are obtained by means of two different waveforms generated by an external source; the ablation in the nucleus is achieved using a more aggressive waveform, called "Bipolar Turbo," the modulation of the annulus using a smoother waveform "called Bipolar Hemo."

The Bipolar Trigger-Flex probe is flexible and steerable (Fig. 10.13), and consequently can be oriented to operate either in the nucleus or along the posterior annulus. At the same time, the flexible probe allows a more targeted removal of the protruding nucleus, thus relieving tension on the innervated and irritated annulus. The action of the probe on the posterior annulus and its nerve fibers should allow treatments also of patients suffering from purely discogenic back pain.

No RCTs have been published in the literature. Two small observational studies are available [53, 54].

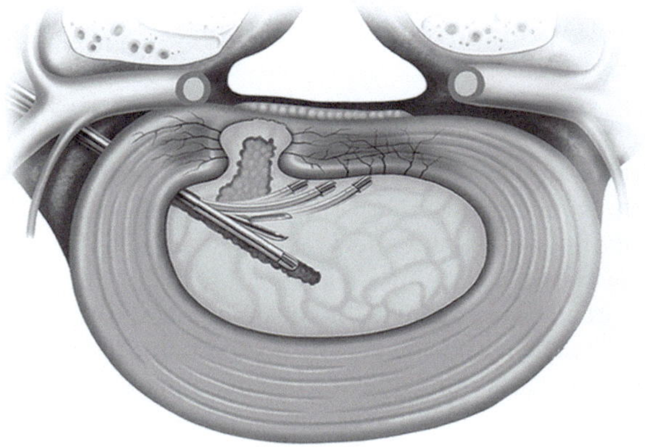

**Fig. 10.13** A schematic drawing of the action of the Disc-FX thermal-radiofrequency device; the steerable probe allows topographic nuclear material removal at the site of internal annular disruption and thermal modulation of the nerve fibers in the posterior annulus, using a less aggressive waveform

### 10.4.3 Coblation

Coblation, or plasma RF-based discectomy, with commercial name Nucleoplasty (ArthroCare, Sunnyvale, CA, now Smith & Nephew), was approved for general use in 1999 and initially used to treat symptomatic contained protrusion in the lumbar spine, subsequently proposed and used also for treatment of cervical herniations. It is a controlled, non-heat-driven, process, which uses radiofrequency energy to excite the electrolytes in a conductive medium. It is conducted by using a bipolar radiofrequency-based device, which functions via a plasma-mediated process [55–57], to perform precise removal of disc tissue. In this process, bipolar voltage pulses at 100 kHz are applied to the active electrode at the distal end of the device, which produces a strong electric field region around the electrode. The electrolytes in the surrounding conductive medium (e.g., sodium ions resident within the nucleus pulposus) respond to the electric fields, and if the voltage is sufficiently large, a localized finely focused plasma field (ionized vapor) is produced between the electrode and adjacent tissue [22, 58]. The plasma field (a layer of only 100–200 μm thick) around the active electrode comprises a complex mixture of gas phase radical chemically reactive and nonreactive molecules and a very small fraction of ionized particles (predominately positive ions and electrons), some of which can break molecular bonds in the adjacent tissue by energetic particle bombardment and chemical reactions. The organic molecules in the disc material (particularly long-chain molecules such as collagen) are thought to be susceptible to fragmentation by the plasma particles, resulting in their conversion into liquid and gaseous products that are subsequently desorbed from the targeted site. Water molecules (which compose a significant fraction of most types of tissue) can be fragmented into excited and ground state hydroxyl radicals and hydrogen atoms. Both of these species are chemically active and can cleave long-chain molecules (e.g., collagen) into smaller fragments that are either more easily liquefied or gasified. Moreover, electrons emitted from the electrodes at the distal end of the device when the voltage is applied can develop sufficiently high energies not only to cause the water molecules to fragment but also to directly dissociate the chemical bonds in the nearby targeted tissue structures (in our case disc tissue) into smaller fragments [57]. The net result is a reduction of soft-tissue volume and effective excision of the soft tissues within the nucleus. The plasma radiofrequency-based process has been reported to have minimal histopathological effect on tissues immediately adjacent to the treated site [22, 58], particularly annulus, endplates, neural elements, and nerve roots [58]. Because radiofrequency current does not pass directly through tissue during the coblation process, tissue heating is minimal. Most of the heat is consumed in the plasma layer or, in other words, by the ionization process. The temperature is kept below 70 °C (typically between 40 and 70 °C) to minimize tissue damage and avoid tissue charring. Because of the mechanism of action on hydrated nuclear components, tissue ablation and consequently intradiscal decompression are supposedly higher in younger patients and in hydrated, non-advanced degenerated disks [22]. In fact, an exclusion criterion for lumbar nucleoplasty must be considered a disc height less than 50% [59]. Action of coblation on disc tissues and nuclear herniations seems not only mechanical (in terms of tissue removal and intradiscal pressure reduction) but also chemical. Symptoms of herniations are not only a consequence of pressure against the nerve roots, since inflammation may well be a major mechanism in the pathophysiology of radicular pain, mainly as a result of injury or exposure of nervous tissue to nucleus pulposus material [60]. Alterations in cytokine expression potentially associated with the mechanism of pain relief have been observed after plasma radiofrequency-based discectomy [61]. Moreover, coblation appears to effectively degrade the PLA2 activity in the degenerative intervertebral disks in an animal model, and also this might contribute to reduction of inflammation and thus represent a potential mechanism of action of coblation in relieving symptoms of disk herniations [62]. Thus, we could speculate that the final clinical effect of coblation is partially due to reduction of inflammatory response, never observed after mechanical nucleotomy in our experience. This anti-inflammatory mode of action, stimulated by the plasma radiofrequency-based treatment, would be similar to that proposed with treatment of other chronic pathology [63] (Fig. 10.14). The coblation probe is introduced through a very thin, 17 G cannula (Fig. 10.15), probably the narrower among nonchemical procedures, laser excepted. This also allows for bending of the cannula and probe, for access to difficult L5–S1 levels (Fig. 10.5).

A large experience is available, and since 2000, many tenths thousands of patients have been treated using coblation technique for lumbar disco-radicular pain, and many observational studies are available [27, 64–75]. A randomized controlled trial was published in 2010 [76], comprising 90 patients who had sciatica associated with a single-level lumbar contained disc herniation, randomly assigned to receive nucleoplasty or transforaminal injection; nucleoplasty patients had significantly reduced pain and better quality of life scores, and significantly lower likelihood to undergo a secondary surgical procedure. In a review article published in 2009 [77],

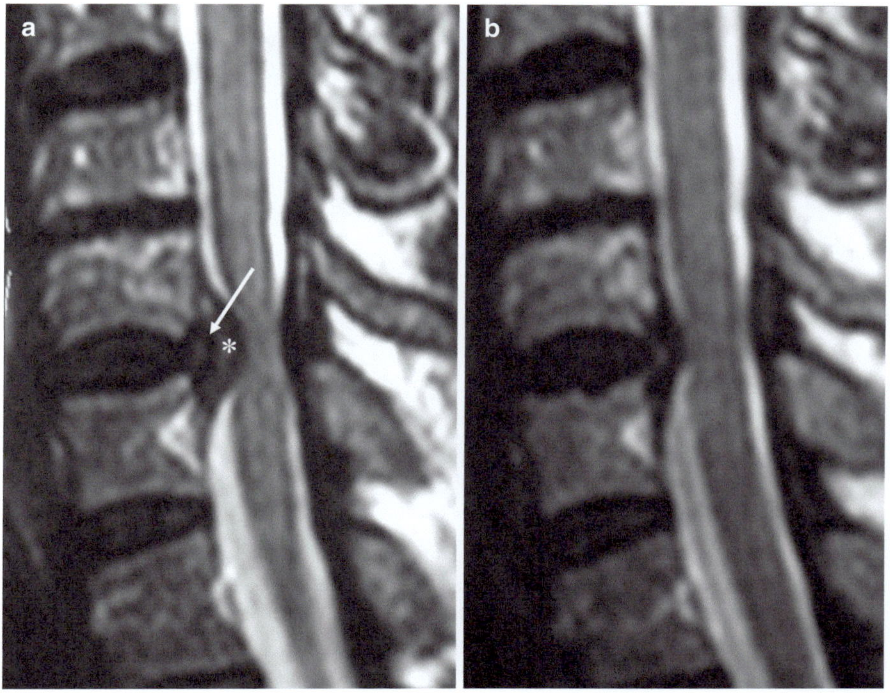


**Fig. 10.14** (**a**) 58-year-old female patient. Magnetic resonance imaging shows a contained central disk (C5–C6) herniation. Compression of the spinal cord is also due to a heavy inflammatory reaction swelling the epidural space (asterisk). In (**b**) imaging follow-up at 6-month post-coblation shows almost complete regression of both herniation and inflammatory epidural reaction; spinal cord is no longer compressed; patient is totally asymptomatic

the level of evidence for clinical effectiveness, based on USPSTF criteria [42], was level II-3 in managing predominantly lower limb radicular pain, with no evidence for axial back pain. In an update of 2013 [78], 37 studies were considered for inclusion; based on USPSTF criteria [42], the level of evidence for nucleoplasty was limited to fair in managing radicular pain due to contained disc herniation. In a 2014 systematic review and meta-analysis [79] examining all study data published in clinical trials, conclusions state that nucleoplasty reduces pain in the long term and improves patients' functional mobility, being an effective, low-complication, minimally invasive procedure used to treat disc herniations.

Three randomized controlled trials are available in the literature for cervical nucleoplasty. A study by Nardi et al. [80] showed complete resolution of symptoms in 80% of all cases ($n = 50$) at 60 days after nucleoplasty compared with only 20% in the control group ($n = 20$). Ten percent had no complete amelioration and

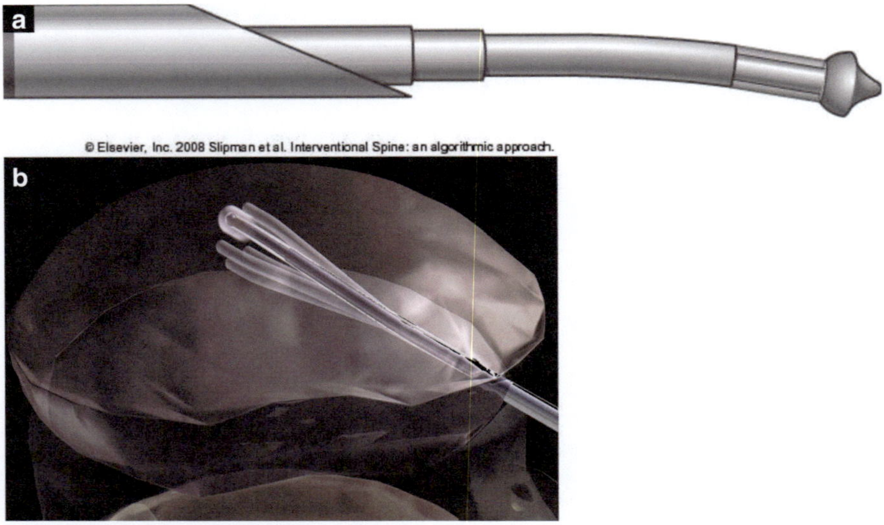


**Fig. 10.15** In (**a**) the active tip of the ArthroCare lumbar coblation probe is shown, introduced in the nucleus pulposus through a beveled 17 G needle; the slightly curved tip allows the creation of multiple coblation channels upon rotating the probe at multiple passes (**b**)

remained under clinical FU with a wait-and-see prospective. The remaining 10% without any clinical improvement were treated with alternative traditional methods. No complications were observed during the study. Overall, at a short term, the nucleoplasty group significantly improved from the baseline ($P \leq 0.001$), unlike the control group ($P = 0.172$). Birnbaum [81] compared 26 patients with a conservative care control group ($n = 30$). Nucleoplasty showed lower VAS pain scores compared with conservative treatment at short-, mid-, and long-term FU. The pain scores (VAS) in the nucleoplasty group were 8.8 (preoperatively), 2.0 (3 months), 2.7 (6 months), and 2.3 (24 months), respectively. No complications were observed during the study. Cesaroni et al. [82] compared 62 patients treated with nucleoplasty to a conservative care control group ($n = 58$). The nucleoplasty group had significant lower VAS pain scores at all FU time points ($P < 0.0001$). The Neck Disability Index (NDI) also improved significantly at 6 weeks ($P < 0.0001$) and 1 year FU ($P = 0.005$), and correspondingly, the SF-36 physical component summary (PCS) improved significantly at 6 weeks ($P = 0.004$), 3 months ($P = 0.0237$), and 1 year FU ($P = 0.0003$). No complications were observed during the study. Overall, the statistical analyses favor Nucleoplasty, mainly at short- and long-term FU. This study was appraised to be of high methodological quality [83]. One of the authors (GB) published a prospective study of nucleoplasty for cervical disc herniation [84]. At 2 months, outcomes were good or excellent in 44/55 (80%) patients; the success rate was similar at 6 months, when 44 (85%) patients ($n = 52/55$) had good or excellent results. Seven patients (14%) never showed improvement. One clinically relevant complication (infectious discitis) occurred, which was successfully resolved. Three patients with clinical myelopathy experienced regression of cord compression symptoms; in two of these patients, MR imaging showed morphological evidence of reduction of cord compression (Fig. 10.14).

A systematic review of cervical nucleoplasty for the herniated disc was published in 2014 and concluded nucleoplasty to be an effective and safe procedure at short-, mid-, and long-term follow-up, with level of evidence moderate [83]. Cervical coblation has been also proposed for treatment of vertigo [85].

### 10.4.4 Laser

Percutaneous laser disc decompression (PLDD) was introduced by Choy et al. [16, 85] in 1986. By 2002, more than 35,000 PLDDs had been performed [87]. The term laser is an acronym standing for light amplification by the stimulated emission of radiation. Laser is a form of light, and light is made up of electromagnetic energy. Laser energy is formed by energizing an active lasing medium. With the introduction of energy from an outside source, the atoms absorb the energy causing the electrons to rise to a higher excited state. When the electron returns to the normal, non-excited state, the energy initially absorbed is given off as a photon, and the photon bundle has unique properties characteristic to that particular medium. Lasers are generally classified according to the medium they use to produce the laser light. Solid state, gas, liquid, and semiconductor are all common types of lasers. The radiant energy of the laser beam can be transformed into heat energy that produces medical and surgical effects in tissue, such as coagulation, vaporization, or cutting. The total power output of a laser is measured in watts, the power density, measured in watts per square centimeter, and it determines the thermal effect in the target tissue; the energy density (measured in power density × time) of joules per square centimeter indicates the total amount of energy put into a given tissue. The majority of surgical lasers fall in the invisible portion of the electromagnetic radiation spectrum. The absorption characteristic of the medium largely determines the extent of penetration in particular tissue types. Application of any laser requires the surgeon to completely understand the characteristics of the specific laser for safe and effective use. The way in which light interacts with a substance largely depends upon its wavelength. Penetration depth at a certain wavelength is mostly affected by absorption by specific molecules, such as water (the principal component of the nucleus pulposus), hematoproteins, pigments, nucleic acids. As a laser is absorbed by the tissue, several surgical effects take place: at 60 °C protein denaturation and coagulation of blood vessels, near 100 °C evaporation of intracellular water causing shrinkage and tissue loss, beyond this point vaporization will occur. In general, the therapeutic effect of a laser significantly depends on penetration depth, in effect determining whether tissue removal or hemostasis will be predominant. Intradiscal decompression is obtained by shrinkage of the water-rich nucleus pulposus by vaporization. The evaporation of water and the increase in temperature cause protein denaturation and subsequent renaturation, causing a structural change of nucleus pulposus, limiting its capability to attract water [16, 87]. An increase of intradiscal volume of only 1.0 mL causes the intradiscal pressure to rise by as much

312 kPa or 2340 mmHg. On the other hand, a decrease of intradiscal volume causes a disproportionately large decrease of intradiscal pressure. Other beneficial effects of the laser action are postulated, such as shrinkage of collagen fibrils with reduction of disc volume [88, 89] and destruction of nociceptors in the annulus or in the granulation, vascularized tissue growing in degenerated discs. Many types of lasers have been reported in the literature for spine applications [90], including the following: Nd:YAG (whose active medium is a crystal of yttrium, aluminum, and garnet doped with neodymium ions, and whose beam is in the near-infrared) at 1054 nm and at 1320 nm, KTP (a beam generated by a neodymium:YAG laser is directed through a potassium titanyl phosphate crystal to produce a beam in the green visible spectrum) at 531 nm, $CO_2$ at 10,600 nm, Ho:YAG (YAG doped holmium) laser at 2100 nm, diode (semiconductor) laser at 810–890–940–980 nm. The Ho:YAG laser is better suited for open or endoscopic surgery, under direct visual control, because of the more mechanical effects and risk of endplate damage from energy scattering [91–93]. Yeung, Casper, Chiu, and Knight further report utility of Holmium laser to remodel extradiscal bony architecture during endoscopic spine surgery [93–95]. Nd:YAG at 1054 nm and KTP 532 are the most popular for intradiscal treatments [16, 96–100]. KTP lasers are similar to Nd:YAG lasers in both action and effects [101, 102], as are diode lasers [103]. The latter have the advantage of a much less expensive and less cumbersome power unit. The advantages of the 980 wavelength (peak absorption of water) of the diode laser are maximum absorption for well-hydrated, soft-tissue like the nucleus pulposus, with great thermal effect and consequent efficient shrinking effect [103, 104], with minimal thermal damage of surrounding tissues (particularly the endplates). Absorption by hemoglobin is lower than KTP 532 nm lasers, but they maintain an acceptable haemostatic effect.

The advantage of the laser discectomy is the tiny access port, the tiniest among the different percutaneous discectomy modalities. For the diode laser, the size of the optic fiber is as small as 220 μm, although the best compromise is obtained with the 360-μm probe (too high concentration of the delivered energy for the 220-μm fiber). Such small fiber sizes, which fits coaxially in 21-G cannulas, allow also a transcanalar/transdural approach to the disc, under CT guidance (personal experience) (Fig. 10.16). Nd:YAG laser fibers have usually a diameter of 400–600 μm. A series of pulsed shots with a maximum of 1-s duration (usually between 0.4 and 0.6 s) at no more than 15 W and at 2 s intervals are delivered to the nucleus pulposus. A minimal saline perfusion through the access cannula prevents the tissue temperature getting higher than 100 °C. No more than 1200 J (but better below 1000, usually between 600 and 800) as total dose are administered to the center of the nucleus pulposus, in two to three different positions of the fiber tip, always under fluoroscopic control of the proper position of the device.

The most frequently described complication of PLDD is spondylodiscitis both aseptic and septic [7, 105–110]. The reported frequency of discitis varies from 0% to 1.2% [105, 111–114]. Aseptic discitis is the result of heat damage to either the disc or the adjacent vertebral endplates [115].

Many observational studies report on the laser disc decompression results [7, 16, 86, 93, 97, 101–103, 105, 107, 109, 112, 113, 116–119]. Neuroradiologist Patrick

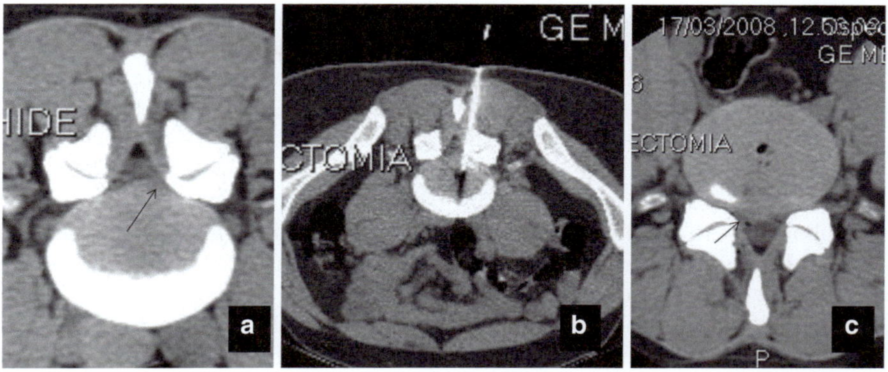


**Fig. 10.16** (**a**) Extruded disc compressing the thecal sac and occupying the radicular recess. (**b**) shows the CT-guided coaxial direct insertion of the laser fiber through a 21 G cannula into the herniation, through a translaminar and transdural approach; note in (**c**) the immediate reduction of the size of the herniation, with partial reopening of the radicular recess (arrow) and clear reduction of the mass effect on the thecal sac. Gas bubbles derive from laser tissue vaporization

Brouwer and coworkers published the first RCT on laser disc surgery in February 2015 [120]. They performed a non-inferiority trial comparing laser disc surgery with conventional disc surgery among 115 patients with a disc herniation, and laser disc decompression proved to be non-inferior to open disc surgery. There was a 38% reintervention rate in the laser group over the course of a year compared with a 16% reoperation rate among patients who underwent conventional discectomy. Overall, at 1 year, a strategy of PLDD, followed by surgery if needed, resulted in non-inferior outcomes compared with surgery. Similar results were found at a 2-year follow-up [121], surgery could be avoided in 48% of those patients that were originally candidates for surgery. A cost utility analysis of the same series [122] showed that PLDD, followed by surgery when needed, results in significantly lower 1-year costs than conventional surgery.

Using CT guidance, and thanks to the minimal size of the optical probe, laser has been also proposed for direct treatment of sequestered or migrated disc fragments [104, 123].

## 10.5 Complications

The main risks associated with these procedures are infection, bleeding, nerve root injury, thecal sac injury, disc endplate injury, injury to the retroperitoneal structures, and colonic perforation. Adherence to a safe technique will dramatically impact the outcome and the probability of realizing a side effect or complication. An incorrect projection means that the cannula and the intradiscal device are actually working away from the place where it is supposed to, not effectively operating on the nucleus or, worse, damaging vital or functionally important structures.

All percutaneous disc procedures harbor a significant risk of disc infection. Absolute contraindication to a disc procedure is local or significant systemic infection. We recommend absolute sterility of the procedure, with particular care in the prep and drape process, strict use of full drape, full gown, gloves, mask, and hat. In addition, we administer the patient an intravenous antibiotic 10 min prior to the procedure for prophylaxis, cefazoline 1 g intravenous, or, in case of allergy to penicillin, ciprofloxacin 400 mg intravenous.

Although there are different policies at different institutions [124], we set our threshold for a safe performance of an intradiscal procedure, to a minimum of 80,000 $mm^{-3}$ platelet count and 1.3 INR. We perform the procedure in patients treated with nonsteroidal anti-inflammatory drugs, including ASA, without special considerations. We recommend withholding the assumption of other anti-aggregants before the procedure, such as clopidogrel (7 days) and ticlopidine (14 days). In case of patients treated with low-molecular-weight heparin (LMWH), we perform the procedure at least 12 h (LMWH prophylaxis regimen) or 24 h (LMWH therapeutic regimen) after the last dose, and we recommend to withhold the LMWH for 24 h after the procedure. Patients treated with unfractionated SQ heparin less than 10,000 units daily can undergo spinal procedures, whereas patients treated with more than 10,000 units daily, and those who receive unfractionated intravenous heparin, can undergo a spinal procedure 4 h after the last dose, provided that the activated partial thromboplastin time is normal, and their heparin can be restarted as early as 1 h after the procedure.

The nerve root is not visualized under fluoroscopy, and this condition could carry the risk of injuring it while approaching the lumbar discs, particularly with the bulkier devices. With the posterolateral paravertebral access to the disc, the needle path is posteromedial to the exiting nerve root. To ensure safe disc access, the needle path has to be lateral but as tangent as possible to the superior articular process of the subjacent vertebral body and with a sufficient degree of obliquity, to avoid the nerve root. Because the radicular pain is a very effective "safety alarm," by no means local anesthesia should be delivered to the region of the neuroforamen. Otherwise, the operator might have the false reassurance of absence of radicular pain while injuring the nerve root. Local anesthetic should be injected to the skin and muscles only, keeping the injection superficial to the articular masses. For the same reason, we strongly recommend the performance of these procedures only under moderate conscious sedation and discourage the use of general anesthesia or heavy sedation. This does not apply to cervical procedures, since the anterior approach to the cervical discs does not cross the path of the roots.

An additional risk at the lumbar levels could be a colonic perforation. A posteriorly placed colon can reside behind the psoas muscle and the spine. For this reason, the preoperative imaging studies, both CT and MRI, must be carefully examined to exclude the presence of such an anatomical condition because bowel in the path of the instruments could be perforated, with the risk of peritoneal or disc infection or local abscess formation.

## 10.6 Postoperative Care and Follow-up

We routinely perform percutaneous procedures on an outpatient basis. At the conclusion of the procedure, observation is needed for about 2 h before discharging the patient home. Prescriptions are provided for a 2-week supply of a nonsteroidal anti-inflammatory agent and for diazepam at bedtime for 10–15 days.

At the end of the procedure, just before needle or cannula removal, we always inject steroids in the void created inside the disc. After nucleus ablation with physical energies (coblation, RF or laser), aspiration with a 20- to 50-mL syringe is needed before steroids injection, to eliminate the space-occupying gaseous or liquid residues. Injection of steroids is helpful in reducing the risk of an aseptic discitis consequent to inadvertent damage of the endplates, also reducing the back pain in the early post-discectomy period. Steroids have also a mild proteolytic and sclerosing action, which could help further reducing the disc volume in the postoperative period. Steroids and local anesthetics can also be injected, during needle removal, in the foramen, around the compressed nerve root.

Patients can stand and walk the same day of the procedure, and they are encouraged to actively move, stand, and walk on day 3. After percutaneous disc decompression, early activity is not only possible but also useful. It is imperative to avoid muscle atrophy and general deconditioning. Repetitive forward flexion, prolonged car driving, prolonged sitting, and lifting heavy weights are nevertheless prohibited for 3–4 weeks. Limb pain resolution may take weeks, owing to "remodeling" of the disc and regression of inflammation at the surgical site. The concept of disc remodeling must also be clarified to the patient. After decompression, reduction of profiles of the outer disc (annulus) is not immediate and is directly related to the residual tissue resilience, the latter depending on both the age of the patient and the pathologic conditions of the disc. Disc remodeling may be fast, taking hour or days, but also much slower, taking several weeks. Consequently, also nerve root decompression may be expected to take the same time lag, and the patient must be aware of that. A procedure that does not result in substantial relief of pain should not be considered a failure until at least 6 weeks have passed. Progressive return to heavy activities or sports is usually possible at 4–6 weeks. During the convalescence phase, rehabilitation measures applied by experienced physical therapists could be important for a good outcome. The patient must be instructed to recognize the difference between symptoms of a residual herniation and those of a healing process and proper biomechanics. The only noteworthy side effect is the possibility of increased back pain. Most patients with a surgical wound have pain and that applies to percutaneous discectomy. The intradiscal wound is more prominent and painful for mechanical procedure, particularly APLD, requiring a longer time for healing. Injury to skin, muscle, fascia, and annulus will occur, while a correct operative technique usually avoids injury to the endplates. Patients are warned that they may experience new back pain for up to 3–4 weeks. Patients should be encouraged to maintain as much mobility as possible despite the presence of this temporary back pain.

## References


1. Anderson GBJ. The epidemiology of spinal disorders. In: Frymoyer JW, editor. The adult spine. New York, NY: Raven Press; 1997.
2. Van de Velden J, de Bakker DH. Basis rapport: morbiditeit in de hui-sartsenpraktijk. Nivel: Utrecht; 1990.
3. Ohnmeiss DD, Vanharanta H, Ekholm J. Degree of disc disruption and lower extremity pain. Spine. 1997;22(14):1600–5.
4. Smith L, Garvin PJ, Gesler RM, Jennings RB. Enzyme dissolution of the nucleus pulposus. Nature. 1963;198:1311–2.
5. Simmons JW, Nordby EJ, Hadjipavlou AG. Chemonucleolysis: the state of the art. Eur Spine J. 2001;10(3):192–202.
6. Nordby EJ, Javid MJ. Continuing experience with chemonucleolysis. Mt Sinai J Med. 2000;67(4):311–3.
7. Choy DS. Percutaneous laser disc decompression (PLDD): twelve years' experience with 752 procedures in 518 patients. J Clin Laser Med Surg. 1998;16(6):325–31.
8. Friedman WA. Percutaneous discectomy: an alternative to chemonucleolysis? Neurosurgery. 1983;13(5):542–7.
9. Hijikata S, Yamagishi M, Nakayama T, Oomori K. Percutaneous nucleotomy: a new treatment method for lumbar disc herniation. J Toden Hosp. 1975;5:5–13.
10. Hijikata S. Percutaneous nucleotomy. A new concept technique and 12 years' experience. Clin Orthop Relat Res. 1989;238:9–23.
11. Kambin P, Gellmann H. Percutaneous lateral discectomy of the lumbar spine. A preliminary report. Clin Orthop. 1983;174:127–32.
12. Schreiber A, Suezawa Y. Transdiscoscopic percutaneous nucleotomy in disc herniation. Orthop Rev. 1986;15:75–8.
13. Yeung AT. The evolution of percutaneous spinal endoscopy and discectomy: state of the art. Mt Sinai J Med. 2000;67(4):327–32.
14. Kambin P, Brager MD. Percutaneous posterolateral discectomy. Anatomy and mechanism. Clin Orthop Relat Res. 1987;223:145–54.
15. Nerubay J, Caspi I, Levinkopf M, et al. Percutaneous laser nucleolysis of the intervertebral lumbar disc: an experimental study. Clin Orthop. 1997;337:42.
16. Choy DS, Michelsen J, Getrajdman G, Diwan S. Percutaneous laser disc decompression: an update–spring 1992. J Clin Laser Med Surg. 1992;10(3):177–84.
17. Bonaldi G. Automated percutaneous lumbar discectomy: technique, indications and clinical follow-up in over 1000 patients. Neuroradiology. 2003;45(10):735–43.
18. Komori H, Shinomiya K, Nakai O, Yamaura I, Takeda S, Furuya K. The natural history of herniated nucleus pulposus with radiculopathy. Spine. 1996;21(2):225–9.
19. Carragee EJ, Han MY, Suen PW, Kim D. Clinical outcomes after lumbar discectomy for sciatica: the effects of fragment type and annular competence. J Bone Joint Surg Am. 2003;85-A(1):102–8.
20. Milette PC. The proper terminology for reporting lumbar intervertebral disk disorders. AJNR Am J Neuroradiol. 1997;18(10):1859–66.
21. Fardon DF, Milette PC, Combined Task Forces of the North American Spine Society, American Society of Spine Radiology, and American Society of Neuroradiology. Nomenclature and classification of lumbar disc pathology. Recommendations of the combined task forces of the North American Spine Society, American Society of Spine Radiology, and American Society of Neuroradiology. Spine. 2001;26(5):E93–E113.
22. Chen YC, Lee SH, Chen D. Intradiscal pressure study of percutaneous disc decompression with nucleoplasty in human cadavers. Spine. 2003;28(7):661–5.
23. Castro WH, Jerosch J, Hepp R, Schulitz KP. Restriction of indication for automated percutaneous lumbar discectomy based on computed tomographic discography. Spine. 1992;17:1239–43.

24. Moon CT, Cho J, Chang SK. Availability of discographic computed tomography in automated percutaneous lumbar discectomy. J Korean Med Sci. 1995;10(5):368–72.
25. Dullerud R, Amundsen T, Lie H, Juel NG, Magnaes B. CT-diskography, diskomanometry and MR imaging as predictors of the outcome of lumbar percutaneous automated nucleotomy. Acta Radiol. 1995;36(6):613–9.
26. Onik GM. Percutaneous diskectomy in the treatment of herniated lumbar disks. Neuroimaging Clin N Am. 2000;10(3):597–607.
27. Sharps LS, Isaac Z. Percutaneous disc decompression using nucleoplasty. Pain Physician. 2002;5(2):121–6.
28. Onik GM, Helms C. Nuances in percutaneous discectomy. Radiol Clin N Am. 1998;36(3):523–32.
29. Hijikata S, Yamagishi M, Nakayama T, et al. Percutaneous discectomy: a new treatment method for lumbar disc herniation. J Toden Hosp. 1975;5:5.
30. Kambin P, Gellman H. Percutaneous lateral discectomy of the lumbar spine. A preliminary report. Clin Orthop. 1983;174:127.
31. Kambin P, Sampson S. Posterolateral percutaneous suction-excision of herniated lumbar intervertebral discs. Report of interim results. Clin Orthop Relat Res. 1986;207:37–43.
32. Suezawa Y, Jacob HA. Percutaneous nucleotomy. An alternative to spinal surgery. Arch Orthop Trauma Surg. 1986;105(5):287–95.
33. Jacobson S. Lumbar percutaneous diskectomy. Bull Hosp Jt Dis Orthop Inst. 1988;48(1):67–74.
34. Maroon JC, Onik G. Percutaneous automated discectomy: a new method for lumbar disc removal. Technical note. J Neurosurg. 1987;66(1):143–6.
35. Onik G, Helms CA, Ginsberg L, Hoaglund FT, Morris J. Percutaneous lumbar diskectomy using a new aspiration probe: porcine and cadaver model. Radiology. 1985;155(1):251–2.
36. Onik G, Helms CA, Ginsburg L, Hoaglund FT, Morris J. Percutaneous lumbar diskectomy using a new aspiration probe. AJR Am J Roentgenol. 1985;144(6):1137–40.
37. Onik GM, Morris J, Helms C, et al. Percutaneous lumbar discectomy using an aspiration probe: initial patient experience. Radiology. 1987;162:129.
38. Krugluger J, Knahr K. Chemonucleolysis and automated percutaneous discectomy–a prospective randomized comparison. Int Orthop. 2000;24(3):167–9.
39. Chatterjee S, Foy PM, Findlay GF. Report of a controlled clinical trial comparing automated percutaneous lumbar discectomy and micro-discectomy in the treatment of contained lumbar disc herniation. Spine. 1995;20(6):734–8.
40. Haines SJ, Jordan N, Boen JR, Nyman JA, Oldridge NB, Lindgren BR. LAPDOG/LEAPDOG investigators. Discectomy strategies for lumbar disc herniation: results of the LAPDOG trial. J Clin Neurosci. 2002;9(4):411–7.
41. Revel M, Payan C, Vallee C, et al. Automated percutaneous lumbar discectomy versus chemonucleolysis in the treatment of sciatica. A randomized multicenter trial. Spine. 1993;18(1):1–7.
42. Berg AO, Allan JD. Introducing the third US preventive services task force. Am J Prev Med. 2001;20(3 Suppl):3–4.
43. Hirsch JA, Singh V, Falco FJ, Benyamin RM, Manchikanti L. Automated percutaneous lumbar discectomy for the contained herniated lumbar disc: a systematic assessment of evidence. Pain Physician. 2009;12(3):601–20.
44. Manchikanti L, Singh V, Falco FJ, Calodney AK, Onyewu O, Helm S II, Benyamin RM, Hirsch JA. An updated review of automated percutaneous mechanical lumbar discectomy for the contained herniated lumbar disc. Pain Physician. 2013;16(2 Suppl):SE151–84.
45. Alò KM, Wright RE, Sutcliffe J, Brandt SA. Percutaneous lumbar discectomy: clinical response in an initial cohort of fifty consecutive patients with chronic radicular pain. Pain Pract. 2004;4(1):19–29.
46. Amoretti N, David P, Grimaud A, et al. Clinical follow-up of 50 patients treated by percutaneous lumbar discectomy. Clin Imaging. 2006;30(4):242–4.

47. Alò KM, Wright RE, Sutcliffe J, Brandt SA. Percutaneous lumbar discectomy: one-year follow-up in an initial cohort of fi fty consecutive patients with chronic radicular pain. Pain Pract. 2005;5(2):116–24.
48. Amoretti N, Huchot F, Flory P, Brunner P, Chevallier P, Bruneton JN. Percutaneous nucleotomy: preliminary communication on a decompression probe (Dekompressor) in percutaneous discectomy. Ten case reports. Clin Imaging. 2005;29(2):98–101.
49. Lierz P, Alo KM, Felleiter P. Percutaneous lumbar discectomy using the Dekompressor system under CT-control. Pain Pract. 2009;9(3):216–20.
50. Singh V, Benyamin RM, Datta S, Falco FJ, Helm S II, Manchikanti L. Systematic review of percutaneous lumbar mechanical disc decompression utilizing Dekompressor. Pain Physician. 2009;12(3):589–99.
51. Manchikanti L, Singh V, Calodney AK, Helm S II, Deer TR, Benyamin RM, Falco FJ, Hirsch JA. Percutaneous lumbar mechanical disc decompression utilizing Dekompressor: an update of current evidence. Pain Physician. 2013;16(2 Suppl):SE1–24.
52. Amoretti N, Gallo G, Nicolas S, Federico T, Theumann N, Guinebert S, Thouvenin Y, Cornelis F, Hauger O. Contained herniated lumbar disc: CT- and fluoroscopy-guided automated percutaneous discectomy-a revival. Semin Intervent Radiol. 2018;35(4):255–60.
53. Kumar N, Kumar A, Siddharth MS, Sambhav PS, Tan J. Annulo-nucleoplasty using disc-FX in the management of lumbar disc pathology: early results. Int J Spine Surg. 2014;1:8.
54. Kumar N, Zaw AS, Kumar N, Sonawane D, Hey HWD, Kumar A. Annulo-nucleoplasty using disc-Fx in the management of degenerative lumbar disc pathology: how long can the effect last? Global Spine J. 2018;8(4):365–73.
55. Woloszko J, Stalder KR, Brown IG. Plasma characteristics of repetitively pulsed electrical discharges in saline solutions used for surgical procedures. IEEE Trans Plasma Sci. 2002;30:1376–83.
56. Stalder KR, Woloszko J, Brown IG, et al. Repetitive plasma discharges in saline solutions. Appl Phys Lett. 2001;79:4503–5.
57. Stalder KR, McMillen DF, Woloszko J. Electrosurgical plasmas. J Phys D Appl Phys. 2005;38:1728–38.
58. Chen YC, Lee SH, Saenz Y, Lehman NL. Histologic findings of disc, end plate and neural elements after coblation of nucleus pulposus: an experimental nucleoplasty study. Spine J. 2003;3(6):466–70.
59. Derby R, Baker RM, Lee CH. Evidence-informed management of chronic low back pain with minimally invasive nuclear decompression. Spine J. 2008;8(1):150–9.
60. Kobayashi S, et al. Pathomechanisms of sciatica in lumbar disc herniation. Effect of periradicular adhesive tissue on electrophysiological values by an intraoperative straight leg raising test. Spine (Phila Pa 1976). 2010;35(22):2004–14.
61. O'Neill C, Liu J, Leibenberg E, Hu S, Deviren V, Tay B, Chin C, Lotz J. Percutaneous plasma decompression alters cytokine expression in injured porcine intervertebral discs. Spine J. 2004;4:115–8.
62. Ren D, Zhang Z, Sun T, Li F. Effect of percutaneous nucleoplasty with coblation on phospholipase A2 activity in the intervertebral disks of an animal model of intervertebral disk degeneration: a randomized controlled trial. J Orthop Surg Res. 2015;10:38.
63. Tasto JP, Cummings J, Medlock V, et al. Microtenotomy using a radiofrequency probe to treat lateral epicondylitis. Arthroscopy. 2005;21:851–60.
64. Singh V, Piryani C, Liao K. Role of percutaneous disc decompression using coblation in managing chronic discogenic low back pain: a prospective, observational study. Pain Physician. 2004;7:419–25.
65. Alexandre A, Coro L, Azuelos A, Pellone M. Percutaneous nucleoplasty for discoradicular conflict. Acta Neurochir Suppl. 2005;92:83–6.
66. Gerszten PC, Welch WC, King JT. Quality of life assessment in patients undergoing nucleoplasty-based percutaneous discectomy. J Neurosurg Spine. 2006;4:36–42.
67. Mirzai H, Tekin I, Yaman O, Bursali A. The results of nucleoplasty in patients with lumbar herniated disc: a prospective clinical study of 52 consecutive patients. Spine J. 2007;7:88–92.

68. Yakovlev A, Tamimi MA, Liang H, Eristavi M. Outcomes of percutaneous disc decompression utilizing nucleoplasty for the treatment of chronic discogenic pain. Pain Physician. 2007;10:319–27.
69. Al-Zain F, Lemcke J, Killeen T, Meier U, Eisenschenk A. Minimally invasive spinal surgery using nucleoplasty: a 1-year follow-up study. Acta Neurochir. 2008;150(12):1257–62.
70. Calisaneller T, Ozdemir O, Karadeli E, Altinors N. Six months post-operative clinical and 24 hour post-operative MRI examinations after nucleoplasty with radiofrequency energy. Acta Neurochir. 2007;149(5):495–500; discussion 500.
71. Kim SH, Kim SC, Cho KH. Clinical outcomes of percutaneous plasma disc coagulation therapy for lumbar herniated disc diseases. J Korean Neurosurg Soc. 2012;51:8–13.
72. Ren DJ, Liu XM, Du SY, Sun TS, Zhang ZC, Li F. Percutaneous nucleoplasty using coblation technique for the treatment of chronic nonspecific low back pain: 5-year follow-up results. Chin Med J. 2015;128(14):1893–7.
73. Cincu R, Lorente Fde A, Gomez J, Eiras J, Agrawal A. One decade follow up after nucleoplasty in the management of degenerative disc disease causing low back pain and radiculopathy. Asian J Neurosurg. 2015;10(1):21–5. https://doi.org/10.4103/1793-5482.151504.
74. Kumar NS, Shah SM, Tan BW, Juned S, Yao K. Discogenic axial back pain: is there a role for nucleoplasty? Asian Spine J. 2013;7(4):314–21. https://doi.org/10.4184/asj.2013.7.4.314.
75. Shabat S, David R, Folman Y. Nucleoplasty is effective in reducing both mechanical and radicular low back pain: a prospective study in 87 patients. J Spinal Disord Tech. 2012;25(6):329–32.
76. Gerszten PC, Smuck M, Rathmell JP, Simopoulos TT, Bhagia SM, Mocek CK, Crabtree T, Bloch DA, SPINE Study Group. Plasma disc decompression compared with fluoroscopy-guided transforaminal epidural steroid injections for symptomatic contained lumbar disc herniation: a prospective, randomized, controlled trial. J Neurosurg Spine. 2010;12(4):357–71.
77. Manchikanti L, Derby R, Benyamin RM, Helm S, Hirsch JA. A systematic review of mechanical lumbar disc decompression with nucleoplasty. Pain Phys. 2009;12:561–72.
78. Manchikanti L, Falco FJ, Benyamin RM, Caraway DL, Deer TR, Singh V, Hameed H, Hirsch JA. An update of the systematic assessment of mechanical lumbar disc decompression with nucleoplasty. Pain Physician. 2013;16(2 Suppl):SE25–54.
79. Eichen PM, Achilles N, Konig V, Mosges R, Hellmich M, Himpe B, Kirchner R. Nucleoplasty, a minimally invasive procedure for disc decompression: a systematic review and meta-analysis of published clinical studies. Pain Physician. 2014;17(2):E149–73. Review.
80. Nardi PV, Cabezas D, Cesaroni A. Percutaneous cervical nucleoplasty using coblation technology. Clinical results in fifty consecutive cases. Acta Neurochir Suppl. 2005;92:73–8.
81. Birnbaum K. Percutaneous cervical disc decompression. Surg Radiol Anat. 2009;31:379–87.
82. Cesaroni A, Nardi PV. Plasma disc decompression for contained cervical disc herniation: a randomized, controlled trial. Eur Spine J. 2010;19:477–86.
83. Wullems JA, Halim W, van der Weegen W. Current evidence of percutaneous nucleoplasty for the cervical herniated disk: a systematic review. Pain Pract. 2014;14(6):559–69.
84. Bonaldi G, Baruzzi F, Facchinetti A, Fachinetti P, Lunghi S. Plasma radio-frequency-based diskectomy for treatment of cervical herniated nucleus pulposus: feasibility, safety, and preliminary clinical results. AJNR Am J Neuroradiol. 2006;27(10):2104–11.
85. Yin HD, Zhang XM, Huang MG, Chen W, Song Y, Du QJ, Wu YN, Yang RB. Curative effect and mechanism of radiofrequency ablation nucleoplasty in the treatment of cervical vertigo. Br J Radiol. 2017;90(1072):20150772.
86. Choy DSJ, Case RB, Ascher PW. Percutaneous laser ablation of lumbar disc. Ann Meet Orthop Res Soc. 1987;1:19.
87. Choy DSJ. Percutaneous laser disc decompression: a practical guide. New York, NY: Springer; 2003.
88. Hellinger J. Technical aspects of the percutaneous cervical and lumbar laser-disc-decompression and -nucleotomy. Neurol Res. 1999;21(1):99–102.
89. Hilbert J, Brawn A, Papp J, et al. Erfahrungen mit der perkutanen Laserdiscudekom–pression bei lumbalem banscheibenschaden. Orthop Prax. 1995;31:217–21.

90. Camper D. Current concepts in minimally invasive approaches to treating the lumbar spine using laser energy. Oper Tech Sports Med. 1998;6(3):174–81.
91. Miriutora NF. Laser therapy in the treatment of discogenic neurological manifestations of spinal osteochondrosis. Vopr Kurortol Fizioter. 2000;3:30–3.
92. Hellinger J. Holmiun-YAG-assistierte offene nukleotomie. Laser Med Surg. 1995;11:86–7.
93. Casper GD. Results of a prospective clinical trial of the holmium-YAG laser disc decompression utilizing a side-firing fiber: four year follow-up (abstract). Fifth Intern Cong IMLAS. 1998;4:22–5.
94. Chiu JC. Endoscopic lumbar foraminoplasty. In: Kim D, Fessler R, Regan J, editors. Endoscopic spine surgery and instrumentation. New York, NY: Thieme Medical; 2004. p. 212–29.
95. Yeung AT, Yeung CA. Posterolateral selective endoscopic discectomy, the YESS technique. In: Kim D, Fessler R, Regan J, editors. Endoscopic spine surgery and instrumentation: percutaneous procedures. New York, NY: Thieme; 2005. p. 201–11.
96. Hellinger J, Linke R, Heller H. A biophysical explanation for Nd:YAG percutaneous laser disc decompression success. J Clin Laser Med Surg. 2001;19(5):235–8.
97. Brat H, Bouziane F, Lambert J, et al. CT guided percutaneous laser-disc-decompression (PLDD): prospective clinical outcome. Laser Med Sci. 2003;18(Suppl 2):16.
98. Turgut M, Açikgöz B, Kilinç K, Ozcan OE, Erbengi A. Effect of Nd:YAG laser on experimental disc degeneration. Part I. Biochemical and radio-graphical analysis. Acta Neurochir. 1996;138(11):1348–54.
99. Hellinger J, Stern S. Nonendoskopiche PLDN-Nd-YAG 1064nm-Eine 10-Jhres-bilanz als megastudie und metaanalyse. Dornier Med Tech. 2000;Newsletter:S2.
100. Choy DS, Ascher PW, Ranu HS, et al. Percutaneous laser disc decompression. A new therapeutic modality. Spine. 1992;17(8):949–56.
101. Knight M, Patko JA, Wan S. KTP 523 laser disc decompression—6 years experience (abstract). Sevilla: Fifth Intern Congress. IMLAS; 1998.
102. Liebler WA. Percutaneous laser disc nucleotomy. Clin Orthop Relat Res. 1995;310:58–66.
103. Paul M, Hellinger J. ND-YAG (1064) versus diode (940 nm) PLDN: a prospective randomized blinded study. In: Brock M, Schwarz W, Wille C, editors. Spinal surgery and related disciplines. Bologna: Monduzzi; 2000. p. 555–8.
104. Menchetti PPM, Longo L. Diode laser treatment of migrated disc-case report. Laser Med Sci. 2003;18(Suppl 2):S1–S29.
105. Gangi A, Dietemann JL, Ide C, Brunner P, Klinkert A, Warter JM. Percutaneous laser disk decompression under CT and fluoroscopic guidance: indications, technique, and clinical experience. Radiographics. 1996;16(1):89–96.
106. Steiner P, Zweifel K, Botnar R, et al. MR guidance of laser disc decompression: preliminary in vivo experience. Eur Radiol. 1998;8(4):592–7.
107. Schatz SW, Talalla A. Preliminary experience with percutaneous laser disc decompression in the treatment of sciatica. Can J Surg. 1995;38(5):432–6.
108. Ascher PW. Laser trends in minimally invasive treatment: atherosclerosis, disk herniations. J Clin Laser Med Surg. 1991;9(1):49–57.
109. Siebert WE, Berendsen BT, Tollgaard J. Percutaneous laser disk decompression. Experience since 1989. Orthopade. 1996;25(1):42–8.
110. Knight M, Goswami A. Lumbar percutaneous KTP532 wave-length laser disc decompression and disc ablation in the management of discogenic pain. J Clin Laser Med Surg. 2002;20(1):9–13; discussion 15.
111. Ohnmeiss DD, Guyer RD, Hochschuler SH. Laser disc decompression. The importance of proper patient selection. Spine. 1994;19(18):2054–8; discussion 2059.
112. Bosacco SJ, Bosacco DN, Berman AT, Cordover A, Levenberg RJ. Stellabo4e J. functional results of percutaneous laser discectomy. Am J Orthop. 1996;25(12):825–8.
113. Nerubay J, Caspi I, Levinkopf M. Percutaneous carbon dioxide laser nucleolysis with 2- to 5-year follow-up. Clin Orthop Relat Res. 1997;337:45–8.

114. Agarwal S, Bhagwat AS. Ho: Yag laser-assisted lumbar disc decompression: a minimally invasive procedure under local anesthesia. Neurol India. 2003;51(1):35–8.
115. Smuck M, Benny B, Han A, Levin J. Epidural fibrosis following percutaneous disc decompression with coblation technology. Pain Physician. 2007;10(5):691–6.
116. Menchetti PP, Canero G, Bini W. Percutaneous laser discectomy: experience and long term follow-up. Acta Neurochir Suppl. 2011;108:117–21.
117. Zhao XL, Fu ZJ, Xu YG, Zhao XJ, Song WG, Zheng H. Treatment of lumbar intervertebral disc herniation using C-arm fluoroscopy guided target percutaneous laser disc decompression. Photomed Laser Surg. 2012;30(2):92–5.
118. Ren L, Guo H, Zhang T, Han Z, Zhang L, Zeng Y. Efficacy evaluation of percutaneous laser disc decompression in the treatment of lumbar disc herniation. Photomed Laser Surg. 2013;31(4):174–8.
119. Erbas YC, Pusat S, Erdogan E. Percutaneous laser disc decompression: retrospective analysis of 197 cases and review of the literature. Turk Neurosurg. 2015;25(5):766–70.
120. Brouwer PA, Brand R, van den Akker-van Marle ME, Jacobs WC, Schenk B, van den Berg-Huijsmans AA, Koes BW, van Buchem MA, Arts MP, Peul WC. Percutaneous laser disc decompression versus conventional microdiscectomy in sciatica: a randomized controlled trial. Spine J. 2015;15(5):857–65.
121. Brouwer PA, Brand R, van den Akker-van Marle ME, Jacobs WC, Schenk B, van den Berg-Huijsmans AA, Koes BW, Arts MA, van Buchem MA, Peul WC. Percutaneous laser disc decompression versus conventional microdiscectomy for patients with sciatica: two-year results of a randomized controlled trial. Interv Neuroradiol. 2017;23(3):313–24.
122. van den Akker-van Marle ME, Brouwer PA, Brand R, Koes B, van den Hout WB, van Buchem MA, Peul WC. Percutaneous laser disc decompression versus microdiscectomy for sciatica: cost utility analysis alongside a randomized controlled trial. Interv Neuroradiol. 2017;23(5):538–45.
123. Bonaldi G, Brembilla C, Foresti C, Cianfoni A. Transarticular laser discal fragmentectomy. A new minimally invasive surgical approach for challenging disc herniations in the elderly. Interv Neuroradiol. 2014;20(5):555–63.
124. Layton KF, Kallmes DF, Horlocker TT. Recommendations for anti-coagulated patients undergoing image-guided spinal procedures. AJNR Am J Neuroradiol. 2006;27(3):468–70.

# Endoscopic Percutaneous Discectomy

# 11

Ali Guven Yorukoglu, Luigi Manfrè, and Altay Sencer

## 11.1 Introduction

Lumbar disc herniations, being the most common pathology in the lumbar spine, are a major cause of back pain as well as radiating leg pain. Statistics show that about 85% of population has experienced back pain with or without leg pain, at least once in their life [1–8]. A small but significant part of those patients with major or progressive neurologic problems like deteriorating neurologic deficits or symptoms of cauda/conus syndrome or who did not benefit from medical management are candidates for major or minor surgical procedures. Microsurgical discectomy is still accepted as the golden standard of surgical treatment. Nucleoplasties and foraminal injections, laser discectomies, and percutaneous endoscopic discectomies can be described as minor or minimally invasive surgical procedures [1–4, 9–17].

In the last three decades, minimally invasive endoscopic surgical techniques have been widely adopted in different fields of medicine, with the evolution and refinement of surgical endoscope. Minimally invasive procedures to lumbar spine date back to 1948, as Valls et al. described a percutaneous technique for aspiration biopsy in the diagnosis of vertebral body lesions [18]. In 1970s, Hijikata and Kambin, separately, defined a posterolateral approach for percutaneous central nucleotomy [6, 19]. After the first visualization of intervertebral disc space with a

A. G. Yorukoglu
RIWOspine GmbH, Knittlingen, Germany

Istanbul Spine Center, Florence Nightingale Hospital, Istanbul, Turkey
e-mail: ali-gueven.yoeruekoglu@riwospine.com

L. Manfrè
Minimal Invasive Spine Therapy Department, Mediterranean Institute of Oncology, Catania, Italy

A. Sencer (✉)
Department of Neurosurgery, Istanbul University Medical School, Istanbul, Turkey



L. Manfrè, J. Van Goethem (eds.), *The Disc and Degenerative Disc Disease*, New Procedures in Spinal Interventional Neuroradiology,
https://doi.org/10.1007/978-3-030-03715-4_11

modified arthroscope at the first half of 1980s, endoscopic lumbar discectomy techniques showed improvement [4, 20–24]. But introduction of surgical microscope into neurosurgery during this time period and its widely accepted use caused a slowdown or cessation in endoscopic neurosurgical procedures including endoscopic disc surgery. Descriptions of "Yeung Endoscopic Spine System (YESS)" by Yeung and full-endoscopic interlaminar technique by Ruetten mark the comeback of endoscopic disc surgery [25–27]. Today, providing higher postoperative patient comfort, endoscopic lumbar discectomy has become a significant alternative to conventional MD in the management of lumbar disc herniations.

Various techniques have been described, but mainly, minimally invasive endoscopic approaches to the lumbar spine can be classified into two major categories: transforaminal (TF) and interlaminar (IL). IL approaches can be summarized as endoscopy assisted techniques and full-endoscopic techniques. Endoscopy assisted IL approaches have been pioneered and popularized by Destandeu (also called after him) [16]. These systems have been further developed by various companies and are still used. But their main disadvantage is that the operation is performed not through the working channel of the endoscope but through tubular dilators, and the endoscope is used only for visualization, like the microscope. Therefore, these approaches called "endoscopy assisted" and, because the purpose of this chapter is to describe the fully endoscopic technique, they will not be mentioned further.

## 11.2 Indications and Standard Approaches

Common indications for full-endoscopic discectomy do not differ from the widely accepted indications of microdiscectomy [27–32]. Today, all kinds of lumbar disc herniations that need surgical treatment can be operated via using an operating microscope and can also be operated by percutaneous full-endoscopic approach; all lumbar levels, all locations from median to far-lateral and all types from protrusions to sequestered fragments. Therefore, indications for full-endoscopic discectomy will not be discussed here.

The choice between transforaminal and interlaminar approaches for full-endoscopic discectomy is based on the principles previously defined by Ruetten et al. [28, 33–35]. Transforaminal approach, providing direct access to the pathology (disc), is usually considered as first choice but because of anatomic limitations IL approach is recommended to be chosen in cases with the following criteria:

(a) When sequestering material is migrated beyond the lower edge of cranial pedicle or over the middle of the caudal pedicle.
(b) When foramen is overlaid by iliac crest on lateral plain radiographs.

The surgeon's experience and preference also play a major role in this decision (Figs. 11.1 and 11.2) [28, 33, 34].

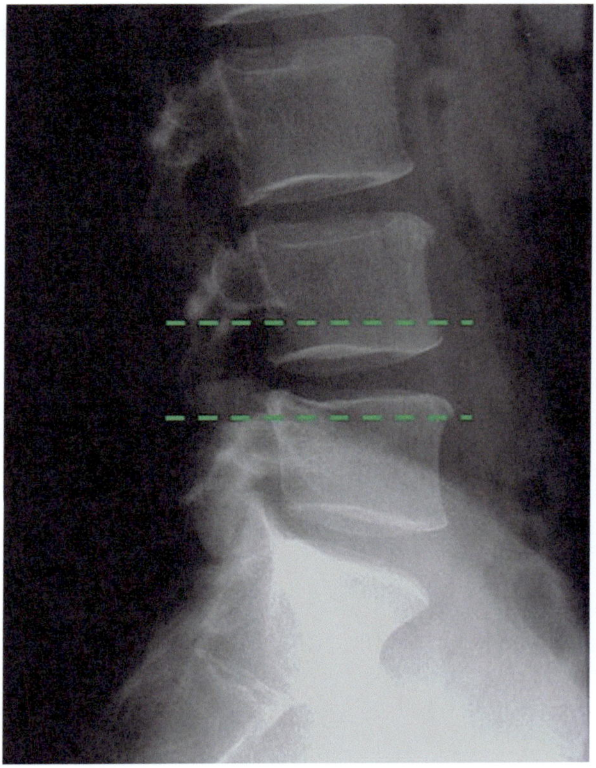

**Fig. 11.1** Easy access area with transforaminal approach

## 11.3 Surgical Techniques

### 11.3.1 Interlaminar (IL) Approach

For the comfort of the patient and surgeon, the operation is performed under general anesthesia, if there are no contraindications. The patient is placed on the operating table in prone position. Shoulders and pelvis are supported by gel cushions to relieve the pressure on the thorax and abdomen (Fig. 11.3). The spine may be slightly flexed for easier access into the interlaminar space. The C-arm is positioned under the radiolucent operating table allowing sterile biplanar X-ray.

Under fluoroscopic control, a skin incision (about 5 mm) is made slightly paramedian to the midline on targeted interlaminar space (actually, as close to midline as possible) and ideally, also through the muscle fascia (Figs. 11.4, 11.5, 11.6, and 11.7).

The dilator is bluntly inserted under fluoroscopic control to the lateral edge of the interlaminar space. An experienced surgeon can directly position the dilator on the lig. flavum, but for inexperienced surgeons, it is safer to head for facet joint and feel bony structures (Figs. 11.8 and 11.9).

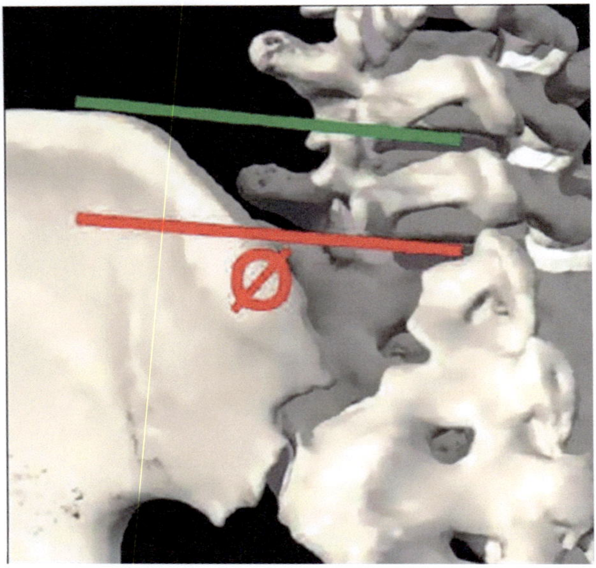

**Fig. 11.2** Iliac crest preventing direct access to L5–S1 (red line)

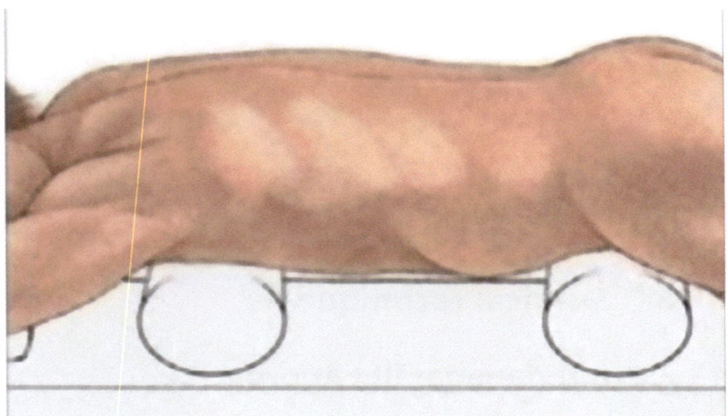

**Fig. 11.3** Patient positioning for IL and TF approaches

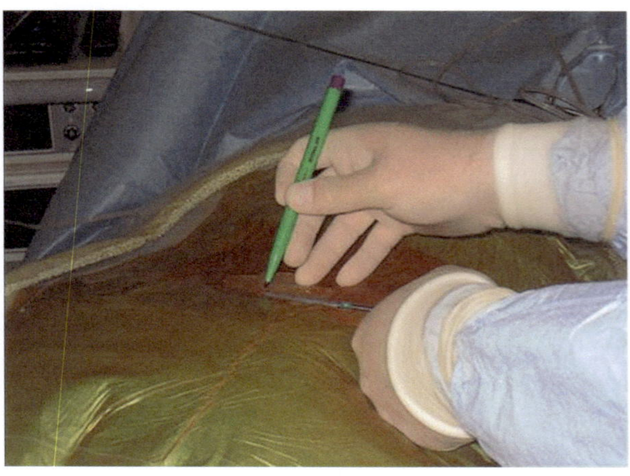

**Fig. 11.4** Marking of skin incision for IL approach

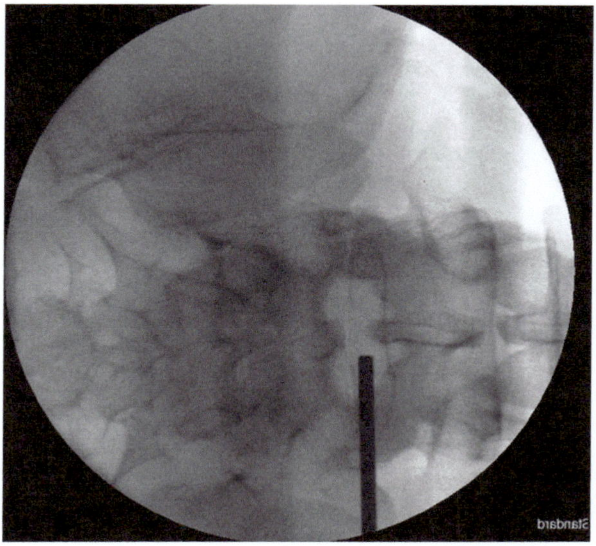


**Fig. 11.5** Ideal entry point from skin on X-ray

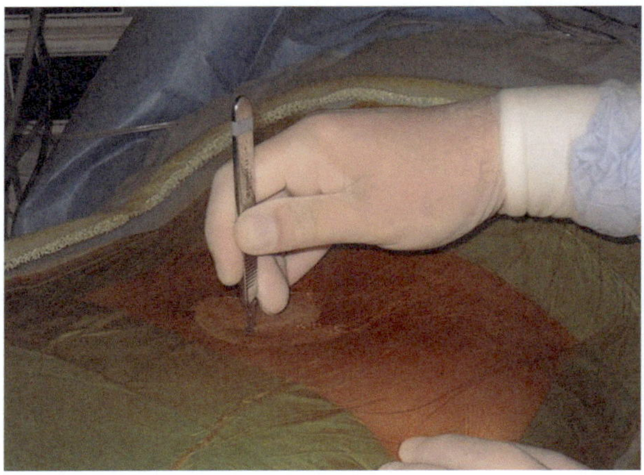

**Fig. 11.6** Making of skin incision

After lateral fluoroscopic control for the avoidance of uncontrolled direct spinal canal penetration through ligamentum (lig.) flavum, the working sleeve with the beveled opening is placed over the dilator with the opening pointing medially (Figs. 11.10, 11.11, and 11.12).

As the next step, dilator is removed, endoscope (usually, a 25° optic) is placed and the operation is continued under direct endoscopic view and continuous high-pressure saline irrigation (Fig. 11.13).

Following cauterization and removal of the surrounding soft tissues, mainly paraspinal muscle remnants, lig. flavum is exposed (Fig. 11.14). Usually, radiofrequency (RF) is used for coagulation; it is safe and effective.

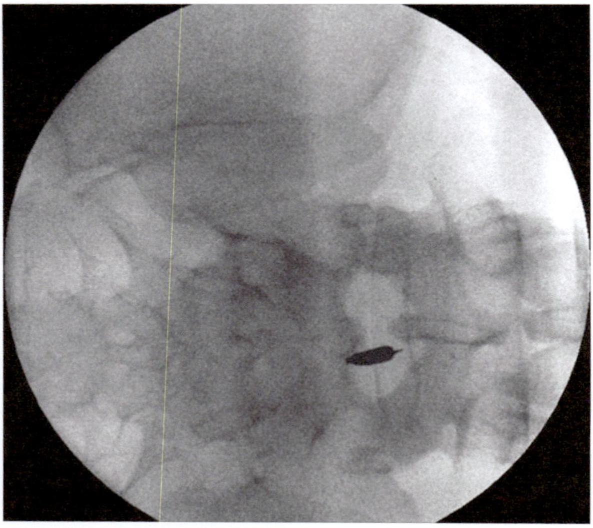

**Fig. 11.7** Making of skin incision (Fig. 11.6) ideally through fascia and its fluoroscopic control

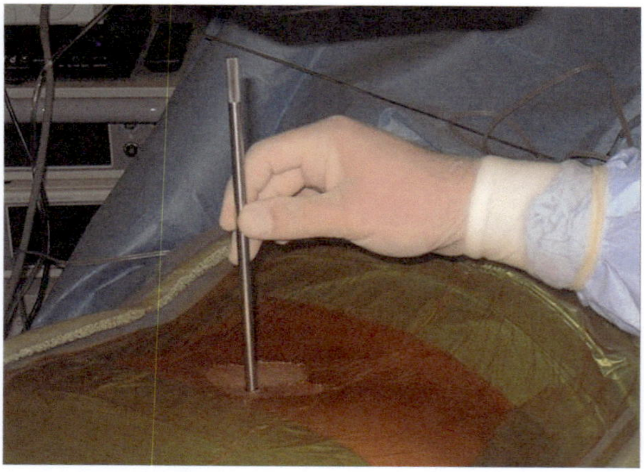

**Fig. 11.8** External view of inserted dilator pointing laterally

A 3–5 mm medial incision of the flavum is adequate. For an easy and safe incision into the ligament, working sheath must be pushed down against the ligament to keep it hard and stretched. After incising, the last layer of lig. flavum, usually a small space, is encountered just under the ligament. This space provides a safe zone when advancing the incision from medial to lateral by using the scissor. Incision should be advanced as laterally as possible to reach the lateral aspects of neural structures and if necessary, bone can be removed by drill or Kerrison rongeurs (Fig. 11.15). Care must be taken to make the first incision into ligament medially because later, if necessary, advancing the incision medially would be technically more challenging.

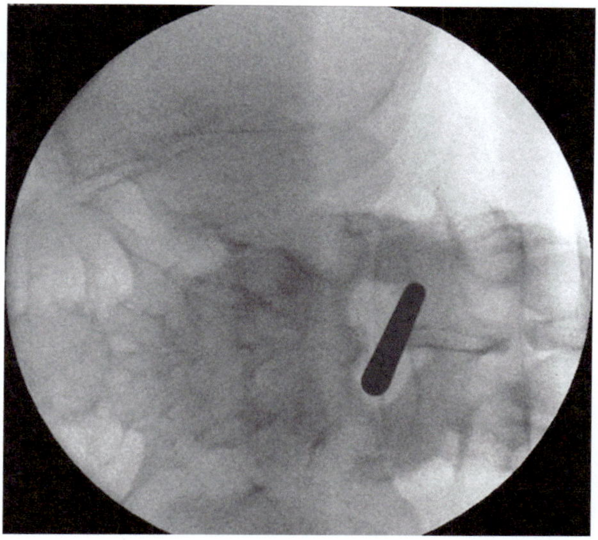

**Fig. 11.9** On X-ray, dilator is on lateral bony structures

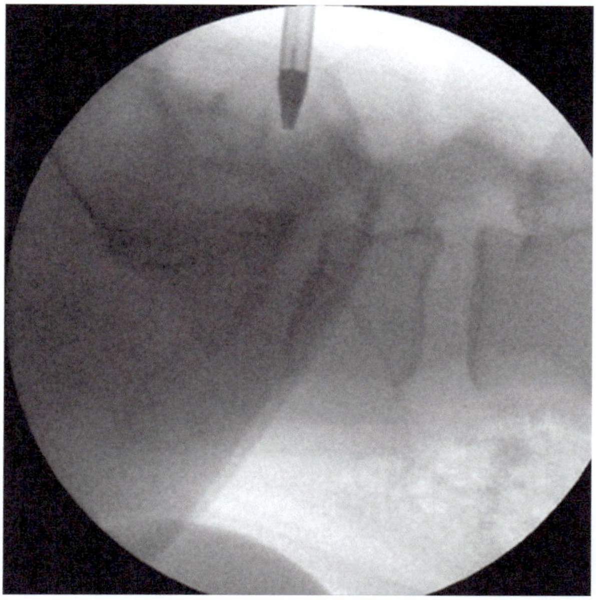

**Fig. 11.10** On the lateral X-ray view, dilator is seen just outside the spinal canal

After accessing the spinal canal and removal of epidural fat tissue, dura mater and nerve roots are visualized (Fig. 11.16).

Retracting nerve root medially by dissector, the beveled opening of the working sleeve is lowered through the incision in the ligament over dissector and rotated 180°, and in this way, the sleeve can be used as a nerve root retractor, retracting the root medially and exposing lateral epidural space and herniation (Fig. 11.17).

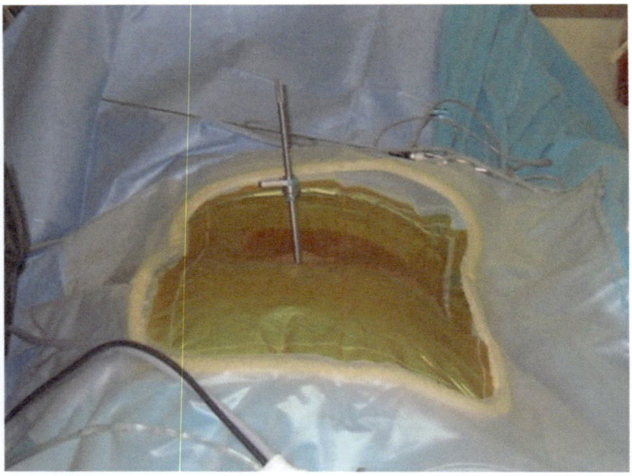

**Fig. 11.11** Insertion of beveled working sleeve

Following the cauterization of the epidural veins, discectomy is performed. After the pressure on the root and dural sac has been relieved, accessing the disc space and removal of the entire disc material is up to the surgeon's choice. When the surgeon is satisfied, the operation can be terminated by taking out the sheath and endoscope.

Use of working sleeve as retractor is rather safe and efficient, but in some cases, for example, if the fragment is very big or if it is located in the axilla, the surgeon may prefer not to lower the working sleeve into the epidural space and do an exploration first with help of dissector or RF probe.

A single suture may be necessary for skin closure. Compared to the TF approach, IL approach provides more mobile access, in which the surgeon can conduct the sleeve and endoscope cranially and caudally, and bony resection can be achieved as necessary with the help of drills to remove migrated fragments [25, 28, 33, 34, 36] (Figs. 11.18 and 11.19). Capture of C-arm images and recording of operation are recommended for educational and medicolegal purposes.

### 11.3.2 Transforaminal Approach (TF)

Usually, we prefer to perform TF approach also under general anesthesia. The patient's position is the same as described for IL approach (Fig. 11.3). Three slightly different techniques are described for TF approach:

#### 11.3.2.1 Posterolateral Transforaminal

In this technique, disc space is accessed by a 45° horizontal angle (Fig. 11.20). Incision is usually made 8 to 10 cm lateral to midline at the targeted disc level [26, 27, 37]. This technique provides adequate access into the disc space, but not to the posterior aspect of disc space, posterior longitudinal ligament (PLL), or anterior epidural space without extensive drilling of facet joint, a major disadvantage for most herniations. On the other hand, this approach is very useful for intradiscal pathologies, like discitis.

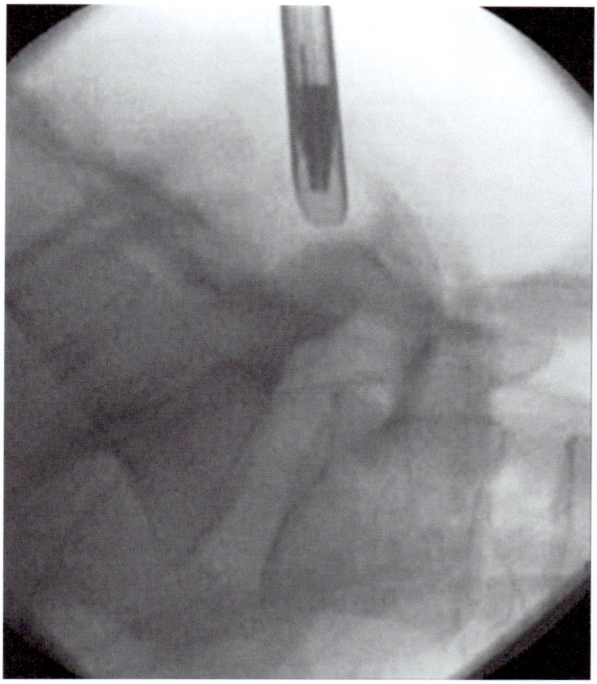

**Fig. 11.12** Lateral X-ray view of working sleeve outside the canal

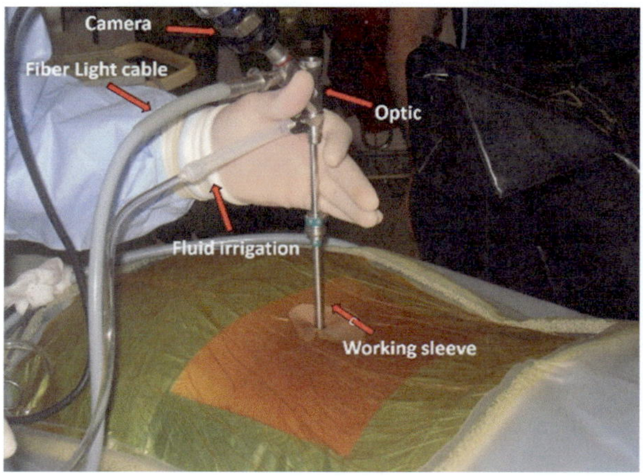


**Fig. 11.13** Working with endoscopic view

#### 11.3.2.2 Far-lateral Transforaminal

Disc space is accessed with a horizontal angle of 15° (Fig. 11.21). First introduced by Ruetten, this approach provides easy access to PLL and anterior epidural space [28, 33, 36]. Because of its convenience (easy and direct access to herniation area, no need for bone drilling), it is the most common applied technique today. Location of incision is determined by anatomic landmarks under fluoroscopic guidance and

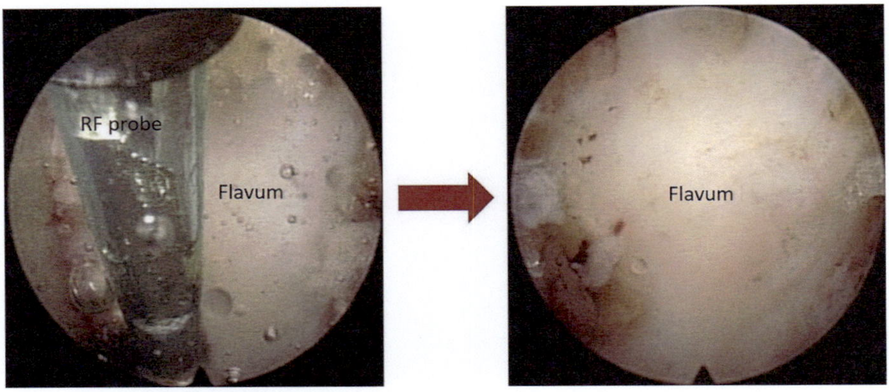


**Fig. 11.14** Coagulation of muscle remnants with RF probe and exposure of lig. flavum

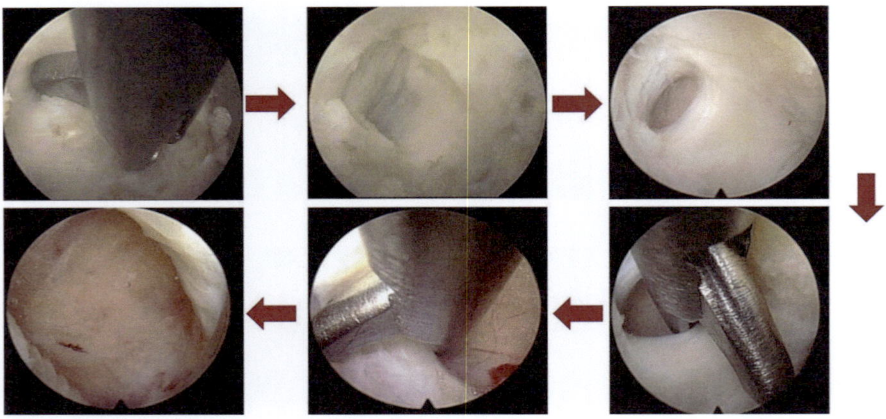

**Fig. 11.15** Making the lig. flavum incision under endoscopic view with scissor. After the last layer of ligament is cut, incision is carried forward laterally

not by measurements. We consider this technique as the golden standard for transforaminal access. Surgical steps for this technique are as follows:

Patient's position and operating room arrangement are the same as for IL approach. First, on lateral X-rays, posterior aspect of facet joints is marked on patient's skin as a vertical line. This line limits the insertion incision anteriorly. More anterior and lateral punctures can cause visceral organ injury (Fig. 11.22).

Then C-arm is positioned in AP view and set parallel to endplates at targeted level. On patient's skin, a horizontal line is drawn from disc level to cross the first line (Fig. 11.23). The crossing point of two lines is marked as an incision point for entry.

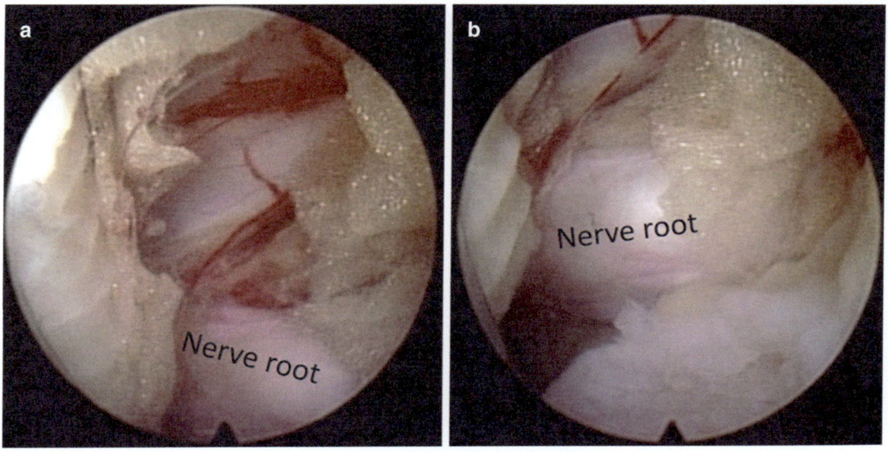


**Fig. 11.16** Visualization of neural structures after removal or mobilization of epidural fat (**a**) and insertion of dissector to retract nerve root exposing herniation (**b**)

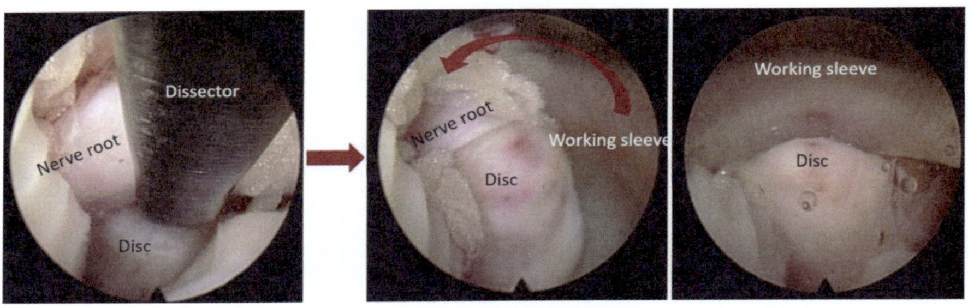


**Fig. 11.17** After retraction of nerve by dissector, beveled working sleeve is lowered into epidural space and rotated 180°, retracting nerve root medially and exposing herniation

Next, a 5 mm incision is made on the skin mark. An atraumatic spinal needle is advanced to the target under fluoroscopic control. The target point is dorsal aspect of annulus fibrosis on lateral view, midpedicular line on AP view (Fig. 11.24).

Next step is advancement of guide wire through spinal needle. Then spinal needle is removed and a cannulated dilator is placed over guide wire (Fig. 11.25). When dilator is placed firmly in the foramen entrance (a hammer can be useful), the wire is removed. Care should be taken to keep the dilator at the foramen during this step because it can easily come off. In this case, the procedure should be restarted all over, otherwise uncontrolled movements with the dilator at the foramen may cause exiting root damage.

After dilator is placed in foramen, a working sleeve with beveled opening is positioned over the dilator and dilator is removed. Working sleeve can be placed laterally or medially according to location of herniation (Fig. 11.26).

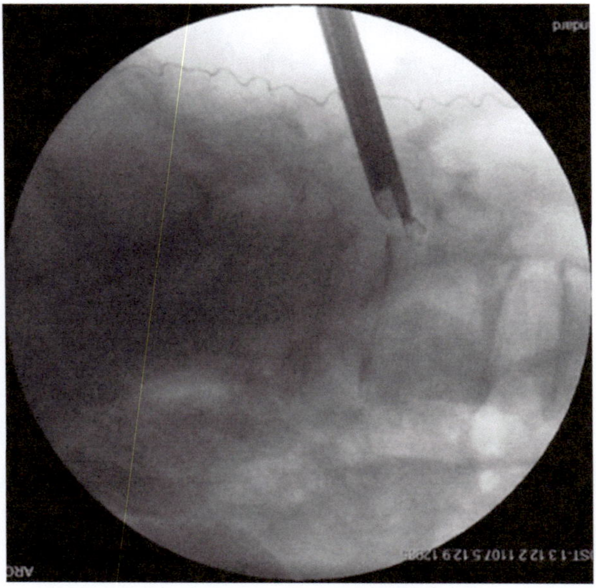

**Fig. 11.18** Exploration for cranially migrated fragment

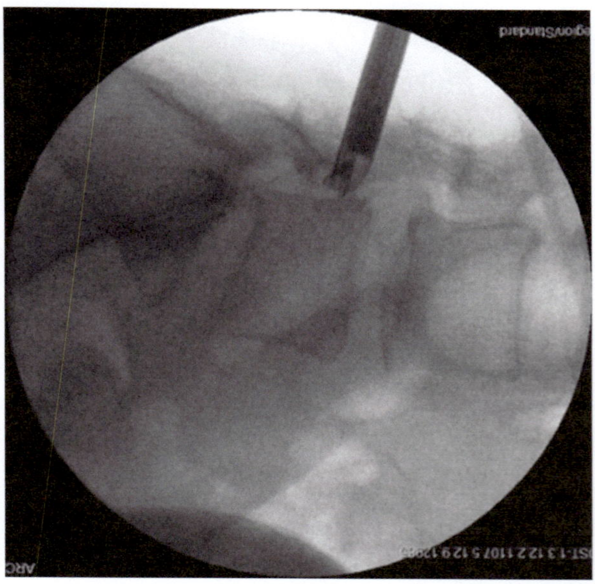

**Fig. 11.19** Exploration for caudal migration

Next, endoscope (25° view) is placed through the working sleeve, and the procedure is continued under direct view with pressurized irrigation. Cauterization of remnants of surrounding tissues with RF provides hemostasis and a clean view, a great help for recognizing anatomic landmarks. Three anatomic landmarks should be identified: epidural space, horizontal fibers and PLL, and disc space (Fig. 11.27).

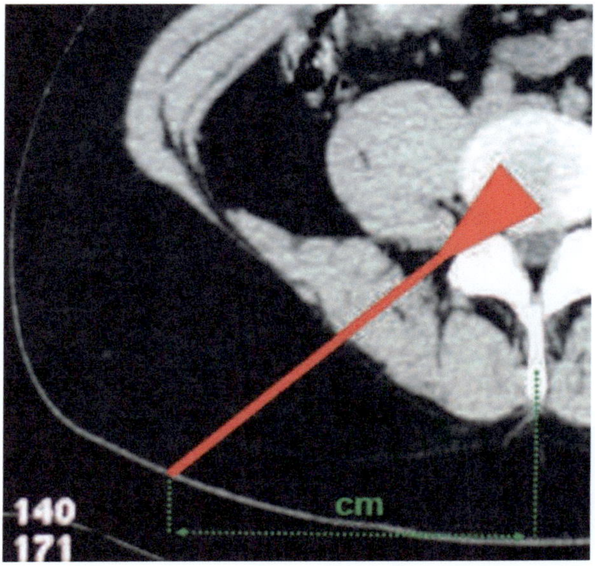


**Fig. 11.20** Easily accessible area by posterolateral approach

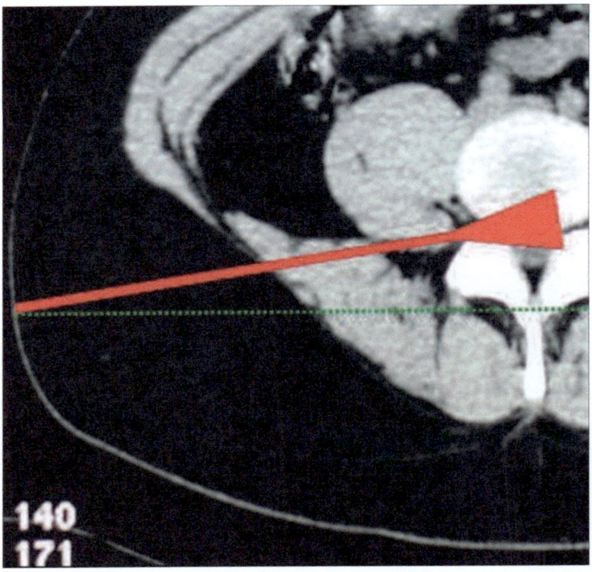


**Fig. 11.21** Easily accessible area by far-lateral approach

Horizontal fibers are cut piece by piece and cauterized with RF allowing a larger view, until herniation is recognized. After annular defect has been found and herniated fragment has been removed, free fluctuation of PLL and direct visualization of epidural space indicate that adequate decompression has been achieved (Fig. 11.28).

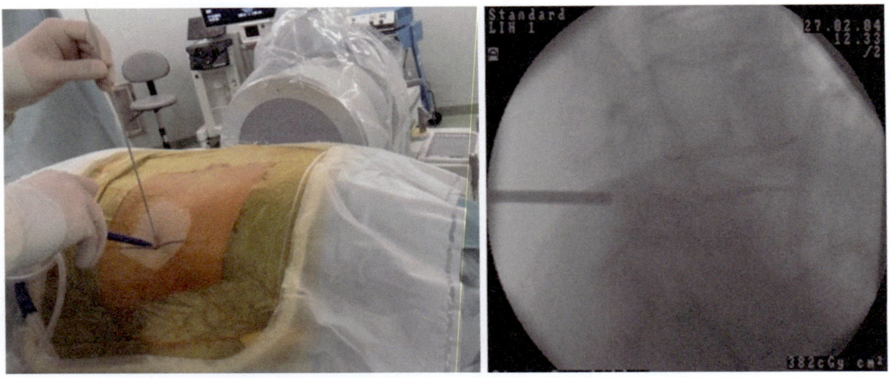

**Fig. 11.22** For marking of incision site, a line is drawn, approximately parallel to posterior margins of facet joints on lateral view

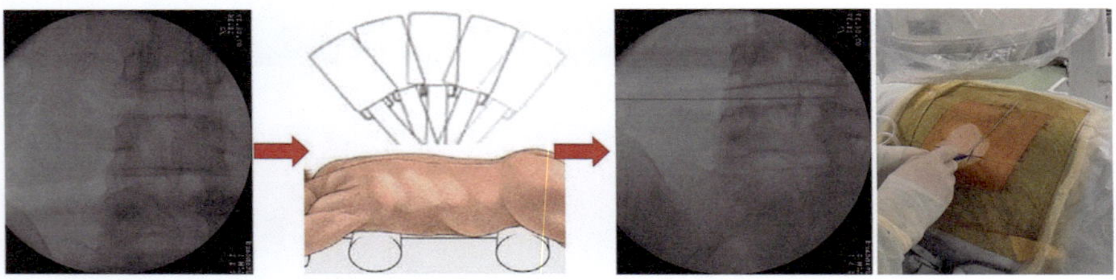

**Fig. 11.23** C-arm is positioned parallel to endplates at targeted level, and a line is drawn from disc level to cross the first line

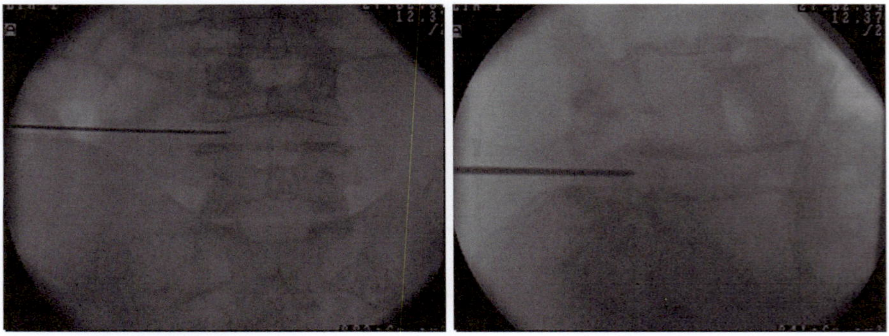

**Fig. 11.24** Target point is midpedicular line on AP view and dorsal margin of annulus fibrosis on lateral view

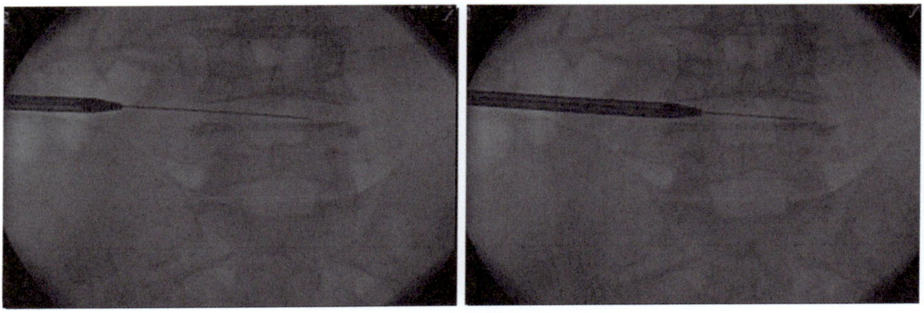

**Fig. 11.25** Placement of dilator in foramen over guide wire

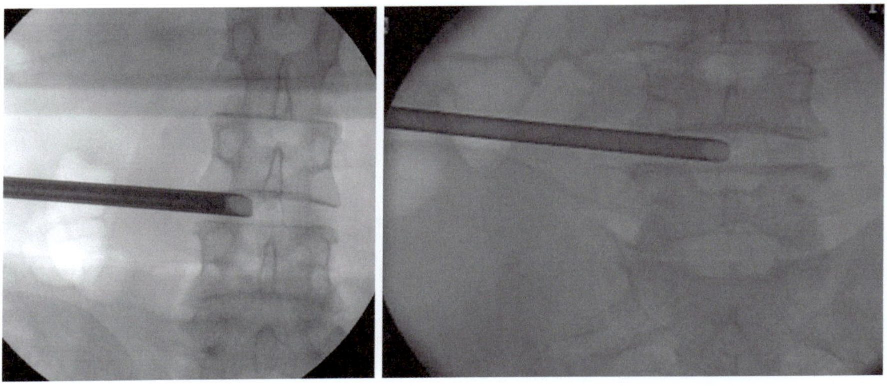

**Fig. 11.26** Working sleeve can be placed laterally or medially according to the location of herniation

### 11.3.2.3 Extraforaminal

At far-lateral (extraforaminal) herniations, herniated fragment may cause the root to relocate in the foramen. In this case, starting the operation directly in the foramen may cause exiting root injury. Therefore, it is safer to start the operation at the caudal pedicle outside the foramen. This should be the target point for insertion of working sleeve. Then, under endoscopic view and with identification of anatomic landmarks, working sleeve is mobilized, and exiting root, together with herniation, is recognized and fragment is removed (Fig. 11.29).

Although full-endoscopic approach can be considered as the least invasive method for far-lateral herniations, extraforaminal technique, where working sleeve cannot be stabilized in the foramen and extensive knowledge of anatomic landmarks are needed, is the most difficult endoscopic technique. Therefore, it should be carried out by experienced surgeons who adequately master lateral transforaminal approach, in order to reduce complication level.

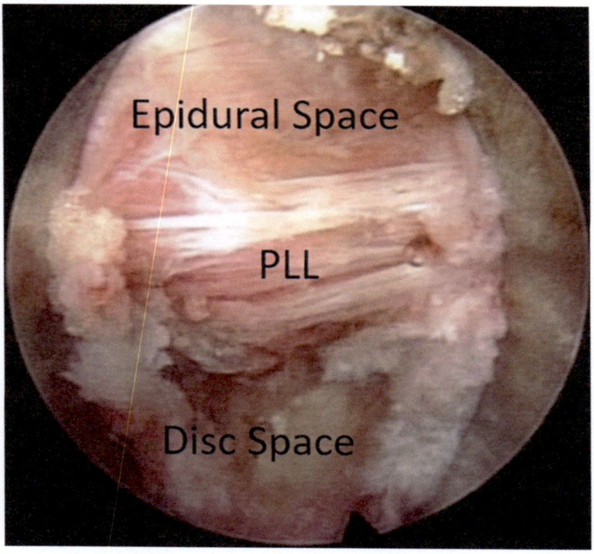


**Fig. 11.27** Epidural space, PLL, and disc on endoscopic view

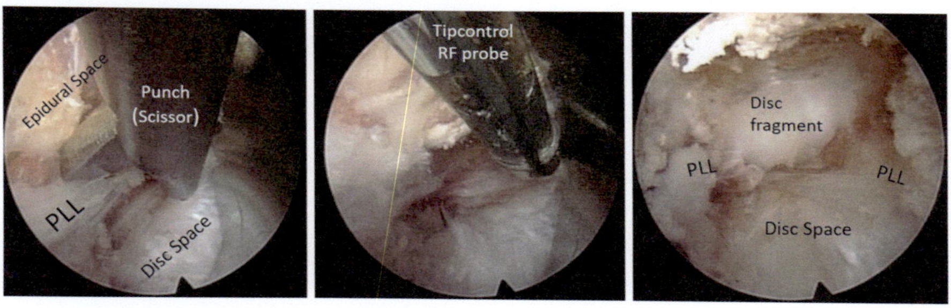


**Fig. 11.28** Cutting of fibers and PLL, exploration with RF probe, and uncovering of herniated fragment

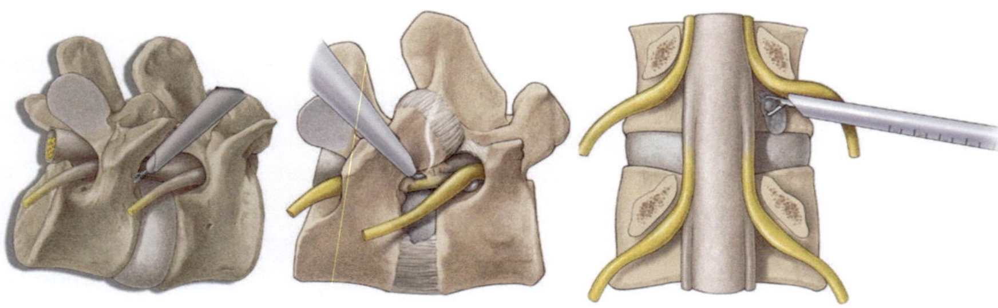

**Fig. 11.29** For extraforaminal herniations, caudal pedicle is targeted, anatomical structures explored, and fragment removed without stabilizing working sleeve in foramen

Although we use the abovementioned criteria for selection between IL and TF approaches, many surgeons worldwide prefer far-lateral TF approach for all kinds of lumbar herniations. Experience, direct access to disc space, and convenience of local anesthesia, if necessary, are the most important factors for this choice. Foraminoplasty techniques like the use of reamers or drills, to enlarge the foramen, are needed to access some fragments through foramen [38–42]. Using a more posterolateral approach to avoid iliac crest and with help of foraminoplasty techniques, L5–S1 discectomies can also be performed by TF approach, but it requires a greater level of expertise. Indeed, the choice between TF and IL approaches depends mostly on the surgeon's experience.

## 11.4 Postoperative Care

Usually, bed rest is not recommended, and patients are discharged on the same day or the day after. Mild pain killers can be initiated.

## 11.5 Complications

Complications of full-endoscopic discectomy are not different than those of microdiscectomy [28, 43, 44]. The learning curve may play an important role, but in experienced hands, rates are the same. Motor and sensorial deficits are reported below 3%. Dural tears may occur, but usually do not necessitate repair. As to our knowledge, major vessel injury, although a possibility, has not been reported with the IL approach, yet.

Recurrence and reoperations, early or late, are reported about 5–10%, and the rate is similar to the microdiscectomies [28, 43, 44]. In a clinical series of 232 patients operated with IL or TF full-endoscopic technique, published by Ruetten et al. in 2007, there was 92% success rate, together with 6% recurrence (patients who needed a reoperation) [28]. In this series, histopathological examination showed that, at least 75% of recurrent disc material was made up by endplates. Recurrence rate in this series is slightly more than in series with extensive disc removal but slightly lower than in series with removal of sequestrated fragment only [28]. To avoid large incisions in PLL or annulus could help to reduce recurrence.

One must keep in mind that, anatomic orientation can easily be lost with misplacement of the working sleeve [45]. With lateral or medial placement, confusion may occur in the identification of the anatomic structures which may lead in prolonged operation time and iatrogenic injury. Also, inappropriate manipulation of neural elements may result in transient or permanent motor deficits [45].

## 11.6 PELD for Recurrent Herniations

Recurrence is one of the most important problems for surgeons dealing with lumbar disc surgery, microdiscectomy, or PELD. Its rate varies from 5% to 20%, about 6–10% from a modern and realistic view [41, 43, 44, 46] and, as abovementioned, there is no difference concerning type of surgery. But another debate is on the selection of type of surgery for recurrent herniation. Although open microdiscectomy may seem more suitable, actually, PELD is equally safe and effective, too, independent from type of previous surgery. Choice of approach (IL or TF) again depends on the experience of surgeon. Both approaches require greater expertise. At IL approach, working sleeve is targeted to bony structures laterally, and epidural space is exposed by drilling of facet joint. For TF approach as well, foraminoplasty techniques may be required. But excellent visualization with 25° optics, chance of rapid rehabilitation, limited anatomic trauma reducing need for stabilization surgery are important advantages of PELD in contrast to its difficult learning curve.

## 11.7 Conclusion

Full-endoscopic surgery is a sufficient and safe supplementation and alternative to microdiscectomy. Similar success rates are reported for both, microdiscectomy and PELD, varying from 75% to 100%. Recurrence rate is similar too, between 5% and 10% [44]. At the same time, there are advantages of reduced traumatization, like greater patient comfort, better wound healing, shorter hospital stay, and of the operation technique, like excellent visualization, direct and easy access at obese patients. The success and advantages of PELD have also been shown in recent studies and meta-analyses [28, 30–32, 35, 36, 44, 47–49].

Clinical and cadaveric studies also indicate that, in near future, PELD will find a greater application area, including decompression of spinal stenosis or treatment of intradural pathologies, like untethering of filum terminale [50–54].

## 11.8 Highlights

- PELD is safe and effective for surgical treatment of lumbar disc disease.
- Results and complication rates of PELD and microdiscectomy are similar in experienced hands.
- Advantages of PELD are excellent visualization, minimal tissue traumatization, postoperative patient comfort, and easy access at obese patients.
- Disadvantages are difficult learning curve and, maybe, cost of new and high-technology equipment.
- Extensive knowledge of anatomy and radiological landmarks is of essential importance for PELD surgery.

## References


1. Fairbank JC, Couper J, Davies JB, O'Brien JP. The Oswestry low back pain disability questionnaire. Physiotherapy. 1980;66:271–73.
2. García-Bach M, López L, Isamat F, Ferrer E. Lumbar microdiscectomy: analysis of 100 consecutive cases. Its pitfalls and final results. Acta Neurochir Suppl (Wien). 1988;43:39–43.
3. Foley KT, Smith MM, Rampersaud YR. Microendoscopic approach to far-lateral lumbar disc herniation. Neurosurg. Focus. 1999;7(5):E7.
4. Forst R, Haussmann B. Nucleoplasty – a new examination technique. Arch Orthop Trauma Surg. 1983;101:219–21.
5. Hermatin F, Peters T, Quartarato I, Kambin P. A prospective, randomized study comparing the results of open discectomy with those of video-assisted arthrosopic microdiscectomy. J Bone Jt Surg Ser A. 1999;81:958–65.
6. Hijikata S. Percutaneous nucleotomy. A new concept technique and 12 years' experience. Clin Orthop Relat Res. 1989;238:9–23.
7. Hirabayashi S, Kumano K, Ogawa Y, Aota Y, Maehiro S. Microdiscectomy and second operation for lumbar disc herniation. Spine (Phila Pa 1976). 1993;18(15):2206–11.
8. Hoogland T, Schubert M, Miklitz B, Ramirez A. Transforaminal posterolateral endoscopic discectomy with or without the combination of a low-dose chymopapain: a prospective randomized study in 280 consecutive cases. Spine (Phila Pa 1976). 2006;31(24):E890–7.
9. Andrews DW, Lavyne MH. Retrospective analysis of microsurgical and standard lumbar discectomy. Spine (Phila Pa 1976). 1990;15(4):329–35.
10. Boyer P, Srour R, Buchheit F, Krause D, Albuquerque M. Lumbar disk hernia. Excision of hernia with or without complementary diskectomy? Neurochirurgie. 1994;40(4):259–62.
11. Cansever T, Kabatas S, Civelek E, et al. Transforaminal epidural steroid injection via a preganglionic approach for the treatment of lumbar radicular pain. Turk Neurosurg. 2012;22(2):183–8.
12. Carragee EJ, Han MY, Suen PW, Kim D. Clinical outcomes after lumbar discectomy for sciatica: the effects of fragment type and anular competence. J Bone Jt Surg Ser A. 2003;85(1):102–8.
13. Carragee EJ, Spinnickie AO, Alamin TF, Paragioudakis S. A prospective controlled study of limited versus subtotal posterior discectomy: short-term outcomes in patients with herniated lumbar intervertebral discs and large posterior anular defect. Spine (Phila Pa 1976). 2006;15;31(6):653–7.
14. Iwa H, Caspar W. A microsurgery operation for lumbar disc herniation (author's transl). No Shinkei Geka. 1978;6(7):657–62.
15. Chiu JC. Evolving transforaminal endoscopic microdecompression for herniated lumbar discs and spinal stenosis. Surg Technol Int. 2004;13:276–86.
16. Destandau J. Technical features of endoscopic surgery for lumbar disc herniation: 191 patients. Neurochirurgie. 2004;50(1):6–10.
17. Ebeling U, Reichenberg W, Reulen HJ. Results of microsurgical lumbar discectomy – review on 485 patients. Acta Neurochir. 1986;81(1-2):45–52.
18. Valls J, Ottolenghi CE, Schajowicz F. Aspiration biopsy in diagnosis of lesions of vertebral bodies. J Am Med Assoc. 1948;136(6):376–82.
19. Kambin P, Gellman H. Percutaneous lateral discectomy of the lumbar spine a preliminary report. Clin Orthop Relat Res. 1983 174 127-132.
20. Hermantin FU, Peters T, Quartararo L, Kambin P. A prospective, randomized study comparing the results of open discectomy with those of video-assisted arthroscopic microdiscectomy. J Bone Joint Surg Am. 1999;81(7):958–65.
21. Kambin P. Arthroscopic microdiscectomy. Arthrosc J Arthrosc Relat Surg. 1992; 3(3 Suppl):60S–64S.
22. Mayer HM, Brock M, Berlien H-P, Weber B. Percutaneous endoscopic laser discectomy (PELD) a new surgical technique for non-sequestrated lumbar discs. Acta Neurochir Suppl (Wien). 2011;54:53–8.

23. Schreiber A, Suezawa Y, Leu H. Does percutaneous nucleotomy with discoscopy replace conventional discectomy? Eight years of experience and results in treatment of herniated lumbar disc. Clin Orthop Relat Res. 1989;238:35–42.
24. Schreiber A, Leu H. Percutaneous nucleotomy: technique with discoscopy. Orthopedics. 1991;14(4):439–44.
25. Ruetten S, Komp M, Godolias G. A new full-endoscopic technique for the interlaminar operation of lumbar disc herniations using 6-mm endoscopes: prospective 2-year results of 331 patients. Minim Invasive Neurosurg. 2006;49(2):80–7.
26. Yeung AT. Minimally invasive disc surgery with the yeung endoscopic spine system (YESS). Surg Technol Int. 1999;8:267–77.
27. Yeung AT, Tsou PM. Posterolateral endoscopic excision for lumbar disc herniation: Surgical technique, outcome, and complications in 307 consecutive cases. Spine (Phila Pa 1976). 2002;27(7):722–31.
28. Ruetten S, Komp M, Merk H, Godolias G. Full-endoscopic interlaminar and transforaminal lumbar discectomy versus conventional microsurgical technique: a prospective, randomized, controlled study. Spine (Phila Pa 1976). 2008;33(9):931–9.
29. Yeung AT, Yeung CA. Advances in endoscopic disc and spine surgery: foraminal approach. Surg Technol Int. 2003;11:255–63.
30. Feng F, Xu Q, Yan F, et al. Comparison of 7 surgical interventions for lumbar disc herniation: a network meta-analysis. Pain Phys. 2017;20(6):E863–71.
31. Kim M, Lee S, Kim H-S, Park S, Shim S-Y, Lim D-J. A comparison of percutaneous endoscopic lumbar discectomy and open lumbar microdiscectomy for lumbar disc herniation in the Korean: a meta-analysis. Biomed Res Int. 2018;9073460.
32. Kim HS, Paudel B, Jang JS, Lee K, Oh SH, Jang IT. Percutaneous endoscopic lumbar discectomy for all types of lumbar disc herniations (LDH) including severely difficult and extremely difficult LDH cases. Pain Physician. 2018;21(4):E401–E408.
33. Ruetten S, Komp M, Godolias G. An extreme lateral access for the surgery of lumbar disc herniations inside the spinal canal using the full-endoscopic uniportal transforaminal approach-technique and prospective results of 463 patients. Spine (Phila Pa 1976). 2005;30(22):2570–8.
34. Ruetten S, Komp M, Merk H, Godolias G. Use of newly developed instruments and endoscopes: full-endoscopic resection of lumbar disc herniations via the interlaminar and lateral transforaminal approach. J Neurosurg Spine. 2007;6(6):521–30.
35. Siepe CJ, Sauer D. Technique of full-endoscopic lumbar discectomy via an interlaminar approach. Eur Spine J. 2018;27(Suppl 4):566–67.
36. Ruetten S.The Full-endoscopic Interlaminar Approach for Lumbar Disc Herniations. In: Mayer H.M. (eds) Minimally Invasive Spine Surgery. Springer, Berlin, Heidelberg. 2006;38:346–55.
37. Yeung AT. The evolution of percutaneous spinal endoscopy and discectomy: State of the art. Mt Sinai J Med. 2000;67(4):327–32.
38. Sairyo K, Chikawa T, Nagamachi A. State-of-the-art transforaminal percutaneous endoscopic lumbar surgery under local anesthesia: discectomy, foraminoplasty, and ventral facetectomy. J Orthop Sci. 2018;23(2):229–36.
39. Choi G, Lee SH, Lokhande P, et al. Percutaneous endoscopic approach for highly migrated intracanal disc herniations by foraminoplastic technique using rigid working channel endoscope. Spine (Phila Pa 1976). 2008;33(15):E508–15.
40. Li Z, Hous S, Shang W, Song K, Zhao H. Modified percutaneous lumbar foraminoplasty and percutaneous endoscopic lumbar discectomy: instrument design, technique notes, and 5 years follow-up. Pain Physician. 2017;20:85–98.
41. Kapetanakis S, Gkasdaris G, Angoules AG, Givissis P. Transforaminal percutaneous endoscopic discectomy using transforaminal endoscopic spine system technique: pitfalls that a beginner should avoid. World J Orthop. 2017;8(12):874–880.
42. LEE S-H, KANG HS, CHOI G, et al. Foraminoplastic ventral epidural approach for removal of extruded herniated fragment at the L5-S1 level. Neurol Med Chir (Tokyo). 2010;50(12):1074–8.

43. Yörükoğlu AG, Göker B, Tahta A, et al. Fully endoscopic interlaminar and transforaminal lumbar discectomy: analysis of 47 complications encountered in a series of 835 patients. Neurocirugia. 2017;28(5):235–241.
44. Ruetten S, Komp M, Merk H, Godolias G. Recurrent lumbar disc herniation after conventional discectomy: a prospective, randomized study comparing full-endoscopic interlaminar and transforaminal versus microsurgical revision. J Spinal Disord Tech. 2009;22(2):122–9.
45. Wang B, Lü G, Patel AA, Ren P, Cheng I. An evaluation of the learning curve for a complex surgical technique: the full endoscopic interlaminar approach for lumbar disc herniations. Spine J. 2011;11(2):122–30.
46. Kogias E, Franco Jimenez P, Klingler JH, Hubbe U. Minimally invasive redo discectomy for recurrent lumbar disc herniations. J Clin Neurosci. 2015;22(9):1382–6.
47. Ahn Y, Lee U, Kim WK, Keum HJ. Five-year outcomes and predictive factors of transforaminal full-endoscopic lumbar discectomy. Med (United States). 2018;97(48):e13454.
48. Casimiro M. Short-term outcome comparison between full-endoscopic interlaminar approach and open minimally invasive microsurgical technique for treatment of lumbar disc herniation. World Neurosurg. 2017;108:894–900.
49. Markovic M, Zivkovic N, Spaic M, et al. Full-endoscopic interlaminar operations in lumbar compressive lesions surgery: prospective study of 350 patients. "Endos" study. J Neurosurg Sci. 2016;64(1):16–24.
50. Yörükoğlu AG, Tahta A, Akçakaya MO, et al. Percutaneous fully endoscopic interlaminar approach to the filum terminale: a cadaveric study. World Neurosurg. 2016;92:402–6.
51. Komp M, Hahn P, Oezdemir S, et al. Bilateral spinal decompression of lumbar central stenosis with the full-endoscopic interlaminar versus microsurgical laminotomy technique: a prospective, randomized, controlled study. Pain Physician. 2015;18(1):61–70.
52. Komp M, Hahn P, Merk H, Godolias G, Ruetten S. Bilateral operation of lumbar degenerative central spinal stenosis in full-endoscopic interlaminar technique with unilateral approach: prospective 2-year results of 74 patients. J Spinal Disord Tech. 2011;24(5):281–7.
53. Ruetten S. Full-endoscopic operations of the spine in disk herniations and spinal stenosis. Surg Technol Int. 2011;21:284–98.
54. Ruetten S, Komp M, Merk H, Godolias G. Surgical treatment for lumbar lateral recess stenosis with the full-endoscopic interlaminar approach versus conventional microsurgical technique: a prospective, randomized, controlled study. J Neurosurg Spine. 2009;10(5):476–85.

# 12 Regenerative Options to Restore the Disc

Stephan Becker

## 12.1 Clinical Problem

The mobility and stability of the spine are crucial for movements. Both aspects are highly depending on discal integrity.

However, since the Second World War, most surgical options are focusing on removal of the disc and fusion.

Degenerative disc disease is the most common indication for fusion in the United States. Comparing the back pain rates with the physiological loss of glycosaminoglycan (Fig. 12.1), it is clear that there is a missing link. The missing biochemical link is the change of intradiscal biochemistry with increased acidity, which has been described in other chapters in this book.

Fusion rates for degenerative disc disease have increased by 220% over the last decades in the United States [3]. In the same time, four randomized trials showed poorer outcome after fusion in degenerative disc disease [4]. It was postulated that we need to have a better understanding of the origin of discogenic back pain which should result in decreased fusion rates [5].

It is well known that removal of the disc and fusion causes adjacent segment disease and SI joint disease. Therefore, attempts to restore the natural disc with an artificial disc (total disc replacement—TDR) have been performed since the late 1980s. All those different artificial discs have never shown to be clinically better than fusion, independent of the material. Lumbar artificial discs so far have never met the expectancies and are not reimbursed in most of the countries around the world. Besides the fact that TDR never exactly mimics natural mobility, normal biologic discs are subjected to aging. The slow loss of water and GAG is effectively decreasing the individual motion of the Junghans motion segment whilst the motion

S. Becker (✉)
Vitalzentrum, Salzburg - Grödig, Austria
e-mail: stephan.becker@vitazen.at



L. Manfrè, J. Van Goethem (eds.), *The Disc and Degenerative Disc Disease*,
New Procedures in Spinal Interventional Neuroradiology,
https://doi.org/10.1007/978-3-030-03715-4_12

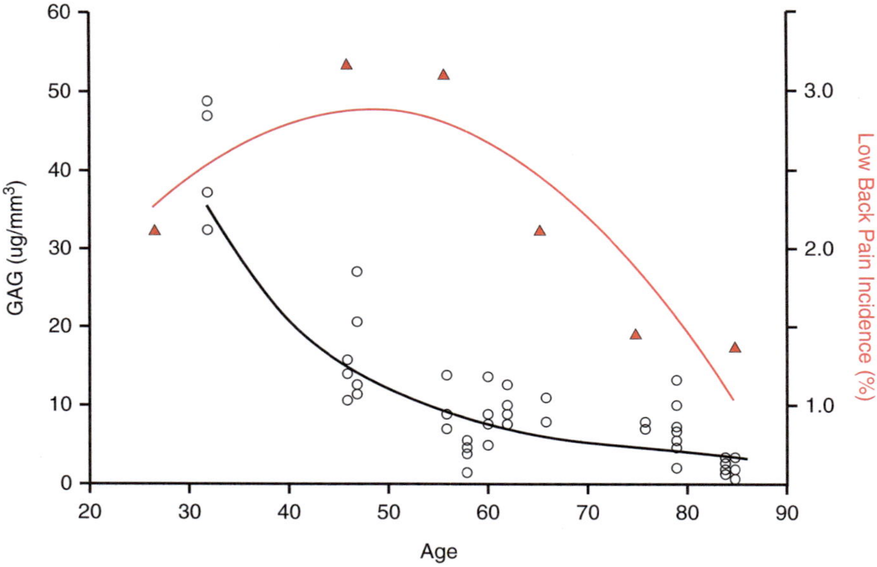


**Fig. 12.1** Loss of glycosaminoglycans (GAG) related to aging of the disc. The back pain incidence, which peaks between the 40th and 50th year is obviously not related to the loss of GAG. It has been described that acidity of the disc is the main factor in back pain in this age group [1, 2]

of an artificial disc remains the same. Those imbalances are the cause of failure of TDR and back pain; they lead to biomechanical stresses of adjacent segments, especially the biggest "facet" joint of the spine, the sacroiliac joints.

Therefore, researchers and doctors worldwide are looking into restoring the natural anatomy of the disc using advances in tissue engineering and biology versus implanting TDR, etc. mainly based on metals.

Especially, the worldwide criticism of increasing surgical rates without increased patient benefits has forced the system to look for alternatives. Public option is challenging surgeons/hospitals which are generally regarded as operating mainly for their own benefits.

Developments of biological solutions as well as imaging (see Chap. 6) are now offering the treating physician a lot of biological options for disc restoration and maintenance of the motion segment instead of "amputating" a degenerative disc.

The aim of a doctor should be to walk along the patient in his or her year-long journey of normal disc aging performing occasionally minimal-invasive treatments and not performing an irreversible, mainly destructive, surgical solution which only leaves as options more and bigger surgical interventions in the future.

Whilst adapting biological techniques/options to the age, physical, mental and social environment of an individual patient, we can always choose the best minimal-invasive regenerating/augmenting or pain mediating technique to allow a normal lifestyle.

The approach not only benefits the individual patient much better than any "heavy metal" surgery but also reduces the financial strain to medical and social insurance systems.

The causes of back pain are so variable that the treating physician should always look at the least invasive and individually best technique without sacrificing normal anatomy and changing the biomechanical environment.

Fusions as well as artificial discs are immediately severely changing this environment, and the body has no time to adapt. The human body can slowly adapt to a lot of challenging external or internal changes, but the body cannot react and adapt to sudden changes created by invasive surgery, especially in the most important part of human biomechanics, the spine.

This chapter gives an overview about minimal-invasive possibilities to treat degenerating discs as one of the main causes of instability and back pain.

Augmentating solutions are looking at the restoration of stability and of a normal environment (mainly buffering the lactate acid, see also Chap. 6) whilst regenerating techniques aim at local cell growth. As both actions are linked, those techniques are more and more used in combinations.

## 12.2 Anatomical and Pathophysiological Update and Possible Implications for Regeneration

### 12.2.1 Basivertebral Nerve

Besides the mentioned MRI developments allowing a much better assessment of disc biology, recent anatomical discoveries are also allowing a much better local treatment without sacrificing the normal or damaged disc.

It is well known that the sinuvertebral nerve innervates the long posterior ligament, the dorsal annulus, the anterior dura mater and the posterior vertebral periosteum [6]. However, it was not known until 1998 that a branch of that nerve, the basivertebral nerve, is entering the vertebral body next to the basivertebral vein and actively innervating the endplates [7] (Fig. 12.2).

Intraosseous sources of pain have been well known for a century or more and would include intraosseous tumours, bone infarcts and stress fractures. There is also some evidence that elevated intraosseous pressure can cause back pain [8, 9]. Periendplate MRI signal changes (Modic changes) are indicative of intraosseous oedema or inflammation, well correlated with clinical low back pain [10, 11]. The basivertebral nerve itself is a substance P positive nerve indicating its role in back pain [12, 13] and opening whole new treatment opportunities [14], which will be demonstrated later. Lactate is sensitizing this nerve resulting in enhanced sprouting of the nerve into the endplate sensitizing the disc even more [15]. Any intradiscal changes therefore affect the basivertebral nerve. The description of this pathway has filled a gap in spinal pain therapy demonstrating an intravertebral receptor of discogenic and vertebrogenic pain.

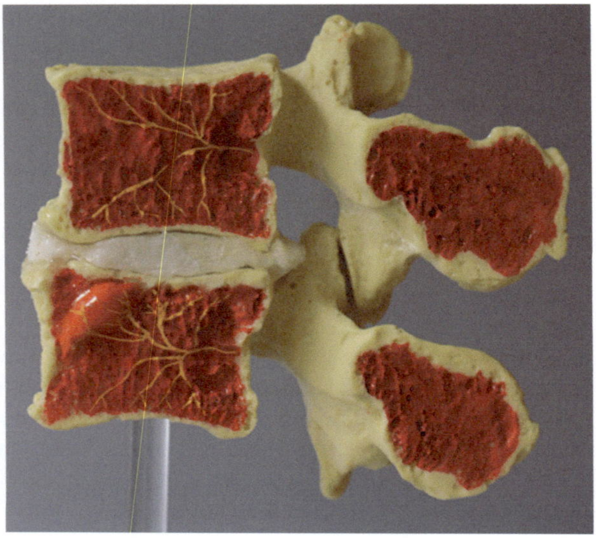

**Fig. 12.2** Basivertebral nerve innervating both endplates (image courtesy of Dr. Jerome Fryer, Dynamic Disc Designs Corp.—www.dynamicdiscdesigns.com). The figure also shows Modic changes on the anterior–superior endplate of the inferior vertebra

However, why is the growth of the basivertebral nerve stimulated by a degenerative disc and for what purpose?

Nature never does anything without a broader meaning. Mechanistic medical thinking explains the changes in the disc and the increased innervation as: pain is helpful in protecting overload. In my opinion, this is only partially true. Why should nature cause the basivertebral nerve superior and inferior to the endplate to increase nociceptors? Would not one-sided growth be enough? Nature never wastes resources, so, in my opinion, there is a deeper meaning in that fact which could be important.

It is known since the 1960s [16], that regeneration of tissue is dependent on microcurrents, especially negative microcurrents. Direct neuroepidermal links have been shown to regenerate whole limbs in amphibia, and new developments in quantum medicine and quantum therapies are supporting those findings [17]. Furthermore, neurotropic cells have been shown to play important roles in heterotopic bone formation [18], and neural stem cells can differentiate into osteoblastic and endothelial cells [19]. Therefore, the increased innervation of the disc could not be a natural regeneration stimulus to regenerate the disc via “neurodiscal” links, similar to proven neuroepidermal connections. As Becker showed [16], negative microcurrents result in tissue regeneration and positive microcurrents cause fibrotic changes. It has been shown that lactate with its low pH causes back pain and induces nerve growth [15]. Is therefore the pure mechanistic medical idea of pain = protection mechanism too trivial for the complex potential of natural regeneration? As a hypothesis, it could well be that the positive microcurrents in acidic tissue is causing the fibroblastic degeneration of the disc whilst the “neurodiscal” interaction via the basivertebral nerve is trying to regenerate the disc.

Therefore, any inversion of positive to negative microcurrent environments should have a potential of regeneration disc tissue. This hypothesis is combining mechanistic medical with modern quantum state/electrical findings. I think by using buffering agents (hydrogels/PRP, etc.) in the disc, we are leaving all options open regarding biochemical and modern quantum medical theories based on Max Planck's and Albert Einstein's discoveries and provide the best environment for possible regeneration.

Later in this chapter, I will further describe minimal-invasive treatment options based around the pain perception by the basivertebral nerve.

### 12.2.2 *Propionibacterium acnes*

Subclinical infections with *P. acne* bacteria have been shown to be associated with back pain. *P. acne* is the most commonly found intradiscal pathogen amongst others [20–22]. Treating this bacterium with antibiotics over several months resulted in decreased back pain in a double-blind controlled trial [23]. However, the discussion of the impact of *P. acne* on Modic changes and back pain is still ongoing, as an antibiotic treatment for back pain is causing various side effects such as destroying the gut microbiome and iatrogenic contamination during sampling could not be ruled out.

New investigations as MRI spectroscopy (MRS—see Chap. 6), however, are able to find pathogens in previously untreated vertebra which opens up another viable treatment path.

Infection of a disc with *P. acne* may be furthermore a contraindication for the local use of intradiscal stem cells.

This chapter is describing viable alternatives to a month-long antibiotic treatment course of a *P. acne* infected disc. Disinfecting agents like DiscoGel® (Gelscom SA) and methylene blue are indicated, as well as platelet-rich plasma (PRP, especially as HD—LR—PRP, see below), and open up another ambulatory, low-cost solution to either a long-term antibiotic treatment or open surgery.

## 12.3 Treatment Options

The aim of this chapter is not to give an overview about possible conservative treatment options nor does it show an overview about disc removal operations such as total disc replacement or fusion. New imaging possibilities (e.g. above shown MRI spectroscopy) allow us to consider disc maintaining for restoring treatment techniques.

### 12.3.1 Nucleus Replacement

Even before developing a total artificial disc, researchers were looking into replacing the nucleus since 1950. Various implants have been developed over the years ranging from polymer/hydrogel cushions, PEEK implants, balloon-shaped implants and spiral-shaped implants (Regain® by Biomet, NuBac® by Pioneer, PDN® by Ray Medica, Newcleus® by Zimmer, Aquarelle® by Stryker and NeuDisc® by Replication Medical). All of the implants, however, demanded a complete removal of the nucleus and invariably failed over time (dislocation, breakdown/resorption, end-plate erosion, subsidence) [24, 25]. The primary idea of limiting disc destruction whilst maintaining better biomechanics than an artificial disc could not be proven. The primary damage of the annulus at insertion of the implant proved to be too invasive for implant stability.

The idea of replacing the nucleus was a typical surgical idea in replacing biological tissue with artificial tissue, whereas the artificial tissue proved again to be vastly inferior to biological tissue. However, experience with water-retaining and memory-shaped implants, especially the NeuDisc® (Replication Medical, Inc.), led to the idea of not completely removing, but just augmenting an otherwise intact disc/annulus.

Before realizing this step, ideas of injectable substances into the disc emerged. The author himself was involved in several of those trials which basically consisted of injecting various substances into the defect created by a microscope-assisted partial discectomy.

The substances consisted of in situ curable silicone and polyurethane with the idea of less damaging the disc, being more elastic and being able to fill all defects and cracks in the nucleus. The author has worked with a product of bovine albumin and glutaraldehyde (BioDisc® by CryoLife). The mixture did cure in situ whilst providing non-covalent direct binding to the annulus. Other approaches involved curable polyurethane and a recombinant amino acid copolymer (Dascor® by Disc Dynamics). In situ curing proved to be partially toxic for surrounding tissue, early breakdown and dislocation occurred through the big defect created by the primary discectomy and incoherent binding to the annulus [26].

Other substances in trials included fibrin-based approaches (Biostat®—Spinal Restoration) trying to avoid those problems.

However, none of the injectable products could achieve either to exit the trial phase or to get a hold on the market, and they are not available anymore.

Recent studies focus therefore on just closing the annular defect with gels in order to limit reherniation [27]. This cannot be seen as a disc regeneration but may have some impact in the future regarding reducing reoperation rates.

Until now, no perfect biomaterials have been found to withstand the biomechanical stresses and the physiologic aging of a disc as well as the changing biomechanics and the weakness of the annulus, respective of the annular defect, created either by a hernia or by a surgical approach.

As mentioned, the experience with nucleus replacement trials has finally led to the idea of not replacing the disc tissue but just augmenting the disc tissue. This mindset followed the experiences gained by vertebroplasty and balloon kyphoplasty where vertebroplasty as an augmenting method of physiological structures showed to be superior than crushing physiological structures by a balloon and replacing it with inadequate materials [28, 29].

### 12.3.2 Augmentation Techniques

In general, it has been proven to be more beneficial to patients to augment damaged tissue instead of completely replacing physiological tissue, especially in biomechanical critical situation or inadequate biomaterials (vertebroplasty versus balloon kyphoplasty, augmenting bone cysts versus amputation and implants, various plastic surgery techniques, etc.).

This mindset was also developed for intradiscal material, especially after developing memory-shaped hydrogels, such as the NeuDisc® (Replication Medical, Inc.).

The problem with the NeuDisc occurred after an insertion defect of an 8–10 mm in the annulus. Even more problematic was the denucleation of the disc space across the annular defect into the centre of the disc. This effectively created a channel for the NeuDisc to herniate into. Since there was immediate pressure on the NeuDisc under load, it was likely that the annular defect never really completely healed. Eventually, the implant started to "herniate" into the annular defect. Most of the implant remained in the disc space and did not completely dislocate like many other implants, but partial herniation made it obsolete in clinical use.

The logical next step was creating a much smaller, completely injectable device (GelStix® by Replication Medical), which got CE approval and is used regularly in Europe since 2010 (http://www.replicationmedical.com/products/gelstix).

It is currently the only augmenting device available on the market. It consists of a hydrogel stick in a dehydrated state (3 cm × 0.8 mm) consisting of HPAN 90. Hydrolysed polyacrylonitrile hydrogels are called "biomimetic". The main advantage of the structural similarity to the nucleus is similar physical (such as swelling pressure and permeability) and mechanical properties. Chemical composition is different, however, HPAN hydrogel is biostable and is not hydrolytically degradable. It consists of multiblock acrylic copolymer, alternating blocks of hydrophilic and hydrophobic groups on a carbon–carbon backbone. The groups are physically crosslinked via crystalline clusters and show an amphoteric polymer with net negative charge at physiological conditions (https://patents.google.com/patent/CA2386265A1/en).

It is implanted in a dehydrated state via an 18-gauge needle into the nucleus, where it resorbs water and swells over the next hour to its final, flexible state of 3.5 cm × 2.5 mm (Fig. 12.3).

The figure shows the continuous swelling of the implant under physiological conditions in the nucleus.

The physical properties of the implant are: high equilibrium swelling, binding more water than the surrounding tissue, responding dynamically to load and to rapidly bind and express fluid.

From a surgeon perspective, the main advantage of the implant is the fact, that it is inserted via an 18-G needle and swells within the disc, hence is too large to herniate through the insertion hole. The overall added volume to the disc can be changed by adding one or more implants, each implant adding 0.33 ml to the disc. On average, 1–2 implants are used per disc.

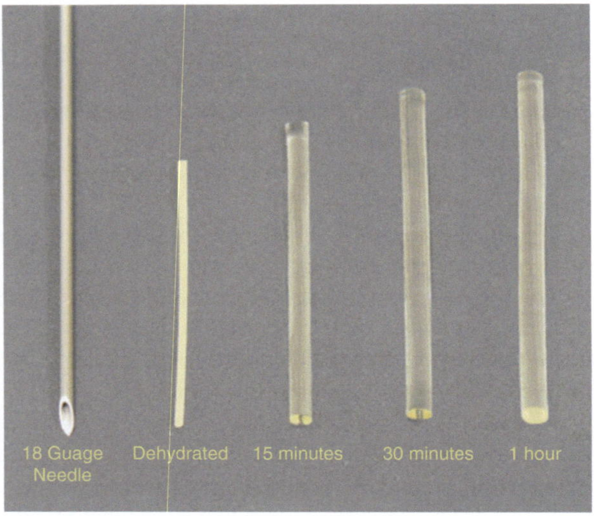


**Fig. 12.3** Gelstix® (image courtesy of Replication Medical Inc.)

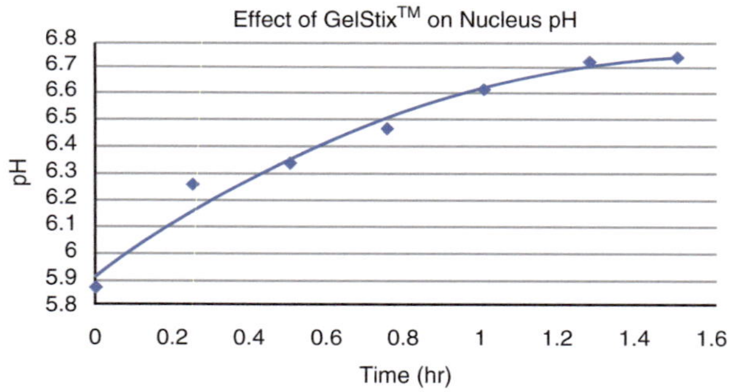


**Fig. 12.4** pH behaviour of a disc augmented with GelStix® (courtesy of Replication Medical Inc., after Yue Literature 33)

However, the indications have to be strictly followed which mainly focus on an intact annulus.

From a regenerative aspect, this implant is able to buffer the pH in the disc, hence allows not only a normal disc physiology but can serve as a platform for later cell therapies such as stem cells (Fig. 12.4).

The implant itself is radiolucent and is only visible on a regular MRI (Fig. 12.5).

It is not unusual for regenerative outpatient minimal-invasive techniques to have only limited clinical data. So far, the implant has been used in over 3000 cases times in Europe, with only a small number (three reported complications) recorded by the supplier.

The first 21-patient post-market clinical study was reported in 2011 [30] to evaluate the potential for GelStix® to reduce back pain in patients diagnosed with DDD. DDD was confirmed with radiographic imaging and provocative

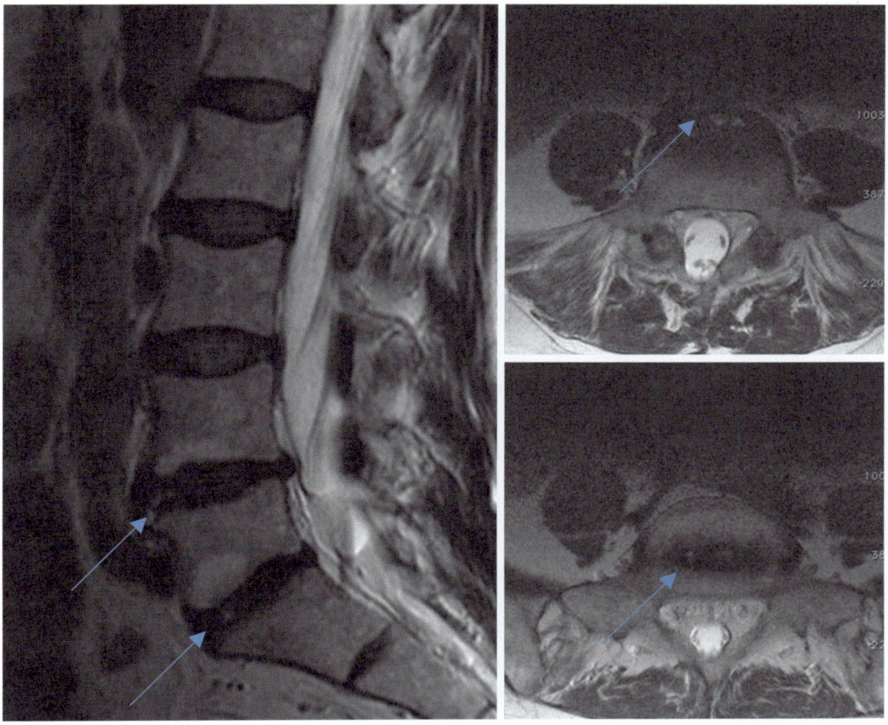

**Fig. 12.5** Fifty-six years old female, hemilaminectomy L4–L5 right side, post-op chronic lumbar pain. Insertion of two GelStix in the disc L4–L5 and L5–S1 each (arrows) in 2011. Pre-op VAS 7.8, post op 6 weeks 1.5, 12 months 0.5, 24/36 months 0.5 and 60 months 0.5. The patient still does not complain about any lumbar pain after the last follow-up 8 years after the operation

discography. Patient enrolment was divided into two phases, with broader inclusion criteria in the first one and stricter criteria in the second one, including restrictions on previous surgeries and Modic changes greater than 1.

At the time of reporting, a total of 21 patients had been enrolled: 11 in the first phase and 10 in the second phase and had been followed up to 12 and 6 months, respectively.

Of the 11 patients treated in the first phase, four were presented with multilevel disease and were treated at both the affected levels. Two patients had previous surgeries (one endoscopic and one microdiscectomy) and were treated at the affected level which had become painful several years after the operation. One patient had a previous dual-level fusion and was treated with GelStix® at the level adjacent to the fusion. Several others had varying levels of disc bulge (<3 mm) and endplate degeneration. In addition to back pain, seven patients (64%) experienced mild-to-moderate radicular pain, and one patient had Grade 1 spondylolisthesis. More than 90% of patients on follow-up showed a significant decrease in back pain quantified with ODI and/or VAS at the latest time points evaluated. Six of the 11 patients treated in the first phase had a post-procedure follow-up >1 year and continued to show significant reduction in back pain. The patient that did not show significant improvement was diagnosed with Grade 1 spondylolisthesis in conjunction with DDD pre-procedure. Somewhat unexpectedly, six of the eight patients (75%) with leg pain had complete leg pain relief following the treatment.

Our own experience in 2011 confirmed the findings in 22 patients after 4 weeks (reduction of VAS from 8.5 to 3, ODI from 25.1 to 10.2 [31].

A randomized prospective controlled clinical trial of GelStix® is currently underway in two centres—one in the Netherlands and the other in Switzerland. The study has been underway for over 2 years and is still recruiting patients.

Inclusion and contraindication for intradiscal hydrogel augmentation are shown in Tables 12.1 and 12.2.

So far, all data shows that this simple and innovative technology is a safe and effective treatment for lumbar pain.

### 12.3.3 Regenerating Techniques

Regeneration or delaying aging is a long-sought after dream of humanity. Regenerating the disc or delaying further damage was the focus of treatments over the last 20 years. However, as the disc has some special pathophysiological properties unseen in other joints, approaches to regenerate the disc until now mainly did fail. The special environment with high lactate, decreased oxygenation, sclerosed endplates and until recently unknown neurological innervation made it impossible to use cell approaches. In the early years of this millennium, clinical trials have been performed using aspirated nuclear intradiscal cells from a patient, expanding them in a lab and reinjecting the cells into the nucleus [32].

**Table 12.1** Inclusion criteria for intradiscal hydrogel augmentation

| |
|---|
| • Lumbar pain without radicular pain |
| • DDD confirmed by MRI |
| • Elevated biomarkers confirmed by MRS |
| • Intact annulus |
| • Modic 1 |
| • Max 50% of disc height collapse |
| • HIZ (high intensity zone) or non-HIZ patients |

**Table 12.2** Contraindications for intradiscal hydrogel augmentation

| |
|---|
| • Radiculopathy |
| • Disc herniations, protrusion >3 mm |
| • Severe central, foraminal or lateral spinal stenosis |
| • Spondylolysis |
| • Fractures |
| • Severe facet degermation |
| • Bechterew's disease |
| • Spondylodiscitis |
| • Spinal claudication |

It was discussed that harvesting cells from a degenerative disc is too invasive and risky and that there is no ethical or medical foundation to do that [33]. Good early results have been demonstrated using cells harvested from sequesters after sequestrectomy [33]. However, the technique is still in its infancy, and long-term results are missing. The company sponsoring the study nowadays uses a similar technology exclusively for cartilage regeneration of large joints.

The environment overall in the disc does not support the survival of external cells. The environment in the disc can be compared with a desert, e.g. acidified soil and no nutrition (e.g. no water). Then when you try to plant a young tree, this approach will fail.

However, if you create an "oasis" meaning adding nutrition, simulators, fertilize and buffer the soil, then the young tree has a choice to survive.

This in my mind is the big difference in using stem cells (e.g. the young tree) versus using platelet-rich plasma (e.g. the fertilizer and buffer) in order to treat disc degeneration.

#### 12.3.3.1 Platelet-Rich Plasma

PRP (platelet-rich plasma) is the longest existing cell therapy worldwide. Attempts to treat disease with blood ingestion/transfer or injections is thousands of years old. With the development of more biochemical tests, and better understanding of cell functions of the blood, it became evident, that thrombocytes play the major role in healing and regeneration.

Physicians understood that healing and regeneration do need a kick-start to occur. After injury/damage, the body is reacting with "fertilizing the soil", e.g. releasing thrombocytes and leucocytes in order to attract other cells and kick-start healing with a large variety of factors. Hence, PRP is the optimal autologous "fertilizer" of a degenerative disc.

First trials with PRP were published as early as 1974 demonstrating an anabolic effect on muscle cells [34], thus describing the healing/regeneration of PRP for the first time. Witte et al. [35] isolated a healing factor in 1978 which they named platelet-derived growth factor (PDGF). Clinical use in the 1980s in veterinary medicine with great results was quickly adopted by dentistry in the early 1990. Dentists realized the huge potential of growth factors to regenerate fragile tissue/bone around the teeth.

Early use in traumatology and plastic surgery focusing on bone healing, infected wounds and pressure sores started in the mid-1990. Our group has used PRP and derivates successfully since that time and reported great result in pressure sores in para- and tetraplegic patients [36]. We used PRP furthermore as an adjunct to surgery or to enhance biomaterials ingrowth [37]. We also developed a standardized approach in order to optimize PRP separation and to increase cell count [38]. This approach has been adopted by various producers of PRP systems worldwide.

For over 10 years now, the indications of the use of PRP have grown significantly. PRP is now used more widely starting from beauty injections, sports medicine, etc. to disc regeneration. Several formulations like leucocyte-rich PRP (LR-PRP), leucocyte-poor PRP (LP-PRP), high-density PRP (HD-PRP (see below)) and platelet-rich fibrin (PRF) are used nowadays. The systems for PRP separation have been further refined, so that we, for instance, use only one single system to create all of those formulations. PRP offers the physician a whole armamentarium for individual treatment in a large variety of indications.

The effect of PRP on disc regeneration has been studied extensively [39]. The regulation effects on the discs are shown in Table 12.3.

We know now a lot more about healing factors released from PRP such as TGF beta, and more and more factors and interactions are found every year. We are by far not fully realizing the PRP potential yet; we just know that nature has developed a highly sensible and effective "fertilizing" cell in order to heal and survive. Therefore, it still is stunning, that the easy technique of PRP preparation and injection has not been adapted by reimbursements systems around the world. This may be due to the fact that research and use of stem cells are better funded with the prospects of bigger financial gain. Individual PRP production is cheap, fast and easily being done in outpatient clinical practices.

Clinical evidence of PRP in general is bountiful, however, also papers negating the effect of PRP do exists. There are so many systems on the market nowadays that it is difficult for the individual physician to choose the best system without training. There are large differences between the systems [40].

Going back to basic considerations, we have to realize that nature is not only giving us platelets for regeneration but also leucocytes. If we can consider PRP as anabolic "fertilizers", leucocytes can be regarded as downregulating and catabolic factors. Only the combination of both factors, like being presented by nature, does have the desired effect. Industry has only partially realized the fact and has produced PRP systems which are not adaptable to clinical setting.

Comparing studies between PRP systems, e.g. comparing a leucocyte-rich PRP system by Biomet Inc. with a leucocyte-poor system of Arthrex Inc. is one of the studies underlining the necessity to combine leucocytes with PRP [41].

Finally, nature again is showing us why PRP is vastly superior to stem cells in having established a bactericidal effect in platelets, which is logical [42–44]. Platelets exist since millions of years and have healed open wounds since those times. The bactericidal effect is not fully understood but is certainly a viable argument for the use of PRP. In my opinion, the future will show that, if stem cells are

**Table 12.3** Effects of activated PRP on a degenerated disc [39]

| Factor | Name | Origin | Effect |
|---|---|---|---|
| PDGF | Platelet-derived growth factor | Activated PRP | Annulus cells: Apoptosis ↓<br>Annulus and nucleus: Proliferation ↑ |
| TGF beta | Transforming growth factor | Activated PRP | Nucleus: Proteoglycan and collagen II synthesis ↑<br>Annulus: Proliferation and matrix synthesis↑ |
| IGF | Insulin-like growth factor | Activated PRP | Disc/nucleus: Proliferation and cell synthesis ↑<br>Annulus: Apoptosis ↓ |

used regularly in medicine in our field, probably only stem cell/PRP combinations will provide the best results in healing whilst reducing infection rates.

Clinical studies of the effect of PRP on disc regeneration are still scarce and summarized on Table 12.4.

A double-blind prospective randomized controlled study showed a beneficial effect in disc [49]. After one injection of 1 ml PRP into a degenerated disc, a positive effect was found after 8 weeks which maintained over 12 months follow-up. This study confirms the findings of Alexandre et al., which reported an ongoing healing of the disc over the next 3–12 months after in the injection of 1 ml PRP just once into the disc over the next months up to 2 years [48]. The result confirms our own experience 10 years ago; however, we were able to speed up healing time by using HD-PRP (see below).

In our own experience with PRP for treating degenerative disc disease since 2010, one of the main aspects is the limited amount of injectable volume. I talked about augmentation of the disc above, hence we are injecting the PRP into an intact disc without any real space. Therefore, it is mandatory to use a system to optimize PRP concentration. The systems on the market vary widely, from threefold concentration to 6–7 times concentration. We use a system with the highest concentration. After generating LR-PRP for optimal healing, we further concentrate the PRP by using a nanofiltration derived from dialysis. Removing only water from the PRP, the

**Table 12.4** Overview of PRP studies in disc regeneration

| Disc | *n* | Control | Results |
|---|---|---|---|
| Intradiscal injection of autologous platelet-rich plasma for the treatment of lumbar disc degeneration [45] | 6 prospective | X | 6 months FU: Sign. Improvement |
| Intradiscal PRP study and MRI predictors of outcome [46] | 42 prospective rand. Double blind | 26 only discogram, 6 cross—After 8 weeks | 8 weeks FU: 58.3% versus 3.3%,<br>1 year/2 year FU: 57% of treatment group and 100% of cross—over improved |
| Intradiscal platelet-rich plasma injection for chronic discogenic low back pain: Preliminary<br>Results from a prospective trial [47] | 22 prospective | X | Success:<br>1 month: 14%<br>2 months: 32%<br>6 months: 47% |
| Intradiscal injections of platelet-enriched plasma for degenerative disc disease: Degenerative aspects on MRI follow-up [48] | 24 prospective | X | Excellent and good:<br>3 months: 24%<br>6 months: 56%<br>12 months: 72%<br>24 months: 88% |
| Lumbar ntradiskal platelet-rich plasma (PRP) injections: A prospective, double-blind, randomized controlled study [49] | 29 prospective rand. Double blind | 18 only discogram | 8 weeks FU: Significant improvement of pain, function and patient satisfaction in treatment group |

microfiltration allows us to create a HD-LR-PRP (high-density-leucocyte-rich PRP) with cells volumes up to10 micro cells/µl, hence up to 66 times concentration. From this HD-LR-PRP, we inject 1 ml into the disc. Combining this HD-LR-PRP with advanced imaging like discussed before (e.g. MR spectroscopy), we are confident to provide an improved approach to our patients, which our early results confirm (see examples below). We are encouraging other physicians to follow our approach to study a HD-LR-PRP for degenerative disc disease.

For interested readers, it is highly recommended to join one of the PRP teaching courses available worldwide or contact the author for more information regarding his own courses.

## 12.4 Other Injectable Treatments Techniques of Discogenic Pain

Discogenic pain is a worldwide problem; therefore, different approaches have been developed all over the world to avoid large interventions/total disc replacement or fusion.

The most prominent therapies currently are DiscoGel and methylene blue.

### 12.4.1 DiscoGel®

DiscoGel, developed in France and first described by Théron in 2007 [50], consists of a gelified ethanol mixed with tungsten for radiopacity. Whilst pure ethanol was used since a long time, DiscoGel® now is visible and, due to the gelification, more viscous and hence stays better in the disc, and injection could be better controlled to avoid leakage/nerve damage. Its further benefit is the low infection rate due to the antiseptic properties of ethanol.

Studies showed very good pain relief in painful disc in 91.4% of the patients [50] whilst newer studies found a high failure rate in patients with Modic signs [51]. This shows, that in cases with high intradiscal lactate, ethanol seems to be not effective. The downside of the use of ethanol is an intradiscal destruction of nuclear cells and transformation into a scar. Therefore, DiscoGel® is not regarded as a regenerative treatment for the disc. Furthermore, no long-term studies are available.

### 12.4.2 Methylene Blue

Methylene blue has been used in different medical fields since its production in 1877 in Germany. It is one of those forgotten agents with long experience and long use, but overall, too cheap to warrant interest of big medical producers and investors.

This fact alone merits to write a summary about this astonishing "therapeutic agent" [52].

Paul Ehrlich and other researchers described very early its antiseptic properties. It was used worldwide as the first antiseptic in clinical therapy, being the first treatment of malaria in 1891 [53].

Since then, the treatment has been shown to be effective for a whole variety of diseases such as melanoma, lung cancer and congenital or toxic methemoglobinemia [54]. Neurological indications are Alzheimer disease, depression and anxiety, psychosis, cognitive deficits, neuroprotection localized pain and intractable itching. For interesting readers, I recommend the article [54], which gives a complete pharmacological overview about this astonishing and promising substance.

For 20 years, it has been used in China and other Asian countries as a cheap agent against discogenic pain [55]. Without knowing the exact anatomy and endplate innervation at that time, physicians used the right approach with methylene blue. Methylene blue in general destroys nociceptor fibres in the disc, the skin (used, for example for pruritus ani since 1990 [56]) and other indications. Hence, the action of methylene blue seems not to be a regenerating or buffering action but is a pure pain control action by destroying the nociceptors in the disc and endplate. It is a very low-cost agent and has demonstrated its value in various placebo-controlled studies [55, 57] and multicentre studies [58] to be safe. Until today, it is not clear whether it has any regenerative actions on the disc. But, as a well-researched, documented and worldwide used agent with additional antiseptic properties, it is today possibly the best and lowest cost agents for worldwide use in the market of pure discogenic pain without focus on regeneration. Furthermore, the agent may indeed have a regenerative aspect not studied until today, which, comparing DiscoGel and methylene blue, DiscoGel does not have.

Regarding clinical applications of methylene blue based on MRI spectroscopy, please see the treatment scheme below.

### 12.4.3 Ablation of the Basivertebral Nerve

As shown above in the anatomy section, the basivertebral nerve (Fig. 12.2) has been identified as being the main nociceptor of discogenic back pain. As it is a pure sensible nerve, the logical next treatment step was the development of an ablation system with radiofrequency through a transpedicular or extrapedicular approach.

Although this by itself is not a regenerating technique of the disc, it potentially has the same outcome as methylene blue or DiscoGel, e.g. treating discogenic back pain.

The first operation in men was performed by the author in 2008. The description of the technique and the clinical results of an international multicentre study received the Lodwick Award 2017 by Harvard University for the best paper published during the last calendar year in the fields of musculoskeletal radiology, medicine or biology [14].

Out of 17 enrolled patients, in 16 cases, the basivertebral nerve was ablated successfully, and all of those patients showed a significant improvement of the Oswestry Disability Score until the final follow-up at 1 year (Fig. 12.6). In one patient, the

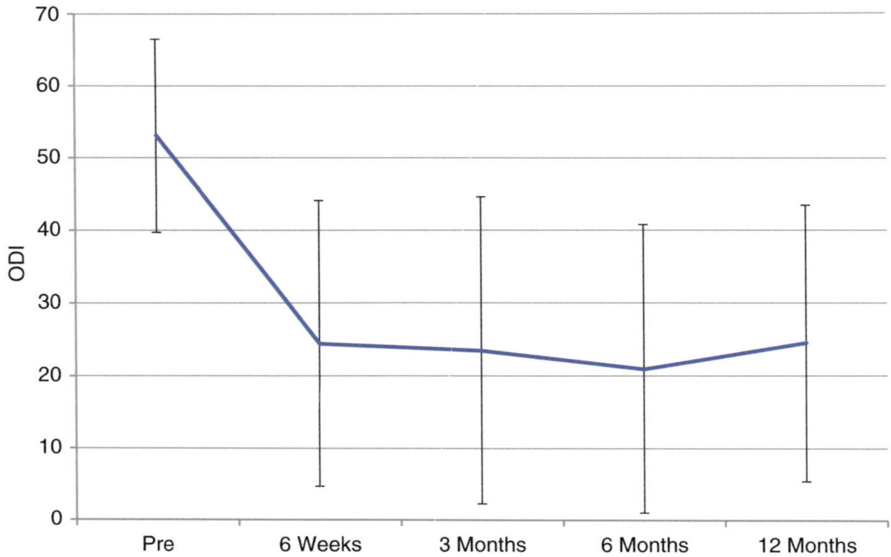


**Fig. 12.6** ODI results of 16 patients treated with BVN ablation. Statistically significant ($p < 0.001$) at each time point compared to the baseline. Minimum clinically significant improvement is ten points of ODI change [14]

basivertebral nerve was missed during the intervention with subsequently no change in back pain. This patient was ultimately fused at the index level. However, none of the successful patients treated by the author were fused until the latest follow-up 8 years after the initial surgery [14].

No resorption of the bone or loss of height was observed during the study (Fig. 12.7).

Since 2008, the author has continued to perform this technique regularly and has never observed any deterioration of bone structures. The positive results were confirmed by a prospective, multicentre, double-blind, sham-controlled (!), FDA-approved investigational device exemption clinical trial in 18 centres [59].

Due to difficulties in obtaining the radiofrequency probe, since 2011 vertebroplasty was used by the author and others in Europe to successfully target the basivertebral nerve with resorbable biocement in Modic patients [60].

Out of 218 treated patients, 172 (79%) showed an immediate significant improvement of ODI/VAS within 4 weeks. Forty-four patients (19%) reached the same clinical improvement after 6 months. Only in 2 cases (1%), no improvement was seen (two patients lost to follow-up [60]).

In all cases, which is also demonstrated by the authors experience, fusion or total disc replacement was avoided. Therefore, ablation of the basivertebral nerve with radiofrequency or vertebroplasty is a potential minimal-invasive option for discogenic pain in patients with discs being too degenerated or too collapsed for intradiscal therapies.

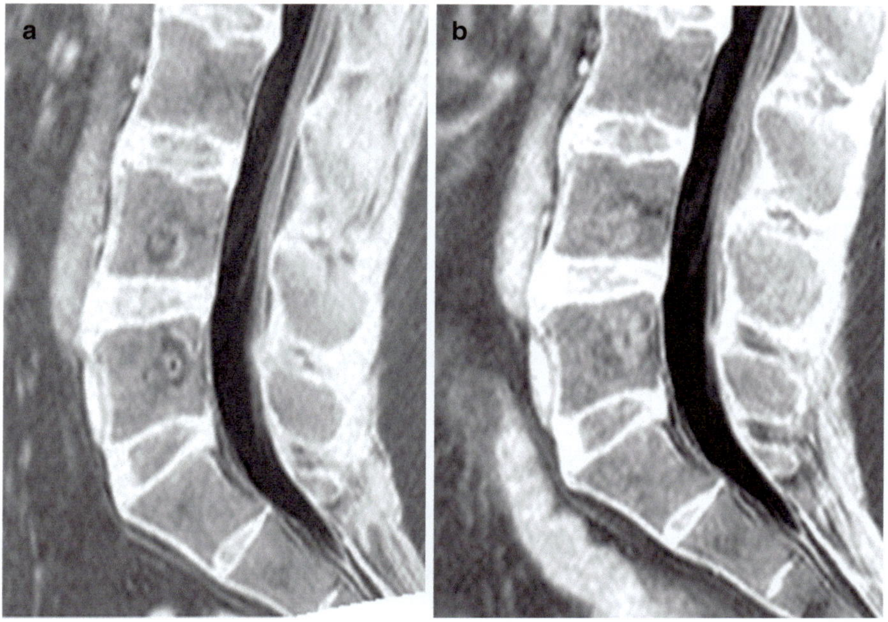


**Fig. 12.7** Forty-nine-year-old male. (**a**) Six weeks after RF ablation of basivertebral nerve L4 and L5. (**b**) 12 months after RF ablation of basivertebral nerve L4 and L5

## 12.5 MRI Spectroscopy-Related Patient Examples and Proposed Treatment Guidelines

This part is showing patient outcomes using some of the abovementioned treatments performed by the author, which exclusively rely on MRI spectroscopy (Nociscan TM), described in Chap. 6.

Like always in medicine, it is beneficial to develop a treatment guideline incorporating new MRI imaging and years of experience with minimal-invasive regenerative techniques.

Therefore, the author developed a staged treatment scheme incorporating the abovementioned regenerative techniques based on the MRI spectroscopy (see Chap. 6.

The treatments described in the guidelines were basivertebral nerve ablation in Modic 1 and 2 situations (performed over the last 7 years as vertebroplasty with resorbable bone cement, intradiscal PRP, intradiscal hydrogels (GelStix, Replication Medical Inc.), conservative treatments (electromagnetic treatments and low laser treatments combined with anti-inflammatory nutraceuticals and disc regenerating nutraceuticals) and finally intradiscal nucleoplasty. Intradiscal nucleoplasty (intradiscal coblation) has not been described in this chapter but is a well-known intradiscal technique used since 1998, initially developed by ArthroCare Inc. to treat contained herniation and has gained a worldwide acceptance [61].

The developed treatment scheme is shown in Fig. 12.8.

The scheme is read as such:

PG pos. Indicates normal proteoglycan levels, e.g. at least >50% as described in the Nociscan™ report. PG neg. means proteoglycan levels <50% in the MRI spectroscopy report.

Lactate pos. signifies any pathological high lactate level and Lactate neg. no increased lactate level in the disc.

The disc height is crucial for many treatments, hence normal disc height means at least 50% of disc height according to adjacent normal levels. Disc height negative means less than 50% according to adjacent normal levels.

Example: A patient with PG pos. Lactate pos., no herniation and normal disc height has an option of treatment 1, e.g. intradiscal PRP, 2 e.g. hydrogel or 5 e.g. conservative treatment.

The scheme should serve as a guideline for inexperienced surgeons and may not contain rare situations. The used approaches are purely chosen after the personal experience of the author. If interested readers have experience with other biomaterials, they are welcome to adapt the scheme. For instance, methylene blue may be used in the indications 1, 2 and 3 as shown in the scheme.

The described treatment scheme was exclusively used in the subsequent examples. Due to very early experience with MRI spectroscopy in Europe, not all of the patients could get re-scanned with spectroscopy prior to printing this book.

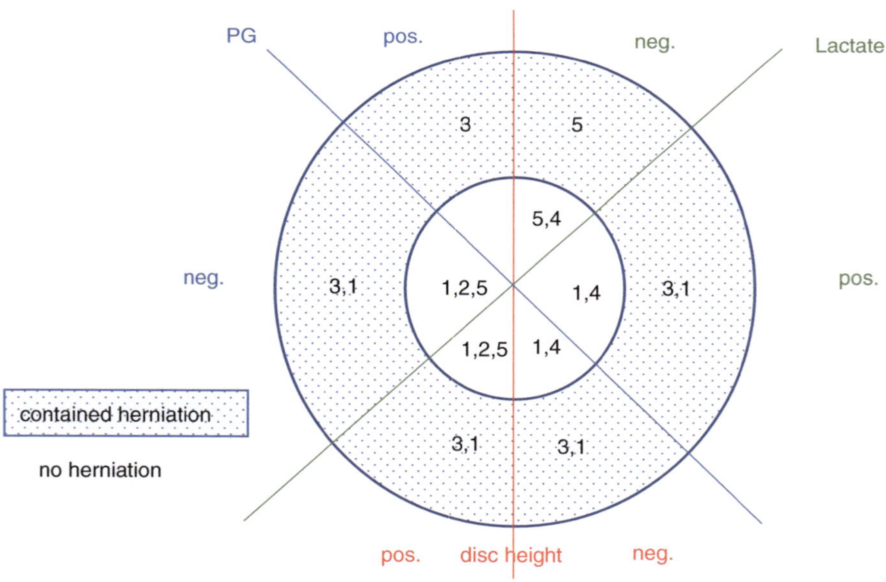


**Fig. 12.8** Treatment scheme developed by the author based on literature and personal experience with the used individual regenerative treatment options and early experience with MRI spectroscopy (Nociscan™). (1) PRP, (2) Hydrogel, (3) Coblation nucleoplasty, (4) Basivertebral RF—Ablation/Vertebroplasty*, (5) Cons. Tx, (asterisk) in Modic 1 and 2 cases

### 12.5.1 **Example 1** (Figs. 12.9a, b and 12.10a, b)

Seventeen-year-old male, Tennis professional, complaining about localized lumbar pain (Vas 6.2) during his sport activities. The regular MRI shows degenerative changes of the L5 disc. Nociscan™ shows in January 2018 positive lactate levels on

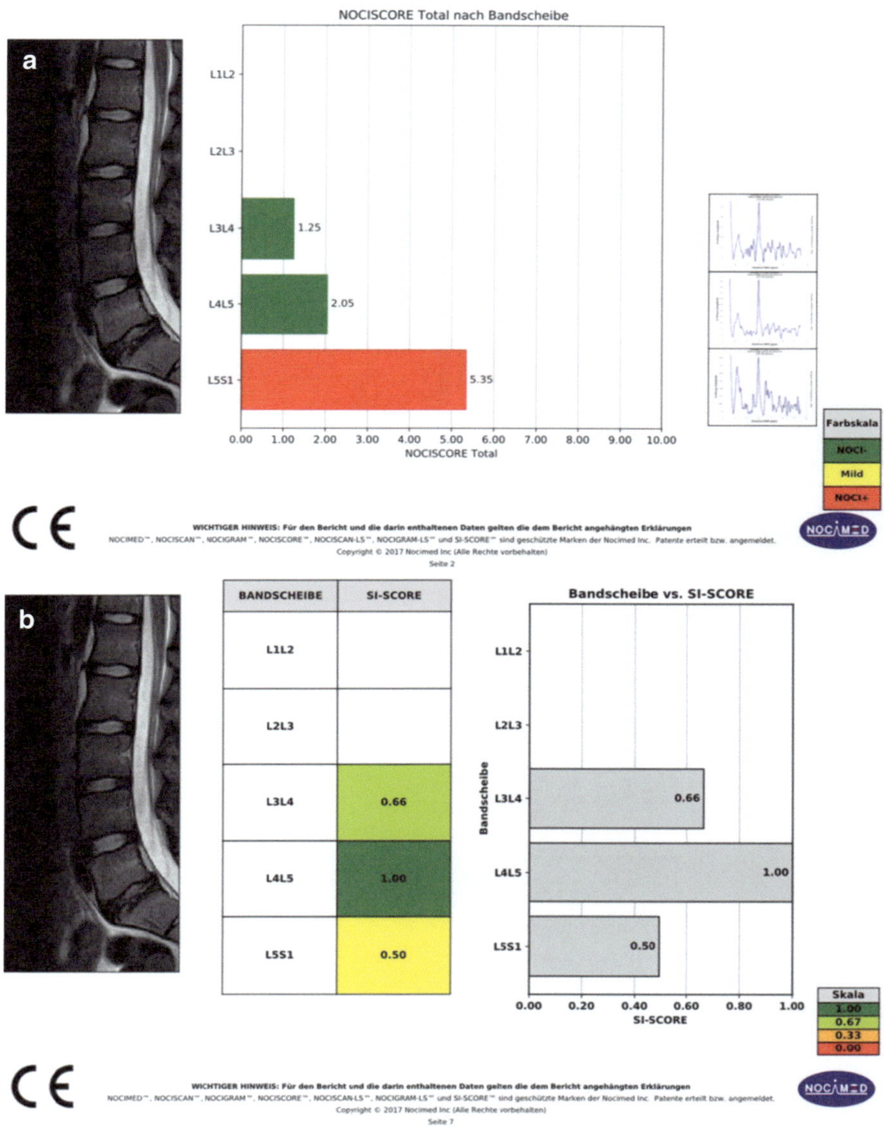


**Fig. 12.9** (**a**, **b**) Example 1

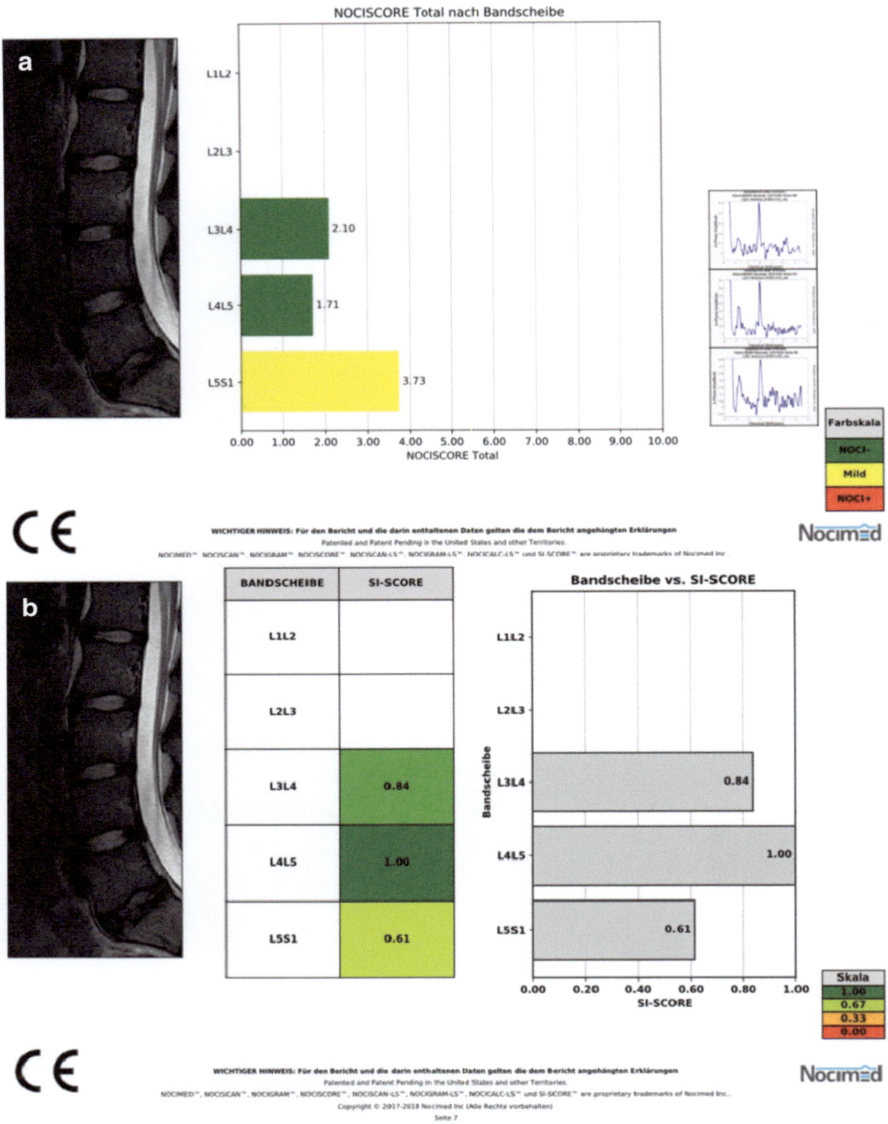


**Fig. 12.10** (**a**, **b**) Example 2

L5 (53.5%) with normal disc biology of L3 and L4. Proteoglycan levels indicating disc stability were normal in L3 and L4 disc whilst reduced (50%) at L5 (Fig. 12.9a, b). According to the treatment scheme (Fig. 12.8), the patient was treated conservatively (electromagnetic field, low laser light treatment, disc focused nutraceuticals, training improvement). The patient was able to play tennis for 6 h per day 3 months after starting the conservative treatment. At the MRI control, 9 months after the treatment, he was pain free whilst continuing to play tennis. The Nociscan™ shows a clear healing of L5 with reduced lactate levels (37.3%) and increased proteoglycan levels on L5 (61%) (Fig. 12.10a, b). The PG levels of L3 also could be increased possibly showing the value of a focused individual nutraceutical disc supplementation. However, we certainly cannot take single cases in order to generalize, but it could well be that the disc is able to regenerative by itself without adding cells if we can reduce the inflammation (e.g. lactate levels as measured in the MRI spectroscopy) in young patients. Time will show whether this trend may also be true for elderly patients; however, it could well be that those patients will need the additional benefit of a cell treatment or, in case of a collapsed disc, just a denervation method (see basivertebral denervation above).

### 12.5.2 **Example 2** (Figs. 12.11, 12.12, and 12.13)

Forty-four-year-old female patient with left-sided radicular pain and focal back pain mid lumbar spine. The MRI shows a medial to slight lateral left-sided herniation of L4 and slight disc degeneration of disc L3 and L4 (Pfirrmann grade 2).

The Nociscan™ was performed in order to assess the intravertebral lactate and proteoglycan levels of the adjacent discs. Lactate levels in the adjacent discs were normal, whilst PG levels were decreased to 29% in L3 (Figs. 12.12 and 12.13).

A microsurgical-assisted nucleoplasty on L4 and a regular nucleoplasty of L3 was performed. The approach in L4 was chosen as coblation nucleoplasty does not only result in an immediate intradiscal loss of pressure [62], but it may also "be capable of initiating a repair response in the disc" [63] and reduce the proinflammatory parameters in the disc [64]. This has a potential to avoid herniation in low proteoglycan discs in the future. The patient was consented that further interventions of the disc L3 (hydrogels / PRP) might be necessary in the event of persisting

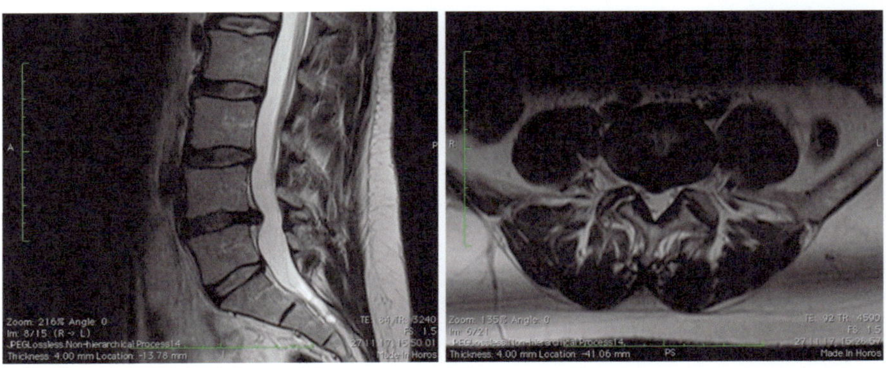


**Fig. 12.11** Example 2

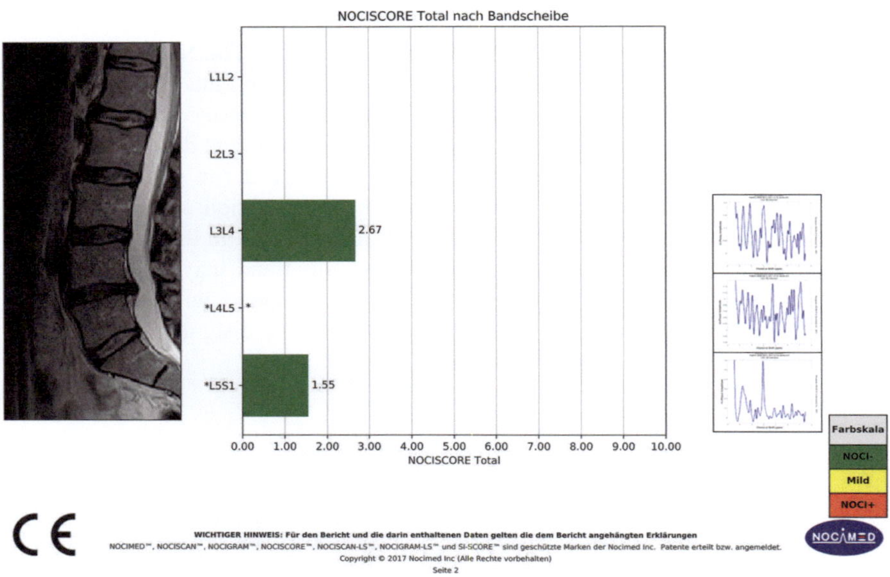


Fig. 12.12 Example 2

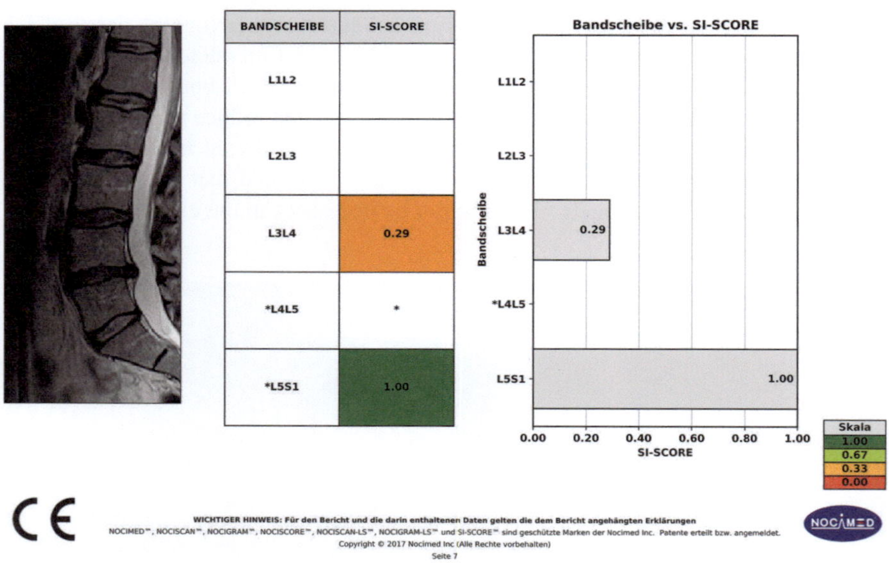


Fig. 12.13 Example 2

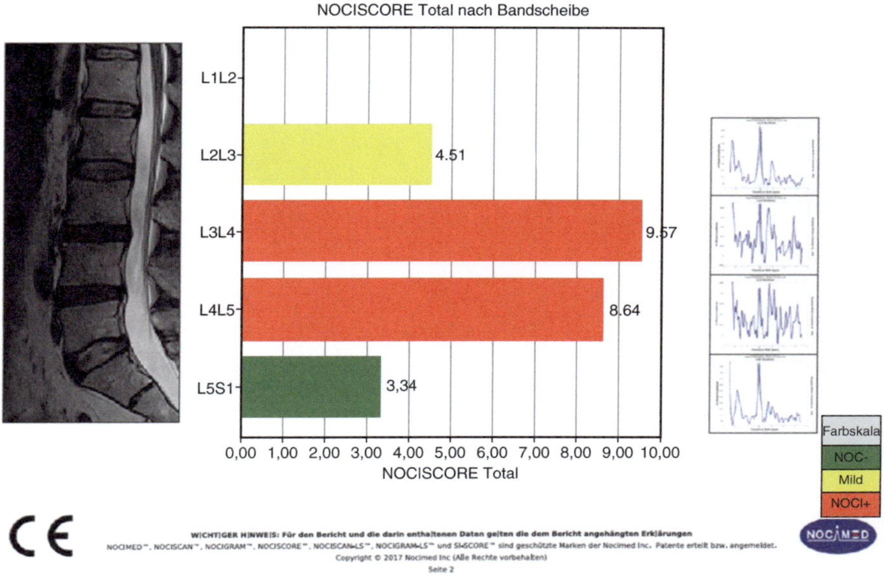


**Fig. 12.14** Example 3

back pain, but the follow-up at 4 weeks showed a significant decrease of back pain and radicular pain (VAS back pre-op 3.4, post-op 0.3, VAS leg pre-op 7.9, post-op 1.2, ODI pre-op 34, post-op 4).

The patient is under constant clinical control, very happy after a successful treatment without deterioration at the time of writing this chapter (12 months after the intervention).

### 12.5.3 Example 3 (Figs. 12.14 and 12.15)

Male, 52 years, chronic back pain. Unemployed because of back pain, on antidepressants. No radicular pain. The MRS shows increased biomarkers in discs L3/L4 and L4/L5 with mildly increased markers on L2/L3 and an intact disc L5/S1 (Fig. 12.14). The stability index assessing the proteoglycan levels shows low levels in L3/L4 and L4/L5 (Fig. 12.15). At the time of discussing, the results with the patient, the patient was very happy, that a cause of his back pain could be established as he had been named a psychiatric case by several physicians and treated accordingly. In order to buffer the increased inflammation biomarkers as well as regenerate the disc, the patient was treated with PRP injections into L3/L4 and L4/L5 (1 ml each, HD-LR-PRP). At the last follow-up 6 months after the treatment, he had stopped the antidepressants and his back pain level dropped to 50% of his

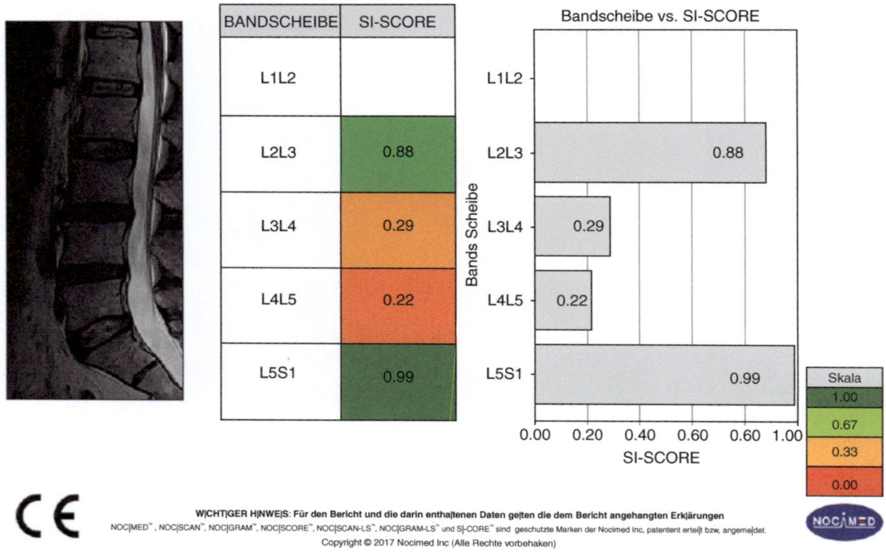


**Fig. 12.15** Example 3

original level. He found new employment and is able to cope with the remaining pain. This case demonstrates the psychological value of MRS in defining the cause of back pain in "psychiatric" cases where MRI alone is not able to describe the origin of pain.

### 12.5.4 Example 4 (Figs. 12.16 and 12.17)

Male 74 years, microdiscectomy L4/L5 right side. Chronic back pain treated with intradiscal ozone injection in L4/L5 in 2015 and 2017. Elevated biomarkers in L3/L4, L4/L5 and L5/S1, decreased proteoglycan levels (SI—spinal stability score) in L4/L5 and L5/S1 (Figs. 12.16 and 12.17). This patient is currently treated conservatively, but it is a good case to demonstrate different options if the conservative treatment fails.

It is clear, that previous physicians did focus only on L4/L5 (also because of the visible Modic changes) as cause of the pain, which obviously has failed, as there is a pain generator in all the lower three disc. According to the treatment algorithm, we have several treatment options. We could of course combine minimal-invasive treatment options, but, lacking long-term outcomes, for a scientific approach it might be best to focus on one treatment.

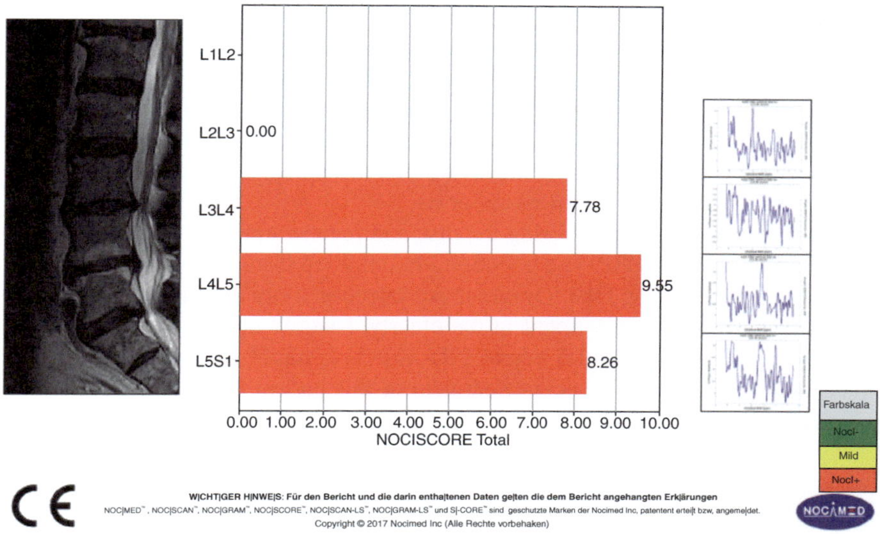


**Fig. 12.16** Example 4

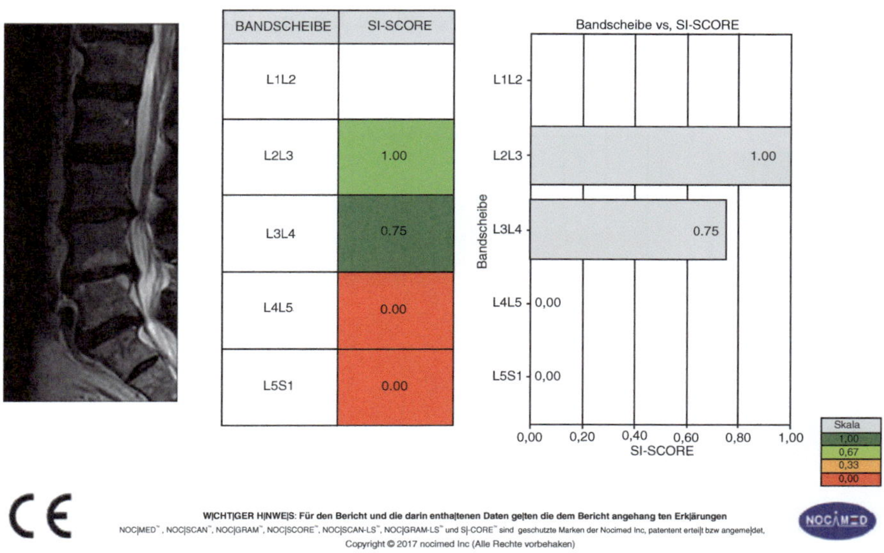


**Fig. 12.17** Example 4

Focusing purely on buffering the elevated biomarkers, hydrogel therapy could potentially be chosen. However, the previously treated disc L4/L5 with scarring and disc collapse is a contraindication for intradiscal hydrogel. Looking at the L3/L4, the disc shows buldging and a hydrogel therapy may disrupt further the annulus. The disc L5/S1 shows to be the most promising disc for a hydrogel treatment but looking at the very low proteoglycan levels with low spinal stability score, again, an inserting of a hydrogel stick might dislocate.

The best candidate for buffering the disc and regenerating the disc in my armamentarium is HD-LR-PRP. The injection into all three discs is possible, whilst the previously operated disc L4/L5 might make injection more difficult. In my experience with basivertebral treatment in the elderly, I would opt for a vertebroplasty, definitely on the levels L4/L5 where PRP injection might not help the patient. I finally will propose the following treatment of this patient if conservative therapy fails: HD-LR-PRP injection into the disc L3/L4 and L5/S1 and vertebroplasty to treat the basivertebral nerve in L4/L5.

### 12.5.5 Example 5 (Figs. 12.18 and 12.19)

Male, 48 years, chronic back pain since more than 10 years, continually increasing. Treating surgeons proposed a multisegmental fusion of the lumbar spine. However, he declined and was able to perform sports till the January 2018. Then lumbar pain during standing, sitting and walking increased significantly. Clinical examination

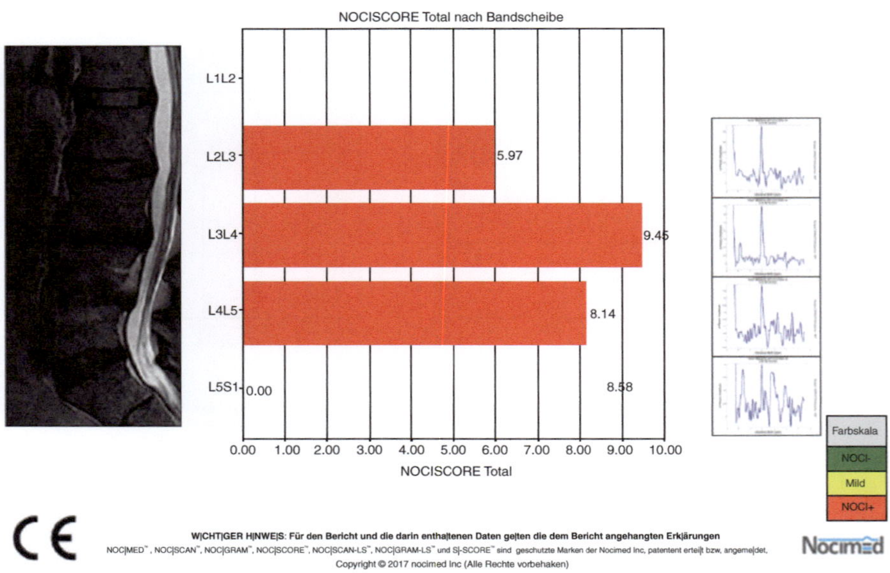


**Fig. 12.18** Example 5

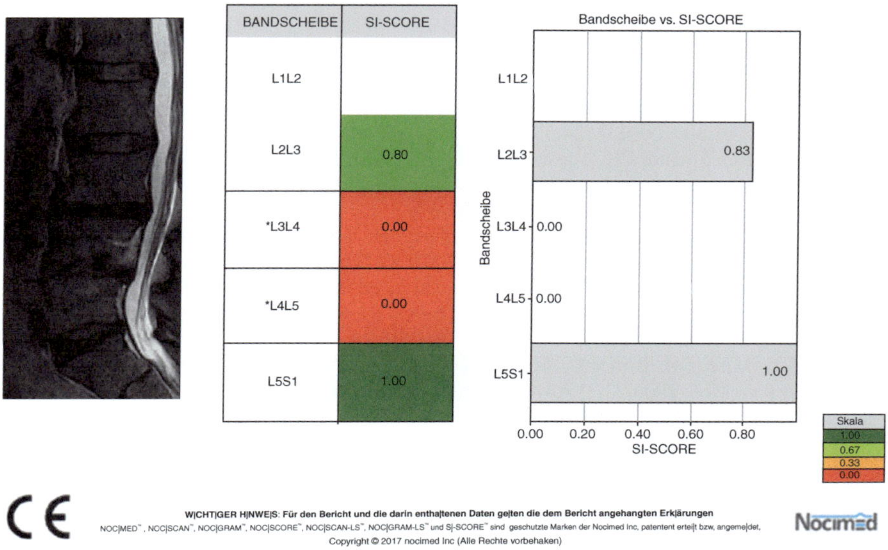


**Fig. 12.19** Example 5

showed an increased tenderness on L3–L5 and SI joint pain on the left side, with most of the pain centred at the lumbar spine. The MRS shows increased biomarkers on disc L2/L3, L3/L4 and L4/L5 (Fig. 12.18). Proteoglycan levels were not detectable in disc L3/L4 and L4/L5 whilst being normal in the adjacent discs (Fig. 12.19).

The patient was treated with a vertebroplasty using a resorbable biocement (Cerament™, Bonesupport Inc.) with injection of 1.5 ml into the vertebrae L3, L4 and L5 at the level of the basivertebral nerve under image intensifier control. Reducing the elevated biomarkers on disc L2/L3, two treatment options were considered, e.g. PRP or intradiscal hydrogel. After discussion, the potentially longer healing course with PRP, the patient opted for the intradiscal hydrogel (GelStix®, Replication Medical, Inc.). The patient is currently at a two-month follow-up. At the 2-week control, he showed an improvement of his VAS score of 70%, at the 2-month follow-up, his lumbar pain was virtually non-existent (less than 0.5) whilst his SI joint pain did not change. Currently he is under SI joint treatment.

Looking at the patient from a spine surgeon's perspective, a two-level fusion L3–L5 would be the most commonly chosen treatment in this case. The MRS showed that the disc degeneration of L2/L3 is much higher than seen on a regular MRI; in this case, an early failure of that disc can be expected after a lumbar fusion. Furthermore, it is known that lumbar fusions increase SI joint degeneration/pain and may lead to SI fusion [65–67]. In this case, the changed biomechanics of the lumbar spine did result in SI joint pain, which would possible have increased after lumbar fusion.

## References

1. Hagen K, Svebak S, Zwart JA. Incidence of musculoskeletal complaints in a large adult Norwegian county population. The HUNT study. Spine. 2006;31(18):2146–50. https://doi.org/10.1097/01.brs.0000231734.56161.6b.
2. Rodriguez AG, Slichter CK, Acosta FL, Rodriguez-Soto AE, Burghardt AJ, Majumdar S, et al. Human disc nucleus properties and vertebral endplate permeability. Spine. 2011;36(7):512–20. https://doi.org/10.1097/BRS.0b013e3181f72b94.
3. Deyo RA, Gray DT, Kreuter W, Mirza S, Martin BI. United States trends in lumbar fusion surgery for degenerative conditions. Spine. 2005;30(12):1441–5; discussion 6–7.
4. Mirza SK, Deyo RA. Systematic review of randomized trials comparing lumbar fusion surgery to nonoperative care for treatment of chronic back pain. Spine. 2007;32(7):816–23. https://doi.org/10.1097/01.brs.0000259225.37454.38.
5. Deyo RA, Mirza SK, Turner JA, Martin BI. Overtreating chronic back pain: time to back off? J Am B Fam Med. 2009;22(1):62–8. https://doi.org/10.3122/jabfm.2009.01.080102.
6. Raoul S, Faure A, Robert R, Rogez JM, Hamel O, Cuillere P, et al. Role of the sinu-vertebral nerve in low back pain and anatomical basis of therapeutic implications. Surg Radiol Anat. 2003;24(6):366–71. https://doi.org/10.1007/s00276-002-0084-8.
7. Antonacci MD, Mody DR, Heggeness MH. Innervation of the human vertebral body: a histologic study. J Spinal Disord. 1998;11(6):526–31.
8. Esses SI, Moro JK. Intraosseous vertebral body pressures. Spine. 1992;17(6 Suppl):S155–9.
9. van Dieen JH, Weinans H, Toussaint HM. Fractures of the lumbar vertebral endplate in the etiology of low back pain: a hypothesis on the causative role of spinal compression in aspecific low back pain. Med Hypotheses. 1999;53(3):246–52. https://doi.org/10.1054/mehy.1998.0754.
10. Weishaupt D, Zanetti M, Hodler J, Min K, Fuchs B, Pfirrmann CWA, et al. Painful lumbar disk derangement: relevance of endplate abnormalities at MR imaging. Radiology. 2001;218(2):420–7. https://doi.org/10.1148/radiology.218.2.r01fe15420.
11. Carragee EJ, Alamin TF, Miller JL, Carragee JM. Discographic, MRI and psychosocial determinants of low back pain disability and remission: a prospective study in subjects with benign persistent back pain. Spine J. 2005;5(1):24–35. https://doi.org/10.1016/j.spinee.2004.05.250.
12. Fras C, Kravetz P, Mody DR, Heggeness MH. Substance P-containing nerves within the human vertebral body. An immunohistochemical study of the basivertebral nerve. Spine J. 2003;3(1):63–7.
13. Bailey JF, Liebenberg E, Degmetich S, Lotz JC. Innervation patterns of PGP 9.5-positive nerve fibers within the human lumbar vertebra. J Anat. 2011;218(3):263–70. https://doi.org/10.1111/j.1469-7580.2010.01332.x.
14. Becker S, Hadjipavlou A, Heggeness MH. Ablation of the basivertebral nerve for treatment of back pain: a clinical study. Spine J. 2017;17(2):218–23. https://doi.org/10.1016/j.spinee.2016.08.032.
15. Lotz JC, Fields AJ, Liebenberg EC. The role of the vertebral end plate in low back pain. Glob Spine J. 2013;3(3):153–64. https://doi.org/10.1055/s-0033-1347298.
16. Becker RO. Cross currents: the perils of electropollution, the promise of electromedicine. Jeremy P Tarcher: Los Angeles, CA; 1990.
17. Kiontke S. Lebende Moleküle. Munsing: VITATEC Verlagsgesellschaft; 2018.
18. Salisbury E, Sonnet C, Heggeness M, Davis AR, Olmsted-Davis E. Heterotopic ossification has some nerve. Crit Rev Eukaryot Gene Expr. 2010;20(4):313–24.
19. Yang SY, Strong N, Gong X, Heggeness MH. Differentiation of nerve-derived adult pluripotent stem cells into osteoblastic and endothelial cells. Spine J. 2017;17(2):277–81. https://doi.org/10.1016/j.spinee.2016.10.002.
20. Agarwal V, Golish SR, Alamin TF. Bacteriologic culture of excised intervertebral disc from immunocompetent patients undergoing single level primary lumbar microdiscectomy. J Spinal Disord Tech. 2011;24(6):397–400. https://doi.org/10.1097/BSD.0b013e3182019f3a.

21. Ohtori S, Koshi T, Yamashita M, Yamauchi K, Inoue G, Suzuki M, et al. Existence of pyogenic spondylitis in Modic type 1 change without other signs of infection: 2-year follow-up. Eur Spine J. 2010;19(7):1200–5. https://doi.org/10.1007/s00586-010-1358-1.
22. Stirling A, Worthington T, Rafiq M, Lambert PA, Elliott TS. Association between sciatica and *Propionibacterium acnes*. Lancet. 2001;357(9273):2024–5. https://doi.org/10.1016/s0140-6736(00)05109-6.
23. Albert HB, Sorensen JS, Christensen BS, Manniche C. Antibiotic treatment in patients with chronic low back pain and vertebral bone edema (Modic type 1 changes): a double-blind randomized clinical controlled trial of efficacy. Eur Spine J. 2013;22(4):697–707. https://doi.org/10.1007/s00586-013-2675-y.
24. Zhang ZM, Zhao L, Qu DB, Jin DD. Artificial nucleus replacement: surgical and clinical experience. Orthop Surg. 2009;1(1):52–7. https://doi.org/10.1111/j.1757-7861.2008.00010.x.
25. Wilke H-J. Principles and mechanical requirements of nucleus implants. Glob Spine J. 2014;4(1 Suppl):s-0034-1376762-s-0034. https://doi.org/10.1055/s-0034-1376762.
26. Hoyland J, Freemont T. Intervertebral disc tissue engineering. Tissue engineering using ceramics and polymers. Amsterdam: Elsevier; 2007. p. 357–78.
27. Scheibler AG, Gotschi T, Widmer J, Holenstein C, Steffen T, Camenzind RS, et al. Feasibility of the annulus fibrosus repair with in situ gelating hydrogels – a biomechanical study. PLoS One. 2018;13(12):e0208460. https://doi.org/10.1371/journal.pone.0208460.
28. Becker S. Surgical options in the osteoporotic spine. In: Mercer's textbook of orthopaedics and trauma. 10th ed. Cleveland, OH: CRC Press; 2012. p. 1046–69.
29. Dabirrahmani D, Becker S, Hogg M, Appleyard R, Baroud G, Gillies M. Mechanical variables affecting balloon kyphoplasty outcome—a finite element study. Comput Methods Biomech Biomed Engin. 2012;15(3):211–20. https://doi.org/10.1080/10255842.2010.522183.
30. Yue JJ, Morgenstern R, Morgenstern C, Lauryssen C. Shape memory hydrogels–a novel material for treating agerelated degenerative conditions of the spine. Eur Musculoskelet Rev. 2011;6(3):184–8.
31. Becker SSH. Lumbar intradiscal treatments: early evaluation of patient satisfaction in disc repair by Nucleus Augmentation (GelStixTM). J Tissue Eng Regen Med. 2012;6(Suppl 1):1–465. https://doi.org/10.1002/term.1586.
32. Meisel HJ, Siodla V, Ganey T, Minkus Y, Hutton WC, Alasevic OJ. Clinical experience in cell-based therapeutics: disc chondrocyte transplantation: a treatment for degenerated or damaged intervertebral disc. Biomol Eng. 2007;24(1):5–21.
33. Hohaus C, Ganey T, Minkus Y, Meisel H. Cell transplantation in lumbar spine disc degeneration disease. Eur Spine J. 2008;17(4):492–503.
34. Ross R, Glomset J, Kariya B, Harker L. A platelet-dependent serum factor that stimulates the proliferation of arterial smooth muscle cells in vitro. Proc Natl Acad Sci. 1974;71(4):1207–10.
35. Witte LD, Kaplan KL, Nossel HL, Lages BA, Weiss HJ, Goodman DS. Studies of the release from human platelets of the growth factor for cultured human arterial smooth muscle cells. Circ Res. 1978;42(3):402–9.
36. Becker S, Weidt F, Röhl K. The role of plasma transglutaminase (F XIII) in wound healing of complicated pressure sores after spinal cord injury. Spinal Cord. 2001;39(2):114.
37. Becker S, Maissen O, Ponomarev I, Stoll T, Meury T, Sprecher C, et al. Osteopromotion with a plasmatransglutaminase on a β-TCP ceramic. J Mater Sci Mater Med. 2008;19(2):659–65.
38. Meury T. Endothelialized tissue engineered 3D-construct for bone repair. Basel: University of Basel; 2005.
39. Wang S-Z, Rui Y-F, Tan Q, Wang C. Enhancing intervertebral disc repair and regeneration through biology: platelet-rich plasma as an alternative strategy. Arthritis Res Ther. 2013;15(5):220.
40. Stoll T, Maissen O, Meury T, Becker S. New aspects in osteoinduction. Materialwissenschaft und Werkstofftechnik: Entwicklung, Fertigung, Prüfung, Eigenschaften und Anwendungen technischer Werkstoffe. 2004;35(4):198–202.

41. Parrish WR, Roides B, Hwang J, Mafilios M, Story B, Bhattacharyya S. Normal platelet function in platelet concentrates requires non-platelet cells: a comparative in vitro evaluation of leucocyte-rich (type 1a) and leucocyte-poor (type 3b) platelet concentrates. BMJ Open Sport Exerc Med. 2016;2(1):e000071.
42. Bielecki T, Gazdzik T, Arendt J, Szczepanski T, Krol W, Wielkoszynski T. Antibacterial effect of autologous platelet gel enriched with growth factors and other active substances: an in vitro study. J Bone Joint Surg. 2007;89(3):417–20.
43. Li H, Hamza T, Tidwell JE, Clovis N, Li B. Unique antimicrobial effects of platelet-rich plasma and its efficacy as a prophylaxis to prevent implant-associated spinal infection. Adv Healthc Mater. 2013;2(9):1277–84.
44. Maeno M, Lee C, Kim DM, Da Silva J, Nagai S, Sugawara S, et al. Function of platelet-induced epithelial attachment at titanium surfaces inhibits microbial colonization. J Dent Res. 2017;96(6):633–9. https://doi.org/10.1177/0022034516688888.
45. Akeda K, Ohishi K, Masuda K, Bae WC, Takegami N, Yamada J, et al. Intradiscal injection of autologous platelet-rich plasma releasate to treat discogenic low back pain: a preliminary clinical trial. Asian Spine J. 2017;11(3):380.
46. Lutz G. Intradiscal PRP study and MRI predictors of outcome. International spine intervention society annual meeting, 30 Jul to 3 Aug 2014, Orlando, FL, 2014
47. Levi D, Horn S, Tyszko S, Levin J, Hecht-Leavitt C, Walko E. Intradiscal platelet-rich plasma injection for chronic discogenic low back pain: preliminary results from a prospective trial. Pain Med. 2016;17(6):1010–22. https://doi.org/10.1093/pm/pnv053.
48. Alexandre A, Giardina G, Caloprisco G, Borean A, Brunori M, Alexandre A, editors. Intradiscal injections of platelet-enriched plasma for degenerative disc disease: degenerative aspects on MRI follow-up 2013. Vienna: European Congress of Radiology; 2013.
49. Tuakli-Wosornu YA, Terry A, Boachie-Adjei K, Harrison JR, Gribbin CK, LaSalle EE, et al. Lumbar intradiskal platelet-rich plasma (PRP) injections: a prospective, double-blind, randomized controlled study. PM&R. 2016;8(1):1–10.
50. Theron J, Guimaraens L, Casasco A, Sola T, Cuellar H, Courtheoux P. Percutaneous treatment of lumbar intervertebral disk hernias with radiopaque gelified ethanol: a preliminary study. J Spinal Disord Tech. 2007;20(7):526–32. https://doi.org/10.1097/BSD.0b013e318033e860.
51. Leglise A, Lombard J, Moufid A. DiscoGel(R) in patients with discal lumbosciatica. Retrospective results in 25 consecutive patients. Orthop Traumatol Surg Res. 2015;101(5):623–6. https://doi.org/10.1016/j.otsr.2015.05.007.
52. Wainwright M, Crossley KB. Methylene blue—a therapeutic dye for all seasons? J Chemother. 2002;14(5):431–43. https://doi.org/10.1179/joc.2002.14.5.431.
53. Guttmann P, Ehrlich P. Ueber die wirkung des methylenblau bei malaria. The Collected Papers of Paul Ehrlich. Amsterdam: Elsevier; 1960. p. 9–14.
54. Oz M, Lorke DE, Hasan M, Petroianu GA. Cellular and molecular actions of methylene blue in the nervous system. Med Res Rev. 2011;31(1):93–117. https://doi.org/10.1002/med.20177.
55. Peng B, Pang X, Wu Y, Zhao C, Song X. A randomized placebo-controlled trial of intradiscal methylene blue injection for the treatment of chronic discogenic low back pain. Pain. 2010;149(1):124–9. https://doi.org/10.1016/j.pain.2010.01.021.
56. Eusebio EB, Graham J, Mody N. Treatment of intractable pruritus ani. Dis Colon Rectum. 1990;33(9):770–2.
57. Peng B, Zhang Y, Hou S, Wu W, Fu X. Intradiscal methylene blue injection for the treatment of chronic discogenic low back pain. Eur Spine J. 2007;16(1):33–8. https://doi.org/10.1007/s00586-006-0076-1.
58. Kallewaard JW, Geurts JW, Kessels A, Willems P, van Santbrink H, van Kleef M. Efficacy, safety, and predictors of Intradiscal methylene blue injection for Discogenic low Back pain: results of a multicenter prospective clinical series. Pain Pract. 2016;16(4):405–12. https://doi.org/10.1111/papr.12283.

59. Fischgrund JS, Rhyne A, Franke J, Sasso R, Kitchel S, Bae H, et al. Intraosseous basivertebral nerve ablation for the treatment of chronic low back pain: a prospective randomized double-blind sham-controlled multi-center study. Eur Spine J. 2018;27(5):1146–56. https://doi.org/10.1007/s00586-018-5496-1.
60. Masala S, Anselmetti GC, Marcia S, Nano G, Taglieri A, Calabria E, et al. Treatment of painful Modic type I changes by vertebral augmentation with bioactive resorbable bone cement. Neuroradiology. 2014;56(8):637–45. https://doi.org/10.1007/s00234-014-1372-9.
61. Eichen PM, Achilles N, Konig V, Mosges R, Hellmich M, Himpe B, et al. Nucleoplasty, a minimally invasive procedure for disc decompression: a systematic review and meta-analysis of published clinical studies. Pain Physician. 2014;17(2):E149–73.
62. Chen YC, Lee SH, Chen D. Intradiscal pressure study of percutaneous disc decompression with nucleoplasty in human cadavers. Spine. 2003;28(7):661–5. https://doi.org/10.1097/01.Brs.0000051920.45671.88.
63. O'Neill CW, Liu JJ, Leibenberg E, Hu SS, Deviren V, Tay BK, et al. Percutaneous plasma decompression alters cytokine expression in injured porcine intervertebral discs. Spine J. 2004;4(1):88–98.
64. Rhyu KW, Walsh AJ, O'Neill CW, Bradford DS, Lotz JC. The short-term effects of electrosurgical ablation on proinflammatory mediator production by intervertebral disc cells in tissue culture. Spine J. 2007;7(4):451–8. https://doi.org/10.1016/j.spinee.2006.07.006.
65. Ha KY, Lee JS, Kim KW. Degeneration of sacroiliac joint after instrumented lumbar or lumbosacral fusion: a prospective cohort study over five-year follow-up. Spine. 2008;33(11):1192–8. https://doi.org/10.1097/BRS.0b013e318170fd35.
66. Ivanov AA, Kiapour A, Ebraheim NA, Goel V. Lumbar fusion leads to increases in angular motion and stress across sacroiliac joint: a finite element study. Spine. 2009;34(5):E162–9. https://doi.org/10.1097/BRS.0b013e3181978ea3.
67. Liliang PC, Lu K, Liang CL, Tsai YD, Wang KW, Chen HJ. Sacroiliac joint pain after lumbar and lumbosacral fusion: findings using dual sacroiliac joint blocks. Pain Med. 2011;12(4):565–70. https://doi.org/10.1111/j.1526-4637.2011.01087.x.

# New Biomaterials for Degenerative Disc Disease

13

Douglas P. Beall, Dereck D. Wagoner, Timothy T. Davis, Timothy Ganey, Edward Yoon, Brooks M. Koenig, Jennifer Witherby, and H. Thomas Temple

## 13.1 Introduction

Degenerative disc disease is one of the main causes of chronic low back pain originating from degeneration of the intervertebral disc and accounts for more patients suffering than any other single cause [1]. Up to 80% of the population will experience low back pain at some point in their lives, and most of them will have pain on many occasions with nearly 20% of the population experiencing low back pain at any given time [2–4]. Back pain is the second leading cause of physician visits next to the common cold and is the greatest cause of disability and lost days from work worldwide [5, 6]. The cost of treating low back pain is extremely high with estimates ranging higher than 100 billion dollars annually [7].

A critically important step in the effective treatment of low back pain is to make an accurate anatomic diagnosis of the exact location of the pain generator. This can

D. P. Beall (✉) · J. Witherby
Oklahoma City, OK, USA
e-mail: db@clinrad.org; jw@clinrad.org

D. D. Wagoner
Interventional Pain, Gershon Pain Specialists, Virginia Beach, VA, USA

T. T. Davis
Source Healthcare, Santa Monica, CA, USA
e-mail: tdavis@sourcehealthcare.com; http://www.sourcehealthcare.com

T. Ganey · H. T. Temple
Vivex Biomedical, Inc., Miami, FL, USA
e-mail: ttemple@vivex.com

E. Yoon
Department of Radiology, Hospital for Special Surgery, New York, NY, USA

B. M. Koenig
305 Hamptonridge Rd, Edmond, OK, USA



L. Manfrè, J. Van Goethem (eds.), *The Disc and Degenerative Disc Disease*,
New Procedures in Spinal Interventional Neuroradiology,
https://doi.org/10.1007/978-3-030-03715-4_13

be challenging but a combination of imaging and diagnostic interventional procedures can reveal the source of back pain in up to 90% of all patients [1].

Discogenic back pain is the most common cause affecting nearly half of the patients with low back pain [1]. Depalma et al. found the prevalence of pain related to the facet joints, sacroiliac joints, and lumbar discs was 31%, 18%, and 42%, respectively [1]. The pain originating from the disc is thought to be due to internal disc disruption (IDD) [8]. This produces the discogenic pain syndrome caused by disc degeneration not related to sciatica or nerve root referred pain. Internal disc disruption has been designated as a separate clinical entity and is thought to account for up to 42% of chronic low back pain [1, 8, 9]. It occurs primarily in younger patients and is separate from other types of degenerative disc entities that will produce pain such as lumbar degenerative disc disease (DDD), segmental instability, and disc herniations [10].

Internal disc disruption is seen as annular disruption on computed tomography (CT) scans after contrast injection or on magnetic resonance (MR) imaging as disc dehydration or high intensity zones, but the findings of disc degeneration along very often do not correlate with either the presence or the severity of the patient's pain [11]. Lumbar X-rays of IDD patients do not have any characteristic signs.

The diagnosis of painful IDD can be supported using provocative and/or anesthetic discography. Discography can be separated into objective anatomic findings on fluoroscopic exam during the procedure and post discogram CT or MRI after injection. Subjective findings constitute recreation of usual and customary pain during pressurization of the suspected disc or alleviation of symptoms after anesthetic infiltration. The use of discography as a method of diagnosing IDD is still debatable, but the authors have found through involvement in numerous intradiscal clinical trials that it is a valid method for assisting in the diagnosis of this anatomic disorder.

The natural history of low back pain due to IDD is chronic and incessant. The treatment for discogenic low back pain has typically been limited to nonsurgical management, disc arthroplasty, or interbody fusion [12]. Despite many treatments available to treat chronic low back pain, there is little consensus among physicians as to which treatment approach is best. Pharmacologic treatment typically includes nonsteroidal anti-inflammatory drugs (NSAIDs) and muscle relaxants, but the literature support for efficacy of treatment is not strong with only minimal improvements in pain and function [13, 14]. Chronic opioid therapy is only marginally effective and is associated with significant side effects and risk of addiction and overdose [14]. Physical therapy with core muscle strengthening along with manipulation has some temporary benefit but the long-term effects are unknown [14]. Epidural injections are performed for patients with discogenic low back pain and have been shown to produce fair results [15]. Intradiscal electrothermal annuloplasty (IDET) was used to treat discogenic low back pain starting in 1996, and a more recent meta-analysis of its effectiveness has shown that this also produces fair results [16]. Over the past two decades, surgical interbody fusion for discogenic back pain has increased significantly but the reported results are mediocre, the postoperative course is difficult, the complication rate is not trivial, and up to 20% of patients will undergo additional surgery within 4 years of lumbar fusion [17–19].

There are therapies that are focused on either treating the inflammatory pathways (i.e., steroid injections) or disrupting the nerve conduction from the painful disc (i.e., methylene blue, ozone, biaculoplasty, etc.) [11]. These types of therapies may be successful in reducing pain but do not have the ability to heal the disc or reverse the degenerative changes suspected to be responsible for the pain. Research efforts have been focusing more on the development of treatments that will repair or regenerate damaged intervertebral discs. Treatments have been focused on restoring the cellular health of the intervertebral disc and on reducing the pain associated with IDD [20].

The benefits of biologic treatments likely originate from tissue repair and changes in cytokine expression following injection of biologic material.

Some of the biologic materials that have been injected into the intervertebral disc include fibrin sealant, isolated growth factors, juvenile chondrocytes, platelet-rich plasma, and mesenchymal stem cells (MSCs) [20, 21]. There have been multiple clinical trials testing MSCs in patients with painful IDD but most of these have had small sample sizes. Despite a lack of firm evidence on the efficacy of stem cell therapy, the trials that have been published suggest a substantial improvement in pain and function [22, 23]. The provisional results of one large phase 2/3 prospective randomized control trial using bone marrow-derived expanded allogeneic MSCs injected into painful lumbar discs has demonstrated significant improvements in pain and function [24].

## 13.2 Intradiscal Biologic Treatments

As mentioned above, there have been many biologic treatments for the intervertebral disc including fibrin adhesives, disc restorative solution, chondrocytes, platelet-rich plasma, bone morphogenic protein, transforming growth factor, disc chondrocytes, and autologous and allogeneic mesenchymal stem cells. Many biologic treatments have been studied and have been found to lack significant efficacy over saline or a placebo. Some of these failed attempts at biologic treatments of the disc have provided guidance for current and future RCTs in this space. Initial studies were focused on MRI changes and 6-month outcomes. We have since learned that MRI changes are not consistent, 6-month results may be too early, and saline treatment to the disc is not a placebo but has up to a 40% responder rate [24]. Biologic therapies still hold significant promise and continue to be studied.

Recent biologic studies for IDD involve injecting directly into the nucleus of the lumbar disc. Risk of discitis has been a concern historically but was found to be between 1 and 4% after discography procedures, but after the introduction of antibiotics the rate of discitis is negligible [25, 26]. Consequently, the use of antibiotics is recommended when injecting any substance into the intervertebral disc.

Discs normally break down their matrix with enzymes such as metalloproteinases, and this degradation is mitigated and/or reversed by certain growth factors such as bone morphogenetic protein-2 (BMP-2), BMP-7 (also known as osteogenic protein-1; OP-1), growth differentiation factor-5 (GDF-5), transforming growth factor-β (TGF-β), insulin-like growth factor-1 (IGF-1), and others [27, 28]. Studies evaluating the use of BMP-7 (OP-1), GDF-5, alpha-2-macroglobulin (A2M), and platelet-rich plasma (PRP) have been conducted to determine the safety and efficacy of these growth factors in treating symptoms from IDD.

### 13.2.1 Fibrin Adhesives

Injection into the disc with fibrin adhesives involves fibrinogen combined with thrombin just prior to injection into the nucleus pulposis with enough volume to fill the potential space of the nucleus and extend into and seal the annular defects from inside (Fig. 13.1). This has been proven in vivo and in vitro [27, 28], and a randomized investigation comparing non-autologous fibrin versus normal saline has shown that significant discal repair occurred along with improvement of the disc's biochemical environment [27]. Although the fibrin sealant initially showed promise, a prospective randomized control trial comparing the fibrin sealant Biostat with a saline injection procedure failed to show statistically significant better results in patients injected with the sealant versus those patient injected when measured at 6 months. This was a rigorous phase III trial with 260 patients including 220 one treatment level subjects and 40 two treatment level subjects who were randomized in a 3:1 ratio. The study has not yet been published.

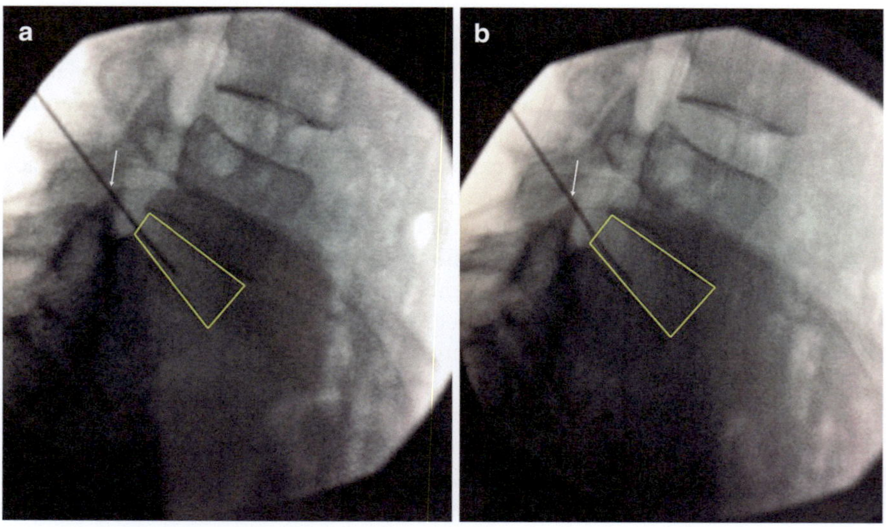


**Fig. 13.1** (**a**, **b**) Lateral fluoroscopic views showing the needle (white arrows in **a** and **b**) in the intervertebral disc. The outline of the disc (yellow lines in **a** and **b**) shows increased disc height after the injection into the nucleus pulposis and adjacent annular fissures (**b**) as compared to the pre-injection disc height (**a**)

### 13.2.2 Bone Morphogenic Protein

A 12-site, double-blind, placebo-controlled RCT with a 3:1 randomization comparing BMP-7 to saline was conducted with 100 patients and a maximum follow-up time of 2 years. The study had patients with less back pain, improved activity levels, better sitting tolerance, and a low crossover to surgery rate; but despite these positive findings, the patients injected with BMP-7 failed to show statistical significance in the primary end points of pain and function improvement. Magnetic resonance imaging of the intervertebral discs also showed no evidence of anatomic improvements. This negative study has not been published at the time of the preparation of this chapter.

### 13.2.3 Growth Differentiation Factor

A phase III trial sponsored by Advanced Technologies and Regenerative Medicine (a Johnson & Johnson affiliate, Raynham, Massachusetts) with 150 patients and 15 clinical sites, including two international sites compared intradiscal GDF-5 with saline. This double-blinded RCT was randomized with half of the patients receiving saline and half receiving GDF-5. The follow-up time points were at 6 months and 1 year but the study was stopped after interim analysis due to lack of efficacy. This study has also not yet been published.

### 13.2.4 Alpha-2-Macroglobulin

In addition to growth factors, alpha-2-macroglobulin (A2M) has been injected into the intervertebral disc [29]. It has been shown that A2M reduces a cartilage degradation product called fibronectin-aggrecan complex (FAC), which has been found in patients with DDD.

A prospective cohort trial with 24 patients with low back pain and MR imaging-concordant DDD were injected with A2M and the Oswestry disability index (ODI) and visual analog scores (VAS) were noted at baseline and at the 3- and 6-month time points [29]. The FAC was also measured in each patient to see if this correlated with the response to A2M injection. It was shown that the patients with FAC-positive in assays were significantly more likely to show pain and functional improvement. The mean VAS improvement in FAC-positive patients was $4.9 \pm 0.9$ and $4.0 \pm 1.0$ at 3- and 6-month, compared to $1.5 \pm 1.2$ and $2.3 \pm 1.3$ in those with negative FAC ($p < 0.0001$). The ODI also improved significantly with an average of $37 \pm 9.3$ and $28 \pm 14$ points at 3- and 6-month in FAC-positive patients compared to $9.4 \pm 11.9$ and $12.6 \pm 11.8$ points at 3- and 6-month in FAC-negative patients ($p < 0.0001$). The authors concluded that A2M may be an important treatment for the pain and dysfunction associated with DDD provided that the FAC biomarker is present. The study was rigorous as the authors used a definition of clinical improvement that was in excess of the minimal clinically important difference (MCID) and an outcome measure that was a combination of the VAS and ODI.

### 13.2.5 Platelet-Rich Plasma

The use of intradiscal PRP has substantially more data than nearly all the other growth factor studies combined (Table 13.1), and all of the observational studies were considered to be of moderate quality as assessed by the Interventional Pain Management Techniques–Quality Appraisal of Reliability and Risk of Bias Assessment for Nonrandomized Studies (IPM-QRBNR) criteria [30]. One RCT of

**Table 13.1** Recent study details and outcomes of the use of Platelet Rich Plasma (PRP) in intervertebral disc degeneration

| Study details | Chronicity of injury and biologic used | Follow-up period | Conclusions |
|---|---|---|---|
| Tuakli-Wosornu et al., 2016 (277)<br>Lumbar discogenic pain<br>Prospective, double-blind, randomized controlled study, $n = 47$ | Chronic<br>PRP injections | 1 year | Intradiscal injections of PRP ×1 showed significant improvement at 8-week follow-up, with maintained improvement compared to controls at 1-year follow-up |
| Monfett et al., 2016 (276)<br>Lumbar discogenic pain, lumbar disc degeneration<br>Prospective trial, $n = 29$ | Chronic<br>PRP injections | 2 years | Intradiscal PRP injections show continued safety and improvements in pain and function at 2 years post-procedure |
| Navani et al., 2018 (274)<br>Lumbar discogenic pain<br>Prospective case series, $n = 20$ | Chronic<br>PRP, single injection, 2 mL injected up to 3 disc levels | 18 months | At 18 months, 15 patients remained for survey compared to 18 patients surveyed at 6 months: >50% relief in VAS in 93% of patients at 18 months ($n = 14/15$) and in 94% of patients ($n = 17/18$) at 6 months [2]. Improvement in SF-36 scores in 93% of patients at 18 months ($n = 14/15$) compared to 100% ($n = 18/18$) at 6 months |
| Akeda et al., 2017 (279)<br>Lumbar discogenic pain<br>Preliminary clinical trial, $n = 14$ | Chronic<br>PRP injections | 12 months | Intradiscal injection of autologous PRP releasate in patients with low back pain was safe with no adverse events observed during follow-up<br>The results showed reduction in mean pain scores at 1 month sustained throughout the observation periods of 6 and 12 months |
| Levi et al., 2016 (275)<br>Lumbar discogenic pain<br>Prospective trial, $n = 8$ | Chronic<br>PRP, single injection | 6 months | Single or multiple levels (up to 5) of discogenic pain injected with PRP showed encouraging improvement, with more patients developing improvement over time. Cohort up to 6 months |

(continued)

**Table 13.1** (continued)

| Study details | Chronicity of injury and biologic used | Follow-up period | Conclusions |
|---|---|---|---|
| Kirchner and Anitua, 2016 (278)<br>Lumbar disc degeneration<br>Observational retrospective pilot study, $n = 86$ | Chronic<br>PRGF-Endoret | 6 months | Fluoroscopy-guided infiltrations of intervertebral discs and facet joints with PRGF in patients with chronic low back pain resulted in significant pain reduction assessed by VAS<br>The results showed reduction of the VAS over time. The study ended at 6 months with 91% of the patients showing an excellent score, 8.1% showing moderate improvement, and 1.2% showing lack of response |

Adapted from: Navani A, Manchikanti L, Albers SL, Latchaw RE, Sanapati J, Kaye AD, Atluri S, Jordan S, Gupta A, Cedeno D, Vallejo A, Fellows B, Knezevic NN, Pappolla M, Diwan S, Trescot AM, Soin A, Kaye AM, Aydin SM, Calodney AK, Candido KD, Bakshi S, Benyamin RM, Vallejo R, Watanabe A, Beall D, Stitik TP, Foye PM, Helander EM, Hirsch JA. Responsible, Safe, and Effective Use of Biologics in the Management of Low Back Pain: American Society of Interventional Pain Physicians (ASIPP) Guidelines. Pain Physician. 2019 Jan;22(1S):S1-S74

*PRP* platelet-rich plasma, *PRGF* plasma rich in growth factors, *VAS* Visual Analog Scale, *SF-36* 36-item Short Form Survey

47 patients followed for 1 year concluded that a single intradiscal injection of PRP showed significant improvement in pain beginning at an 8-week follow-up that was maintained when compared to control patients at the 1-year follow-up. A meta-analysis including all other studies in Table 13.1 with a pooled patient number of 171 was analyzed, five of the studies showed decrease in pain scores following injection of PRP [31–36]. The combined mean difference in pain scores at the 6-month follow-up was 40.29 ± 13.76 points (95% CI: −67.25 to −13.33, $p < 0.001$, $I^2$ 93.3%). Heterogeneity across all of the studies was high ($I^2 = 98\%$). The 12-month follow-up evaluation had three studies with 63 patients and showed a decrease in post-injection pain scores [31–36]. The combined mean difference in pain scores from baseline to 12-month follow-up was 34.405 ± 6.879 points (95% CI: −47.88 to −20.92, $p < 0$ 0.013, $I^2$ 77.2%). Heterogeneity across the studies at the 12-month follow-up was also high ($I^2 = 77\%$). Due to differences in functional measurement and a lack of detailed data meta-analysis results of functional improvement data were not possible.

### 13.2.6 Mesenchymal Stem Cells/Medicinal Signalling Cells

As mentioned, the use of MSCs in the intervertebral disc has been characterized by small clinical trials and RCTs with small sample sizes. A recent meta-analysis by Wu et al. [22] conducted a random effects model analysis to assess outcomes. The initial search identified 1393 articles but only six studies were appropriate for review. The characteristics of these studies are shown in Table 13.2. Three of these studies used MSCs [37–39] and three used chondrocytes [40–42] with five of the six

**Table 13.2** Characteristics of the studies on cell-based therapy for the treatment of discogenic low back pain

| Study | Sample size | Patients age (years) | Population | Cell type | Cell dose and deliver pathway | Follow up (months) | Main evaluation index |
|---|---|---|---|---|---|---|---|
| Mochida | 9 | 20–29 years | Patients with Pfirrmann grade III disc degeneration and posterior lumbar intervertebral fusion | Autologous cultured nucleus pulposus chondrocytes that cocultured with MSCs | One million activated autologous NP cells were injected into the degenerated disc 7 days after fusion surgery | 36 months | JOA and MRI |
| Kenneth Pettine 2015 | 26 | 18–61 years (median 40) | Patients presented with symptomatic moderate-to-severe discogenic low back pain | Autologous bone marrow concentration (non-expanded) | 2–3 ml of bone marrow concentrate was injected in lumbar disc ($1.66 \times 10^6$ ml$^{-1}$) | 24 months | ODI, VAS, and MRI |
| Xiao Dong Pang 2014 | 2 | 41.5 ± 3.5 (mean ± SD) | Patients with low back pain >2 years without lower leg pain and provocative discography (+) | Cultured human umbilical cord tissue-derived mesenchymal stem cells | 1–2 ml of cultured HUC-MSCs ($1 \times 10^7$ ml$^{-1}$) injected into lumbar disc immediately following discography | 24 months | ODI and VAS scores |
| Domagoj Coric 2013 | 15 | 19–47 years (median 40) | Patients with single-level, symptomatic lumbar DDD from L3 to S1 and medically refractory low back pain | Expanded allogeneic juvenile chondrocyte cells | Mean 1.3 ml (1–2 ml, $10^7$ ml$^{-1}$) cells solution was injected in the center of the disc space | 12 months | ODI and NRS scores, 36-item short form health survey and MRI |
| Lluis Orozco 2011 | 10 | 35 ± 7 (mean ± SD) | Patients with degenerative disc disease and persistent low back pain (>6 months; decrease of disc height >50%) | Autologous expanded bone marrow-derived mesenchymal stem cells | $23 \pm 5 \times 10^6$ autologous expanded BMSCs was injected into the nucleus pulposus area | 12 months | ODI and VAS scores and MRI |
| Hans Joerg Meisel 2006 | 12 | 18–75 years | Patients with discogenic pain after repeat discograms. Patients were treated cell therapy at least 3 months post endoscopy | Autologous cultured disc-derived chondrocytes (from surgical treatment of their disc prolapsed) | Cells are injected into disc approximately 12 weeks following discectomy. The cell dose was not mentioned | 24 months | ODI, VAS scores, and MRI |

Adapted from: Wu, T, Song, HX, Dong, Y, Li, JH. Cell-based therapies for lumbar discogenic low back pain: systematic review and single-arm meta-analysis. *Spine*. 2018; 43: 49–57 studies expanding the number of cells. The number of cells injected into the lumbar intervertebral discs varied widely ranging from 1 to 23 million cells ±5 million cells and the follow-up averaged 22 months, ranging from 12 to 36 months.

The VAS or numerical rating scale (NRS) of the studies had a prominent combined mean statistically significant difference in pain from baseline to follow-up of 44.2 points (95% CI: −61.8 to −26.5, $p < 0.001$, $I^2 = 99.4\%$). The ODI also demonstrated a profoundly positive difference with a pooled mean difference from baseline to follow-up of 32.2 points decreased (95% CI: −41.6 to −22.9, $p < 0.001$, $I^2 = 99.5\%$).

A subgroup analysis that evaluated potential heterogeneity in pain scores in respect to the injected cell type (stem cell versus chondrocyte) or the follow-up time period demonstrated that there was no difference in pain scores between either group in the follow-up times. These results, however, showed that the stem cells were more effective than the chondrocytes in giving rise to significantly less pain ($p < 0.001$).

The meta-analysis of Wu et al. also examined the MR imaging evaluation of patients undergoing cell therapy of the intervertebral disc and found some improvements in the contour and height of the disc along with an increase in the signal within the disc at the 12-month follow-up [22]. The increased signal noted at the final follow-up was initially not there at the 6-month follow-up. In the study by Mochida et al., when the degree of degeneration of the treated disc was less than a Pfirrmann grade III, there were no cases where the disc degeneration worsened at the time of the final 3-year follow-up.

The cellular therapy is designed to augment the existing cells within the intervertebral disc. The disc is a relatively acellular tissue with a cell density of only $5.8 \times 10^3$ cells/mm$^3$, and the cell number decreased prominently with age [43]. These cells play an important role in the production of matrix and in the maintenance of health of the intervertebral disc [43]. The process of DDD involves the loss of matrix and nucleus pulposis (NP) cells, so the therapeutic strategy of cellular therapy is to augment this cell population in an attempt to restore the functioning cell population and the matrix that would follow. The cell types that have been investigated include both autologous and allogeneic chondrocytes and MSCs. In one of the largest clinical trial to date, autologous chondrocytes were obtained from the patients after their discectomies, expanded in culture, and given back to them after cell expansion [42]. Despite the success seen in the trial, it was limited to only patients who required surgery for their disc herniation and to apply this harvesting process in patients who did not have surgery would necessitate a separate interventional procedure prior to cell expansion and reinjection. Allogenic cells donated from health donors and tissue banks would overcome this limitation, and as mentioned, the MSC cells had a significantly better outcome in reducing pain than did the chondrocyte cells [22].

Mesenchymal stem cells, also called medicinal signaling cells (MSCs), can be isolated from a number of different tissues and show promise for repairing tissues in the intervertebral disc [22]. The MSCs can renew themselves while maintaining an undifferentiated phenotype but when exposed to certain stimuli they undergo differentiation into certain types of cells such as NP cells or chondrocytes. Bone marrow-derived MSCs are the most commonly used autologous stem cell but only represent a small percentage of the total number of cells present in the bone marrow. This low number further decreases with increasing donor age normally. Recent work with MSCs has shown that if cocultured with NP cells, the MSCs could be differentiated into NP cells [44], so MSCs taken from multiple sources could be induced into the type of cell needed for augmenting the intervertebral disc.

The cell number is also something that may be important but remains controversial as to what is the right cell number to inject into the disc. Pettine et al. used unexpanded bone marrow concentrate in their study with an average CD34 cell concentration of $1.66 \times 10^6$ per mL, and they used 2–3 mL for the injection [37]. The as of yet unpublished phase II study sponsored by Mesoblast (Mesoblast Ltd., Melbourne, Australia), and evaluating Rexlemestrocel-L, reportedly compared the injection of 6 and 18 million MSCs per disc and found that the six million injection worked better for reducing pain. Therefore, it is thought that identifying the optimal number to inject into each disc is important.

In addition to cell number, some authors have advocated for a carrier to keep the MCSs within the intervertebral disc and to assist and support the MSCs until the cells can graft on to the native anatomy [45, 46]. A carrier or scaffold can be important to protect the cells from the harsh environment of the degenerated disc and can restore some of the support and mechanical function of the disc while the regeneration can take place [47].

## 13.3 Level I Data with Allogeneic MSCs

### 13.3.1 Rexlemestrocel-L (Mesoblast)

In addition to the meta-analysis of the completed trials using cellular therapy to treat painful DDD, there are ongoing clinical trials currently being conducted at the time of the writing of this chapter including three open-label single-arm trials and two phase I/II randomized control trials. There have also been two large blinded placebo-controlled RCTs that have been completed. One of these completed trials is coming on the heels of some very positive but as of yet unpublished on the phase II Rexlemestrocel-L trial data and the other large placebo-control RCT is a triple-armed trial with 224 patients that has provisional results that have been reported at multiple conferences [48, 49]. This trial is evaluating a product that contains $6 \times 10^6$ combined with micronized disc material ground to a size of 300 μm that is used as an allograft carrier [49].

The phase I work with Rexlemestrocel-L was performed with an ovine model with STRO-1 and STRO-3 antibody-labelled allogeneic MCSs. The intervertebral discs were injected with chondroitinase at three levels to produce a DDD model, and the discs were treated differently (Fig. 13.2). One level was treated with MSCs plus hyaluronic acid (the carrier), one level was treated hyalgan alone, and the other level received no treatment (Fig. 13.2). An MR imaging exam obtained 9 months

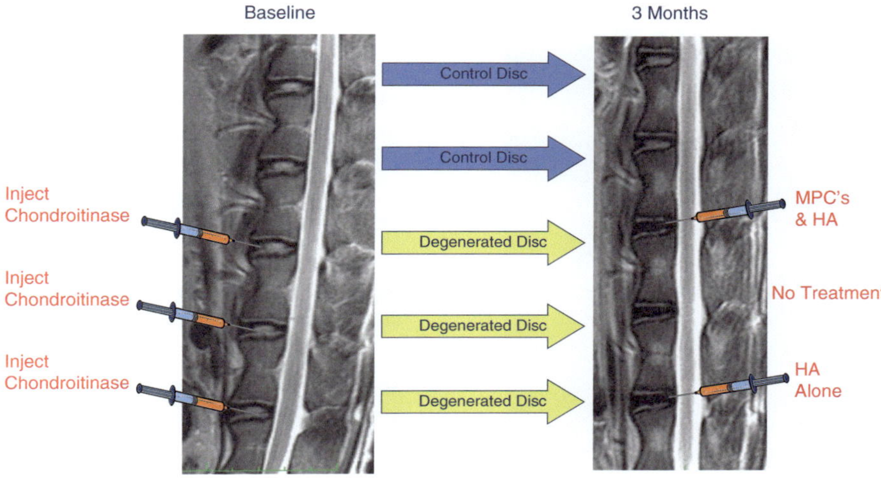


**Fig. 13.2** Lateral STIR MR images of an ovine spine showing the baseline intervertebral discs being injected with chondroitinase (image on the left) and the status of the discs at 3 months (image on the right). The chondroitinase produced degeneration of the intervertebral discs at the three levels where it was injected. The three levels received different treatments with one level treated with MSCs and hyaluronic acid (the carrier), one level treated hyaluronic acid alone and the other level received no treatment

after the initial MRI and 3 months after the chondroitinase injection showed complete restoration of the fluid signal within the intervertebral disc treated with the MSCs and hyaluronic acid but no change in the degenerated absence of fluid signal in the other two discs that were not treated with the MSCs (Fig. 13.3).

The phase II trial studying the allogeneic MSCs produced by Mesoblast was a prospective, multicenter, double-blinded, controlled clinical study of two doses of allogeneic MSCs combined with hyaluronic acid in subjects with discogenic low back pain [24]. This study included patients had back pain for more than 6 months, a visual analog score (VAS) of >40, an Oswestry Disability Index (ODI) score of >30, and had failed at least 3 months of nonoperative care. The patient selection included intervertebral discs with a moderate amount of degeneration (modified Pfirrmann score 3–6) [50] without or with a protrusion that was less than 3 mm. Patients were excluded if they had clinically significant radiculopathy, sacroiliac pain, facet-mediated pain (diagnosed via relief from facet injection or medial branch block), severely degenerated discs, or full thickness tears of the annulus fibrosis.

There were 100 total patients that were randomized to one of four treatment arms receiving intradiscal injection: saline (control), hyaluronic acid (HA), HA and six million MSCs, or HA and 18 million MSCs. The pain (VAS) and disability (ODI) were evaluated at 1, 3, 6, 12, and 24 months [24].

At the 24-month follow-up 60.9% of patients receiving six million MPCs had ≥50% pain reduction ($p = 0.020$) and 47.8% ($p = 0.093$) of those receiving 18 million MPCs had more than a 50% reduction in pain (Fig. 13.4). This was compared

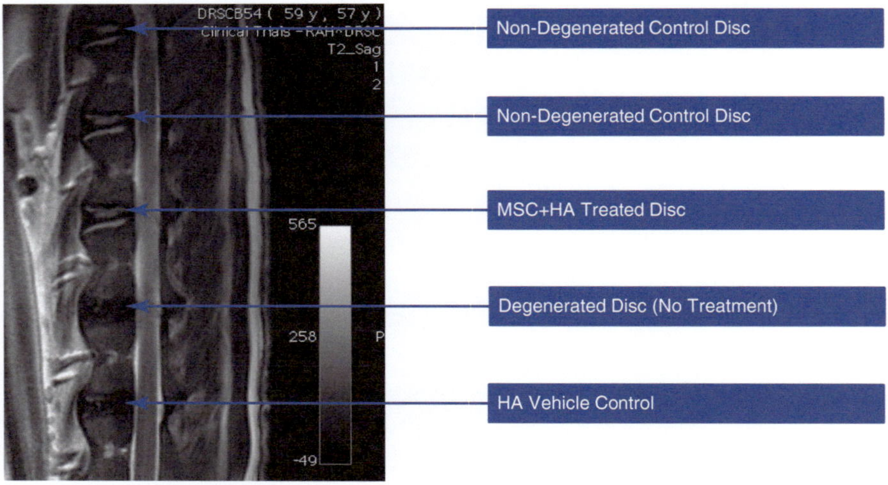


**Fig. 13.3** Lateral STIR MR images of an ovine spine taken 6 months after injecting 0.5 million MSCs shows signal similar to the control discs in the disc treated with MSCs but no change in the appearance in the other discs from the MRI obtained 3 months after injecting chondroitinase

**Fig. 13.4** Percent of patients with ≥50% back pain reduction at 24 months

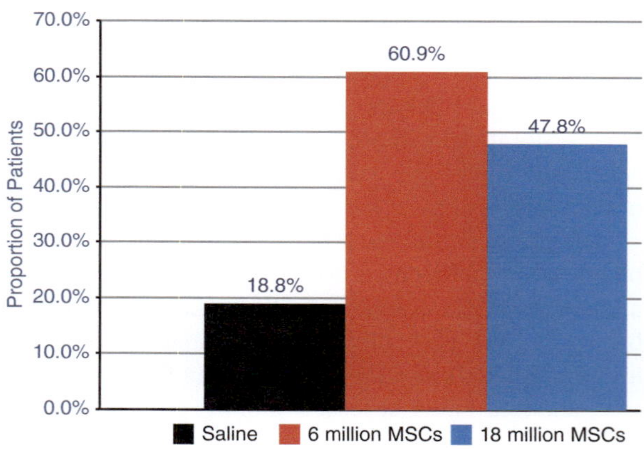


to only 18.8% of controls that had this degree of pain relief. More than half of the patients in the six million MPC arm had complete or near-complete resolution of pain with VAS scores in the range from 0 to 10. The ODI disability scores improved ≥15 points in 56.5% ($p = 0.024$) of the patient injected with six million MSCs and in 60.9% ($p = 0.020$) of the patients in the 18 million MSC arm, compared to only 18.8% in the saline control group (Fig. 13.5) [24].

After a 3-year follow-up, 86% of the patients treated with the six million cell dose that successfully met the 24-month primary end point for pain reduction remained successful at meeting this end point at 36 months (Fig. 13.6) [24]. The

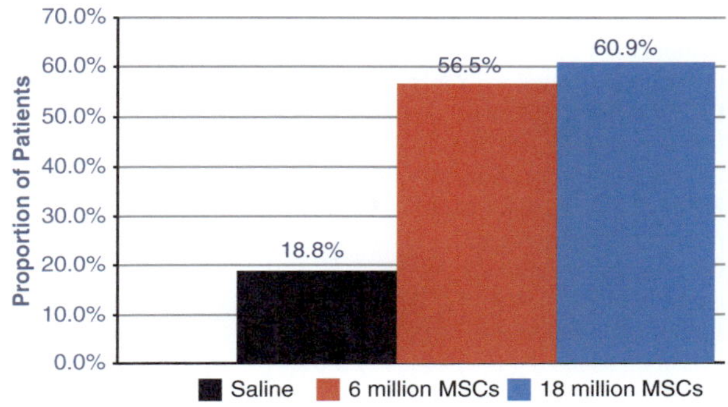


**Fig. 13.5** Proportion of patients that had no subsequent intervention after the initial intradiscal injection with at least a 15 point improvement in the Oswestry Disability Index score at the 24 month follow-up

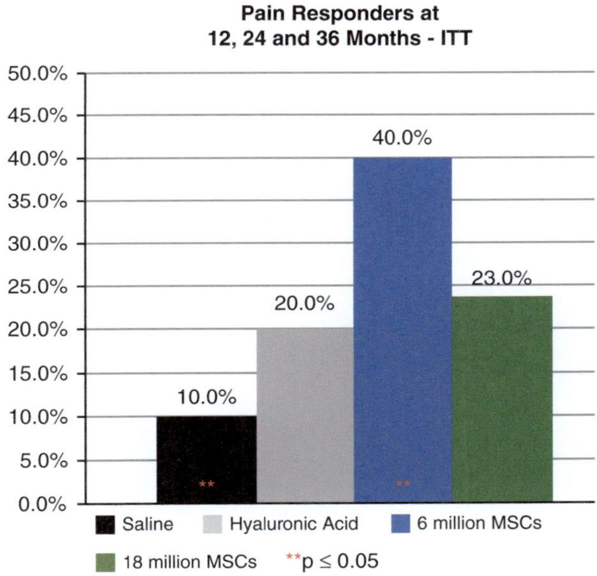


**Fig. 13.6** Bar graph demonstrating that 86% of the patients treated with the six million cell dose that successfully met the 24 month primary endpoint for pain reduction remained successful at meeting this endpoint at 36 months. In this trial a pain responder is classified as having a greater than or equal to 40% reduction in pain and no additional intervention

3-year functional improvement showed that 92% of the patients treated with the six million cell dose that successfully met the 24-month primary end point for disability improvement remained successful at meeting this end point at 36 months (Fig. 13.7) [24].

Given this data from the phase II trial of 100 patients, it was concluded that MSCs cells injected into moderately degenerated discs causing discogenic back pain can demonstrate statistically significant improvement in pain and function at 3 years compared to normal saline controls [24]. The dose of six million MSCs demonstrated statistically significant better pain control but equivalent improvements in disability relative to 18 million MSCs. There were no SAEs reported in this trial.

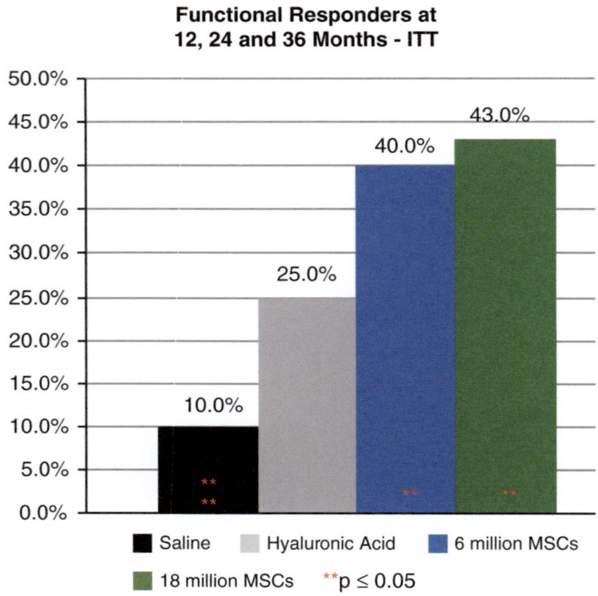


**Fig. 13.7** Bar graph demonstrating that 92% of the patients treated with the six million cell dose that successfully met the 24 month primary endpoint for disability improvement remained successful at meeting this endpoint at 36 months. In this trial a functional responder is classified as having a greater than or equal to a 15 point reduction in ODI and no additional intervention

**Table 13.3** Current trials involving cellular augmentation of the intervertebral disc in patients with internal disc disruption and discogenic back pain

| Sponsor | N | Phase | Design | Cell type | Dosage | Outcomes |
|---|---|---|---|---|---|---|
| Red de Terapia | 24 | I–II | RCT, 2 arms | Autologous BMSC, cultured | 25 M | VAS, ODI, SF-12, MRI, AEs |
| Bioheart | 100 | II | Open label, single arm | Autologous AMSC + PRP | Will vary | VAS, ODI |
| Biostar | 8 | I–II | Open label, single arm | Autologous AMSC | 40 M | VAS, MRI, AEs |
| Inbo Han, CHA University | 10 | I | Open label, single arm | Autologous AMSC | 20-40 M + HA | VAS, ODI, SF-36, MRI, DHI, AEs |
| DiscGenics | 60 | I | DBRCT (HA/Plac) | Allogeneic, cultured | 3 M and 9 M + HA | VAS, ODI, EQ-5D, TUG |

## 13.3.2 Ongoing Clinical Trials

At the time of writing this chapter, there were five ongoing trials evaluating the safety and effectiveness of MSCs for treating low back pain associated with DDD including three open-label single-arm trials and two RCTs (Table 13.3). In addition to the studies evaluated in the meta-analysis by Wu et al. [22] and the phase II trial by Mesoblast discussed above, there is a completed phase III Mesoblast trial and a nearly complete three-arm-blinded RCT evaluating a product called VIA Disc® made by Vivex Biomedical (Atlanta, Georgia, USA) (Table 13.4).

**Table 13.4** Completed randomized control trials of cellular augmentation of the intervertebral disc in patients with internal disc disruption and discogenic back pain

| Sponsor | *N* | Phase | Design | Cell type | Dosage | Outcomes |
|---|---|---|---|---|---|---|
| Mesoblast | 404 | III | RCT, three arms | Allogeneic MSCs | 6MM<br>6MM + HA | VAS, ODI |
| Vivex | 224 | HCTP-361 | RCT, three arms | Viable allograft | 6 MM + micronized disc material | VAS, ODI |

The largest trials are evaluating the use of allogeneic MSCs that are selected through a specific enzymatic reagent and mechanical process either by immunoselection and cell sorting or by isolating and growing intermediate cells into discogenic cells. These cells are already predisposed to in vitro or in vivo differentiation into cells of bone, fat, and cartilage lineages and are not immunogenic. It is the hope that allogeneic MSC therapy can offer "off-the-shelf" treatment with a defined product that has established potency assays and batch-to-batch consistency. In addition to the presence of growth factors, the cellular component is thought to have great promise due to its ability to respond to injury-specific microenvironmental cues by detecting injury, releasing a wide range of biomolecules, increasing proteoglycan synthesis, increasing migration and proliferation of nucleus cells, and by repairing the intervertebral disc [48].

### 13.3.3 Progenitor Stem Cells (VIA Disc® by Vivex)

The largest randomized control with provisional data at the time of writing this chapter is from the Viable Allograft for Intervertebral Disc Supplementation (VAST) Trial. This trial was performed to evaluate the safety and effectiveness of MSCs mixed with allograft disc material in treating patients with painful DDD.

There were 224 patients at five U.S. sites enrolled in the trial which was segmented into a treatment group, an NSM group, and a placebo-control group with a 3.5:1:1 randomization ratio. The first 24 participants were assessed at a 1-month posttreatment visit to assess for safety. There were two co-primary end points including back pain as measured by the visual analog scale (VAS) and function as measured by the Oswestry Disability Index (ODI). The primary end points were evaluated along with safety data and reported adverse events (AEs) and changes in clinical laboratory evaluations. The data was collected at baseline and at 3, 6, and 12 months. Structural evaluation was also performed, and imaging studies including X-rays and MR imaging were performed at 6 and 12 months.

The data on the first 24 patients out to the 1-year follow-up was available at the time of writing this chapter. At the 6- and 12-month time points, VAS back pain improved from 58.13, 60.0, and 59.75 in the allograft, placebo, and NSM subjects, respectively to 16.40, 28.60, and 16.0 at 6 months, and 9.85, 27.0, and 6.0 at 12 months (Fig. 13.8). At 3 months, the VAS of the NSM group was 55.0. There was an option for the NSM patients to crossover to the allograft treatment group at the 3-month time point and all subjects elected to crossover to allograft treatment. At

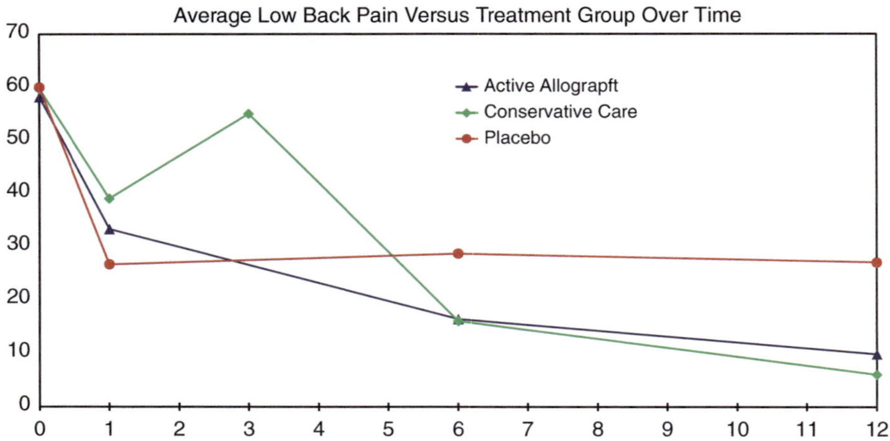


**Fig. 13.8** Visual analog scores as measured from the baseline and at 1, 3, 6, and 12 months. All treated patients experienced pain relief with the allograft patients (blue line) and the conservative care (green line) experiencing the greatest amount of relief and the placebo patients (red line) experiencing the least pain relief. It should be noted that all conservative care patients crossed over to allograft treatment at 3 months

the 6- and 12-month time points, the ODI improved from 54.67, 50.40, and 51.75 in the allograft, placebo, and NSM subjects, respectively to 19.73, 15.25, and 22.50 at 6 months and 12.85, 17.5, and 20.0 at 12 months (Fig. 13.9). At 3 months, the ODI of the NSM group was 65.5 and all subjects crossed over to allograft treatment. At 12 months, there were no AEs in the first 24 participants, and the MRI evaluation showed anatomic improvement of the disc and enhanced nucleus signal (Figs. 13.10 and 13.11).

The first 24 subjects had full data collected at 1 year as part of a safety assessment. This was included as part of this large triple-arm prospective randomized control trial. The safety data showed that a delivery of a viscous cellular allograft can be done safely with no AEs in these initial subjects followed up to 1 year. The patients receiving the allograft had a very high level of pain decrease and functional improvement compared to the placebo and NSM cohorts, and those NSM subjects crossing over to allograft supplementation attained similar pain and functional improvements to those initially randomized to receive the active treatment (Figs. 13.8 and 13.9). The safety data was not powered for statistical significance, but the prominent improvements in pain and function trend towards the possibility of statistically significant differences at the final analysis of the data that will be performed after completion of this chapter.

The cellular disc allograft VIA Disc was originally developed after a cellular bone allograft and was used for an interbody fusion which resulted in a pseudoarthrosis. The pseudoarthrosis was revised, and an incomplete discectomy was determined to be the primary cause of the non-union. The residual disc fragments were sent to pathology for further evaluation, and spheroids of disc regeneration were found in the residual disc tissue surrounding the interbody fusion cage (Fig. 13.12).

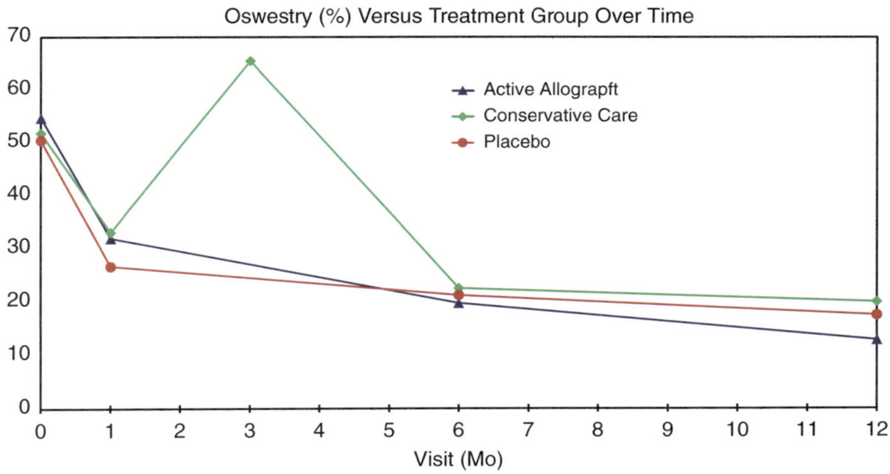


**Fig. 13.9** Oswestry Disability Index scores as measured from the baseline and at 1, 3, 6, and 12 months. All treated patients experienced functional improvement with the allograft patients (blue line) experiencing the greatest degree of functional improvement and the conservative care (green line) and the placebo patients (red line) experiencing functional improvement to a lesser degree. It should be again noted that all conservative care patients crossed over to allograft treatment at 3 months

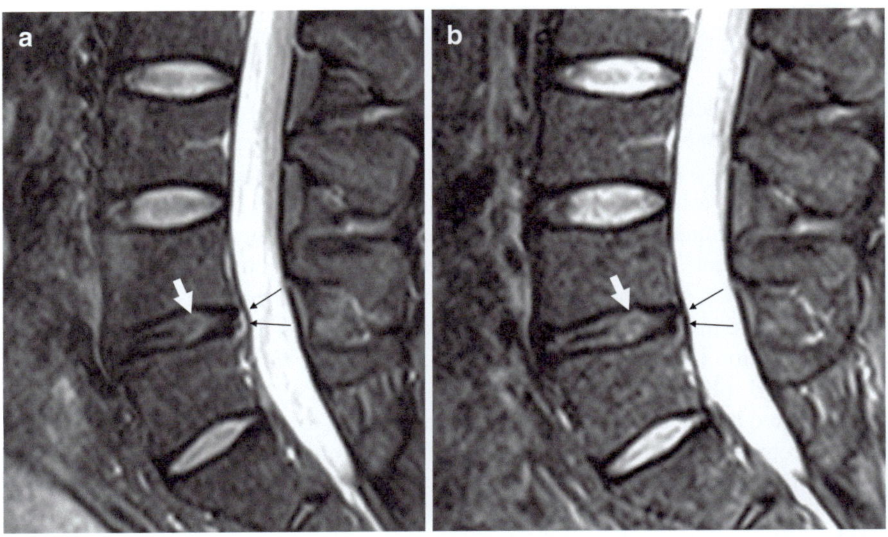


**Fig. 13.10** Lateral STIR MR images of the lumbar spine from the same patient taken at baseline (**a**) and 6 months following injection of ViaDisc (**b**) showing less posterior prominence of the intervertebral disc at the 6 month time point (black arrows) and increased signal within the nucleus pulposis (white arrowhead). The subject's VAS and ODI decreased from 58 and 50 to 0 and 0 respectively at 6 months

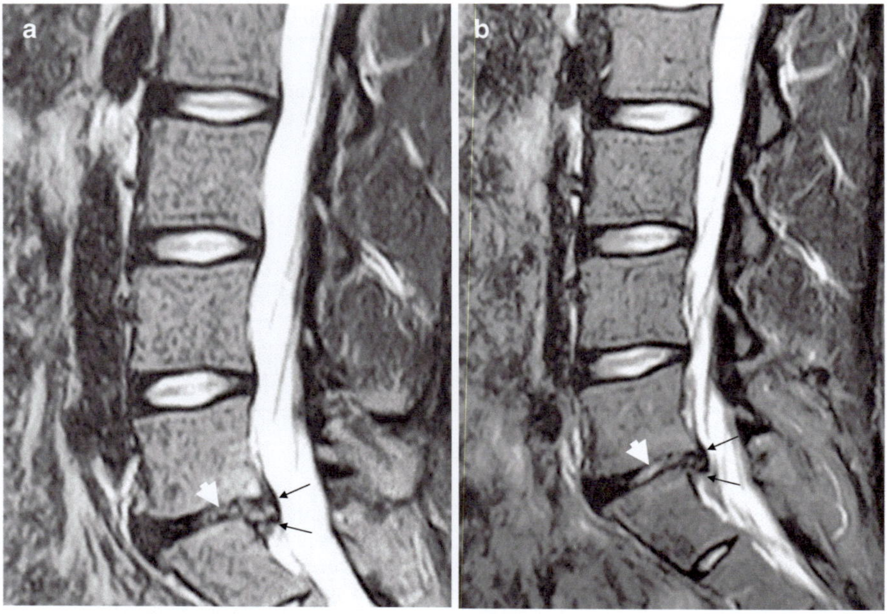


**Fig. 13.11** Lateral STIR MR images of the lumbar spine from the same patient taken at baseline (**a**) and 1 year following injection of ViaDisc (**b**) demonstrates healing of a disc protrusion (black arrows) and increased signal within the nucleus pulposis (white arrowhead). The subject's VAS and ODI decreased from 70 and 58 to 15 and 22 respectively at 1 year

The cells, which are isolated by an enzymatic digestion process from the hypoxic region of the bone marrow immediately adjacent to the vertebral endplate, were then placed into a more concentrated solution, and micronized disc material was used as a carrier when injecting into the intervertebral discs (Fig. 13.13). The components of the liquid MSC solution and the micronized disc material comprise the VIA Disc product. The liquid component contains concentrated cells that are identifiable as MSCs, and the micronized disc material also contains various growth factors that are involved in cell survival and proliferation as well as in suppression of inflammation (Figs. 13.14, 13.15, 13.16, 13.17, and 13.18). The cells are stored in a dimethyl sulfoxide (DMSO)-free cryoprotectant at −75 °C and then thawed and reconstituted before use. The cell viability has shown to be consistently greater than 75% thereby ensuring that the target number of six million viable cells will be available for injection into the disc (Fig. 13.19).

At the time of writing this chapter, the data collection for the VAST trial was continuing. The 1-year data should be collected by the end of 2019 and complete results will be available shortly after that. Based on the previous data as discussed in the meta-analysis by Wu et al., the Rexlemestrocel phase II data and the

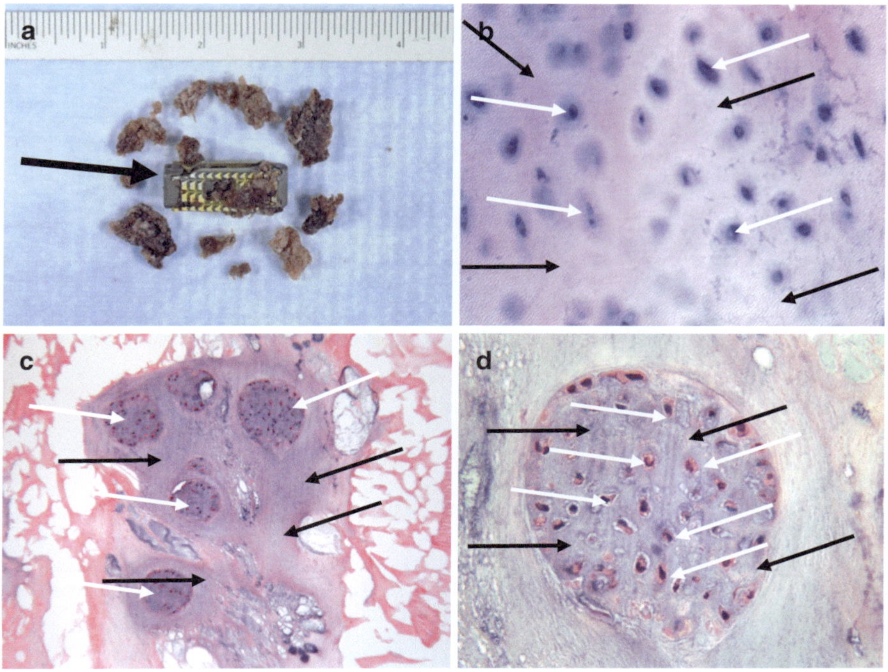


**Fig. 13.12** (**a**) Residual fragments of the residual intervertebral disc removed from the pseudoarthrosis along the the interbody fusion cage (black arrow in **a**). Representative hematoxylin-eosin histophotomicrographs at 400× (**b**), 100× (**c**), and 200× (**d**) show fibrocartilate from the annulus and cloning of the chondrocytes (white arrows in **c** and **d**) surrounded by new matrix (black arrows in **c** and **d**). A high powered view (**b**) shows chondrocytes (white arrows in **b**) from the endplate of the vertebral body producing hyaline cartilage matrix (black arrows in **b**).

**Fig. 13.13** Vial of allogeneic MSCs isolated from the hypoxic region of the bone marrow adjacent to the endplate containing six million cells (vial on left) is mixed with the micronized disc material (powder in small dish on the right) which forms a liquid with a thin paste consistency that can be injected into the intervertebral disc

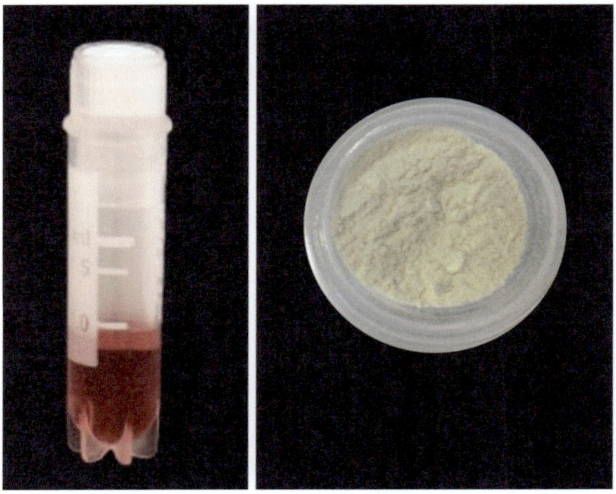

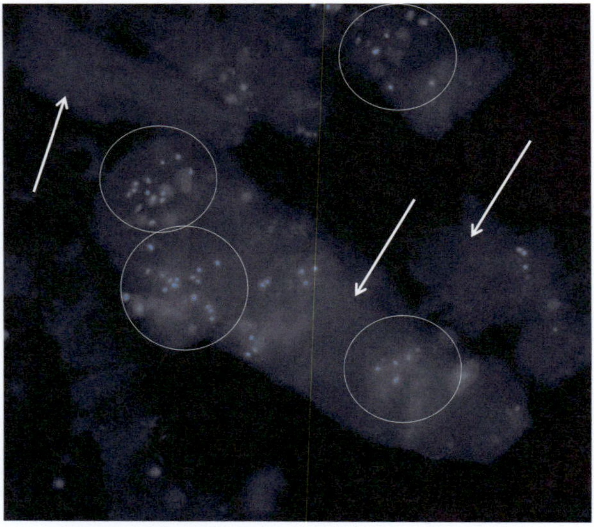

**Fig. 13.14** Histophotomicrograph intervertebral disc material (white arrows) ground to 300 μm and having undergone DAPI staining showing DNA seen as light blue dots (within the white circles) by fluorescence microscopy

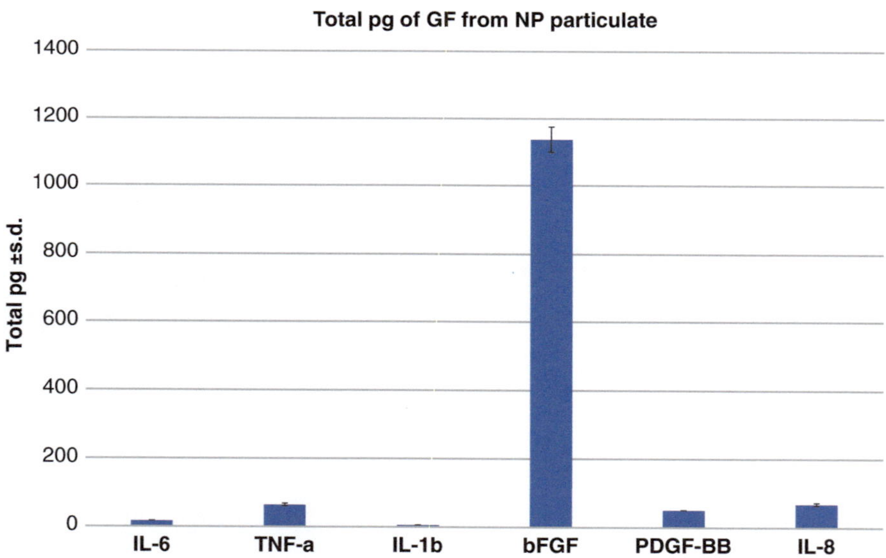


**Fig. 13.15** A bar graph showing the measurements of the amount (in pg) and type of growth factors present in the micronized disc material that is mixed with the bone marrow derived MSCs to make ViaDisc. *IL* interleukin, *pg* pictograms, *TNF* tumor necrosis factor, *FGF* fibroblast growth factor, *PDGF* platelet-derived growth factor, *NP* nucleus pulposis

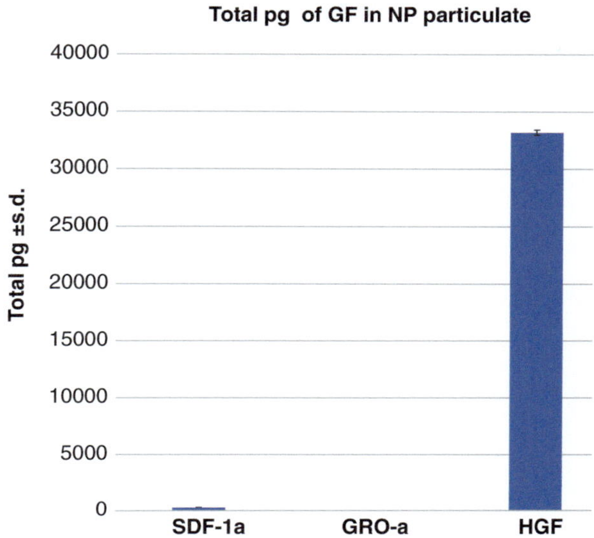


**Fig. 13.16** Bar graph showing the measurements of the amount (in pg) and type of growth factors present in the micronized disc material that is mixed with the bone marrow derived MSCs to make ViaDisc. *SDF* stromal cell-derived factor, *GRO* gro alpha, *HGF* hepatocyte growth factor

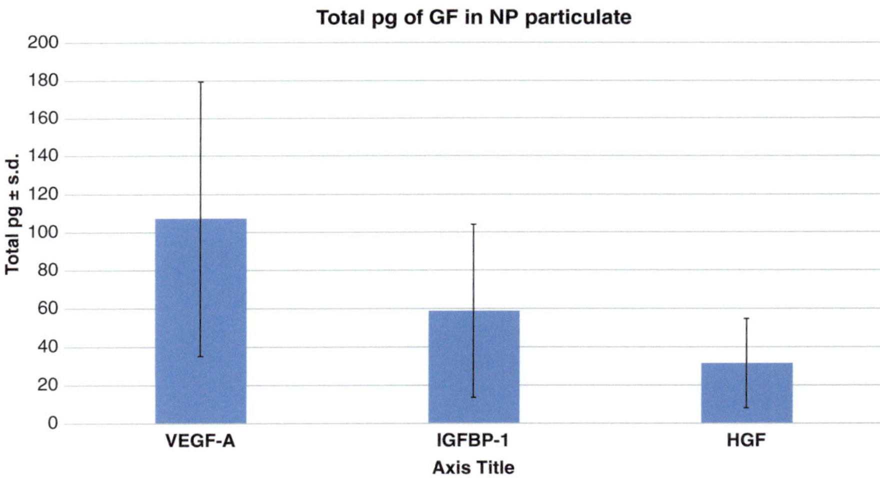


**Fig. 13.17** A bar graph showing the measurements of the amount (in pg) and type of growth factors present in the micronized disc material that is mixed with the bone marrow derived MSCs to make ViaDisc. *VEGF* vascular endothelial growth factor, *IGFBP* insulin-like growth factor-binding protein, *HGF* hepatocyte growth factor

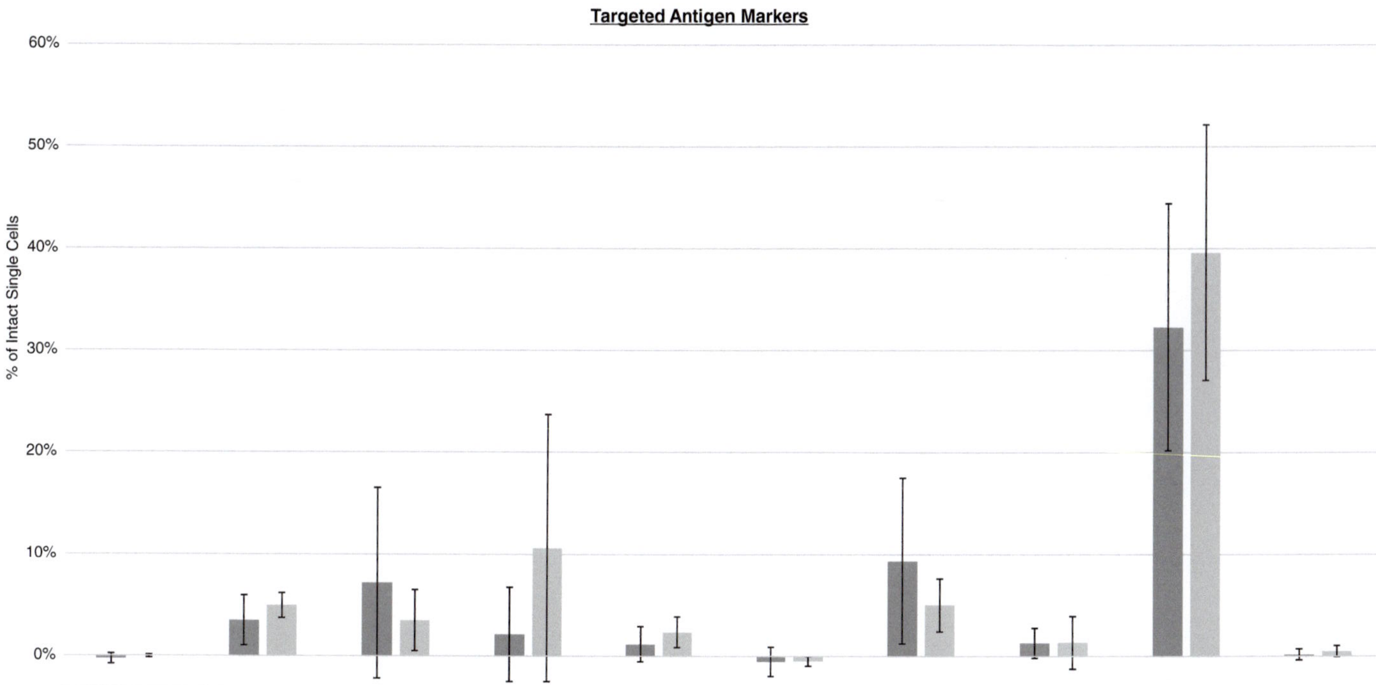


| | CD105-FITC | CD73-APC | CD90-APC | CD44-PE | CD271-APC | CD166-PE | SSEA4-FITC | CD146-488 | LepR-647 | CD106-PE |
|---|---|---|---|---|---|---|---|---|---|---|
| ■LCC | -0.28% | 3.48% | 7.15% | 2.11% | 1.17% | -0.53% | 9.35% | 1.29% | 32.30% | 0.17% |
| ■HCC | -0.03% | 4.94% | 3.49% | 10.60% | 2.35% | -0.48% | 5.01% | 1.33% | 39.62% | 0.49% |

**Fig. 13.18** Bar graph showing the percentage of intact single cells with the antigen markers consistent with MCSs. *CD* cluster of differentiation, *FITC* fluorescein isothiocyanate, *APC* antigen presenting cell, *PE* phycoerythrin, *SSEA* stage-specific embryonic antigen, *LepR* leptin receptor

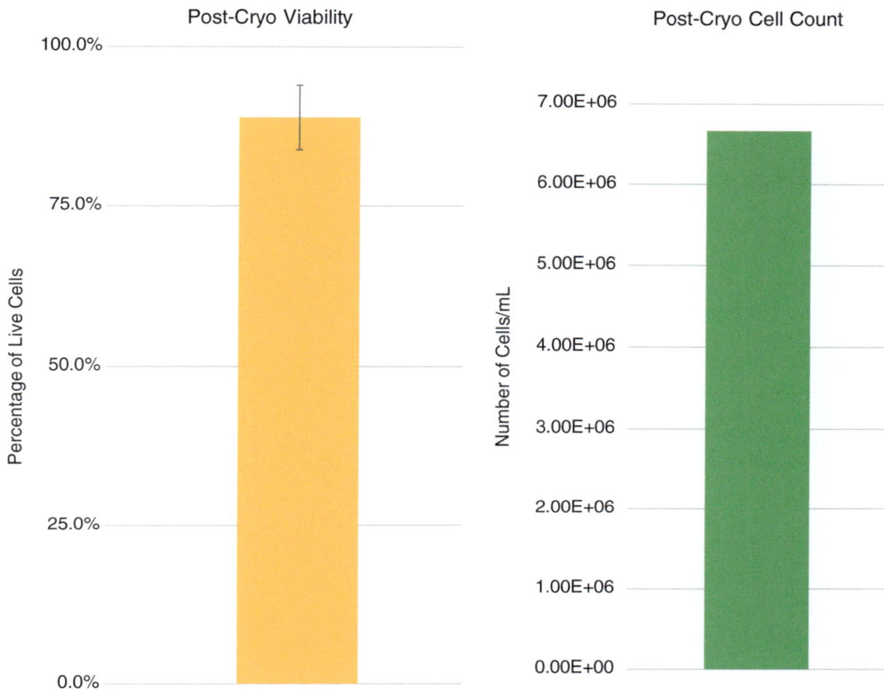


**Fig. 13.19** A bar graph showing the percentage of viable cells (**a**) after the MSCs have been thawed. The cell number available after the thawing process is demonstrated in the bar graph on the right (**b**). The objective is to have consistently greater than 75% cell viability and to deliver at least six million viable cells to the intervertebral disc by injection

provisional data from the first 24 patients in the VAST trial, the final data should be optimal and could usher in an entirely new and highly effective treatment option for patients with stable discogenic back pain [22].

## 13.4 Intervertebral Disc Injection Protocol

### 13.4.1 Eligibility

Patients who are optimal candidates for injection of intradiscal biologics have painful discs that are moderately degenerated and tend to be typically younger and healthier than patients with severely degenerated discs. Most of the trials and use of intradiscal biologics have been in intervertebral discs that are moderately degenerated rather than discs that are severely degenerated due to the assumptions that moderately degenerated discs are capable of regeneration and should be treated at this point prior to when the degeneration can reach a point where the tissue cannot recover and/or be regenerated. There are certain eligibility criteria that are used to

**Table 13.5** Patient eligibility criteria for intradiscal regenerative biologic treatment

| |
|---|
| 1. Age 18 and 60 years inclusive |
| 2. Male or female |
| 3. Body mass index <35 |
| 4. Modified Pfirrmann grade (3–6) |
| 5. Radiographic confirmation by MRI/X-ray of:<br>(a) Translational instability defined as ≤5 mm or<br>(b) Angular instability defined as ≤5 |
| 6. Back pain (with or without radicular leg pain) measured by:<br>(a) ODI of at least 40%<br>(b) VASPI of at least 40 mm |
| 7. Pathologic level between L1 and S1 |
| 8. One or two vertebral level involvement that has been evaluated for at least 6 months and treated with conservative care |
| 9. Psychosocially, mentally, and physically able to fully comply with physician treated with conservative care |
| 10. No history of malignancy or chronic infectious disease (e.g., HIV, hepatitis) |
| 11. Patients with mechanical instability and/or type III Modic changes should be excluded |

determine whether a patient is an optimal candidate for an intradiscal regenerative biologic treatment. An example of a fairly restrictive set of criteria that has been used for intradiscal allogeneic MSC trials is shown in Table 13.5. Clinical application of these criteria can be less stringent than that used for an RCT and should be left to the discretion of the treating physician.

### 13.4.2 Standards for Pre-procedural, Intra-procedural, and Post-procedural Treatment

#### 13.4.2.1 Pre-procedure

The procedure to inject the intervertebral disc should be described to the patient. An example of this is to discuss that the treatment is a human donor (or describe the product origin) product used to repair damaged discs resulting from DDD. Degenerative disc disease arises as the result in loss of hydration and ultimately tissue matrix within the intervertebral discs (IVD). The intradiscal biologic product is intended to replace or supplement the degenerated tissue in the disc in which it is injected. The disc injection procedure is a nonsurgical, minimally invasive procedure. The material is injected under fluoroscopic imaging into the nucleus pulposis of the disc and fills the voids in the damaged disc, providing hydration and supporting the disc to function as intended.

**Risks, Benefits, and Alternatives**

As with any spine injection procedure, the risks include infection, bleeding, nerve damage, localized increase in pain, anxiety, discitis, osteomyelitis, and immune reaction to the injected material. The risk of any of these occurring is quite low, and there were no adverse events recorded in the safety data obtained from the VAST trial, and Wu et al. reported no related adverse events in any of their included study

[22, 49]. There have also been no tumor formation observed in any clinical cases in stem cell transplantation during the observed follow-up period [22].

The potential benefits include improvements in pain, function, and quality of life. In the provisional data collected from the VAST Trial, the visual analog scale (VAS) improvement of 48.3 points and an Oswestry Disability Index (ODI) improvement of 41.8 were profoundly positive [49]. The meta-analysis by Wu et al. reported a mean VAS reduction of 44.2 points and a mean ODI improvement of 32.2 points [22]. Additionally, based on intradiscal stem cell data, the change and improvement appear to be a long-lasting or permanent benefit.

The alternatives to treatment in a patient with painful discogenic back pain include injections of anesthetic and anti-inflammatory agents into the disc, basivertebral nerve ablation, and fusion or disc replacement surgery. Intradiscal biologic treatment is recommended after injection therapies fail to provide durable relief of symptoms and in a disc that is mild to moderately degenerated with a Modified Pfirrmann Grade of 3–6. When there is severe degeneration with degenerative endplate change, either basivertebral nerve ablation or disc replacement surgery can be used if the lumbar segment is stable or surgical fusion if the segment is unstable.

#### 13.4.2.2 Intra-procedure

Injection of the intradiscal biologics is performed with the same technique as any intradiscal injection. Intravenous access is obtained and the patient is given intravenous antibiotics just before the injection. The recommended antibiotics include 1–2 g of cefazolin (Ancef) and 80 to 160 mg of gentamicin. Patients with an allergy to penicillin should be given 600–900 mg of clindamycin in place of cefazolin with the higher dose for all antibiotics given to patients weighing 90 kg or more. Patients with impaired renal function should have the dosage adjusted accordingly. In addition to pre-procedure antibiotics, an injection of the anti-inflammatory medication ketorolac (Toradol) 30 mg intravenously given before and after the injection can help with procedural and post-procedural pain.

Moderate sedation is recommended in these patients as injection into a pain generating intervertebral disc can be painful. Typical agents given for moderate sedation include midazolam and fentanyl, and the dosage for this procedure can range from 1 to 5 mg of midazolam and from 25 to 100 μg of fentanyl. Other sedatives such as ketamine or propofol may be used in certain circumstances such as in an opioid-tolerant patient, if needed, but must be administered carefully by experienced personnel.

The injection into the intervertebral disc is performed the same as traditional lumbar discography with a 22-G spinal needle placed through Kambin's safe triangle into the disc from a posterolateral oblique approach using fluoroscopy or computed tomography (CT) guidance (Fig. 13.20). The needle is placed into the center of the disc (Fig. 13.20). An alternative approach is to use an 18-gauge needle that is placed just outside the intervertebral disc and a 22-G needle is placed through the 18-G needle into the nucleus pulposis of the target disc. The product is then injected through the 22-G needle into the disc using moderate consistent pressure. Following the injection, the needle(s) is/are removed, and the patient is taken

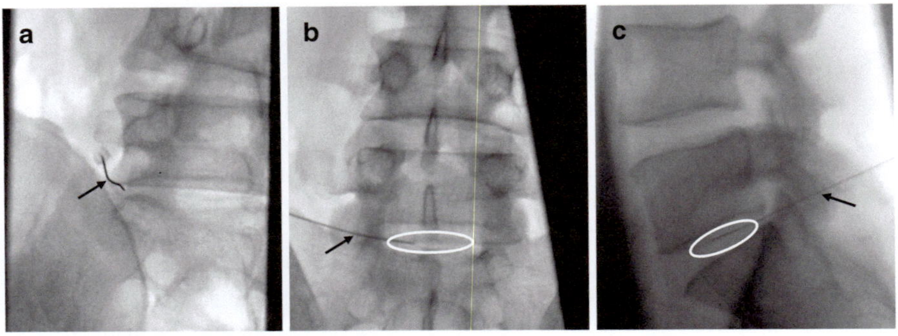


**Fig. 13.20** Fluoroscopic views in the oblique (**a**), anteroposterior (**b**), and the lateral (**c**) views showing a 22 G needle (black arrows) places within the center of the intervertebral disc as confirmed on the anteroposterior and laterl fluoroscopic views (area within the oval in **b** and **c**)

to the recovery area for further observation and/or monitoring is done until they are ready to be released.

#### 13.4.2.3 Post-procedure

The patient is instructed to limit physical activity to the normal activities of daily life and to limit strenuous activity for 72 h. After that they are instructed to resume all normal activities within reason keeping in mind that the regeneration time for the intervertebral disc can be up to 6 months.

Prescriptions are given to the patient for medications to take as needed including a steroid dose pack (i.e., Medrol Dosepak), a muscle relaxer (i.e., metaxalone 800 mg), and a narcotic (i.e., hydrocodone/acetaminophen or oxycodone/acetaminophen 10/325 mg). Although these medications are typically needed sparingly or not at all, there is a subgroup of patients that experience moderate-to-severe pain after injection of an intradiscal substance and oral medications may be needed promptly to treat this post-injection pain and discomfort. An icepack may be given to the patient to place over the injection site in the event of post-injection site discomfort.

A follow-up appointment is made 2–4 weeks after the injection to see how the patient is doing and to assess for significant post-injection discomfort. Additional follow-up appointments can be made at the discretion of treating physicians to assess the patient's treatment progress.

## 13.5 Noninfectious Reactions Seen with Intradiscal Biologics and Other Materials

Pain related to the intervertebral disc has been a known issue in healthcare for decades. The concept of discs that appear similar or just slightly different on imaging but that present with differing clinical presentations of pain is known but still a somewhat difficult concept to grasp. Over the years, there have been many attempts to diagnose and treat discogenic-mediated pain. Discography has been and remains one of the standard diagnostic procedures used to evaluate the disc. Pressurization to create a provocative pain response is an important component of the study as is the assessment of contrast flow and the subsequent response to anesthetic infusion.

When the annulus fibrosis is breached during discography, this gives rise to the possibility of infectious discitis. The infection rate for discography had originally been reported to be 1–4% [25]. This unacceptably high infection rate has subsequently been profoundly reduced by sterile technique, different needle techniques, and pre-procedure IV antibiotics [26]. Modern techniques have resulted in negligible rate of discitis after discography [51].

Reactive changes that mimic infection have previously been reported including changes from seronegative spondyloarthropathies, neuropathic spine, acute cartilaginous nodes, and other conditions [52]. Recently, the authors of this chapter have noted noninfectious reactive changes of the disc associated with injections of many of the intradiscal biologics described above. Just as with some of the other noninfectious entities that can mimic discitis, these post-injection changes associated with intradiscal biologics can look identical to discitis on cross-sectional imaging (Figs. 13.21, 13.22, 13.23, and 13.24).

Anytime there has been a violation of the annulus, whether for discography or biologic treatment, discitis is possible. Differentiating between an infectious cause and a noninfectious cause or biologic immune reaction is of paramount importance. Discitis will most commonly present with an increase in axial back pain with or without radiating pain. There are similar clinical and radiological characteristics for both types of conditions. Timing of this increase in pain can be one of the important differentiating factors that separates infectious discitis from noninfectious inflammatory changes. Regardless of the type of process affecting the disc, a diagnostic workup must be done promptly to include MR imaging and laboratory testing with assessment of WBC (white blood cell count), CRP (C-reactive protein), and ESR (erythrocyte sedimentation rate).

Either form of reactive changed in and around the disc will appear similar on cross-sectional imaging. The T2-weighted images often reveal increased signal approximating the vertebral endplates adjacent to the suspected disc (Figs. 13.21, 13.22 and 13.24). This can be seen with or without endplate erosions or enlarged Schmorl's nodes (Figs. 13.21, 13.22, 13.23, and 13.24). The most common site for these changes will be at the center of the endplate where the endplate cartilage is thin and most nutrient transfer occurs. Laboratory values can be normal in both types of processes, especially if the inflammatory response is confined to the intervertebral disc. The probability of an infectious cause is higher when the laboratory values including the CRP, ESR, and the WBC become elevated, and the probability of a noninfectious process increases when these laboratory values remain either normal or very slightly elevated.

There should be an increased suspicion of infectious discitis, if fluid signal is observed within the nucleus pulposis [53]. Extra annular or paraspinal inflammatory response or fluid signal also elevates suspicion for infection and should increase the urgency to treat [53]. In these cases, antibiotics should be started and a disc

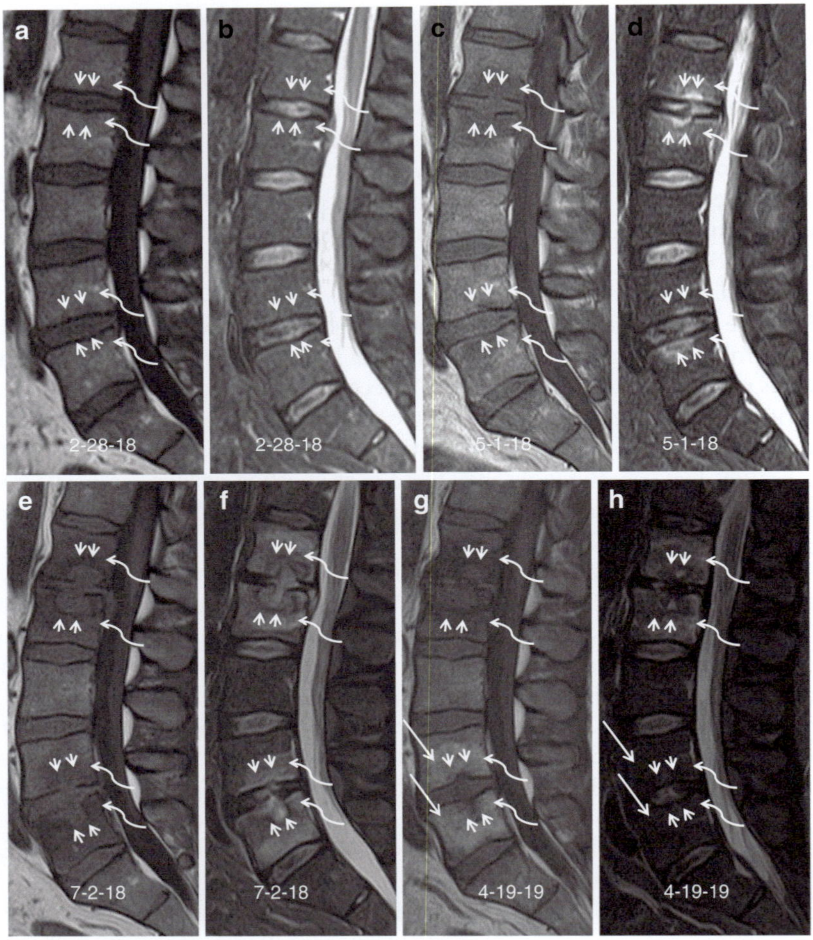


**Fig. 13.21** (**a**–**f**) Lateral T1-weighted (**a**, **c**, **e**, and **g**) and STIR (**b**, **d**, **f** and **h**) MR images taken from a 44 year old male before (**a**, **b**) and after (**c**–**h**) injection of autologous stem cells. The dates are displayed at the bottom of each image. Signal and endplate changes were noted at the injected L1–2 and L4–5 levels progressing from the normal pre-procedure appearance of the endplates (white arrowheads in **a**) and the marrow (curved white arrows in **a**) to erosions of the endplates best seen on the T1-weighted images (white arrowheads **c**, **e**, and **g**) and prominent endplate edema characterized and best seen as increased signal on the STIR images (curved white arrows in **d**, **f**, and **h**). The edema was first noted when the patient initially presented with pain just over 2 months after injection (curved white arrows in **c** and **d**) and the edema progressed to its maximal amount approximately 4 months after injection (curved white arrows in **e** and **f**) and began to normalize approximately 13.5 months after injection (curved white arrows in **g** and **h**) with regions surrounding the L4–5 endplate resembling Modic type 1 endplate changes (straight white arrows in **g** and **h**) with fat signal on the T1-weighted images (straight white arrows in **g**) which is isointense to the surrounding marrow on the STIR images (straight white arrows in **h**). The patient's sed rate and C-reactive protein levels were never greater than 22 and 1 respectively and the patient was treated expectantly with medication for pain and no antibiotics due to a provisional diagnosis of non-infectious reactive changes rather than discitis primarily due to the time course of appearance of symptoms and the normal sed rate and C-reactive protein

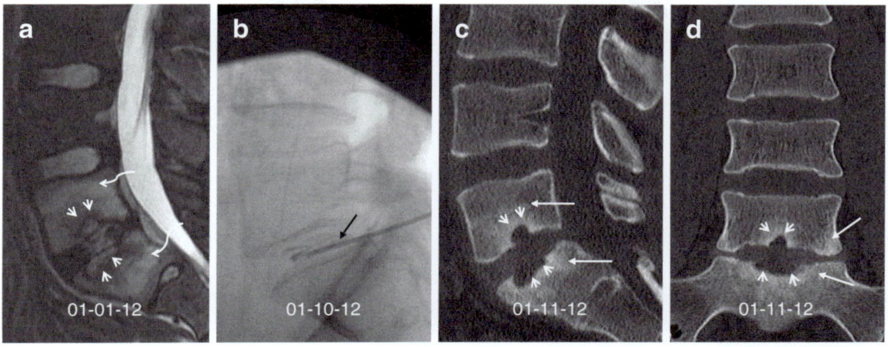


**Fig. 13.22** (**a–d**) Lateral T2-weighted MR image (**a**), lateral fluoroscopic image (**b**) and sagittal and coronal CT reconstructed images (**c** and **d** respectively) from a 23 year old male taken after injection of fibrin sealant (Biostat) on 08-05-11 show edema in the L5 and S1 vertebral bodies (curved white arrows in **a**) along with endplate erosions (white arrowheads in **a**, **c** and **d**). The CT images also show reactive osseous sclerosis around the endplate erosions (straight white arrows in **c** and **d**). The lateral fluoroscopic image shows a needle and auger device (black arrow) sampling the disc tissue. The dates are displayed at the bottom of each image and the patient's symptoms began approximately 4 months after injection of the MSCs. Disc biopsy showed no evidence of discitis with a negative gram stain and culture and the patient's sed rate and C-reactive protein levels were never greater than 22 and 1 respectively. He was treated expectantly with medication for pain and no antibiotics due to a provisional diagnosis of non-infectious reactive changes rather than discitis primarily due to the time course of appearance of symptoms and the normal sed rate and C-reactive protein

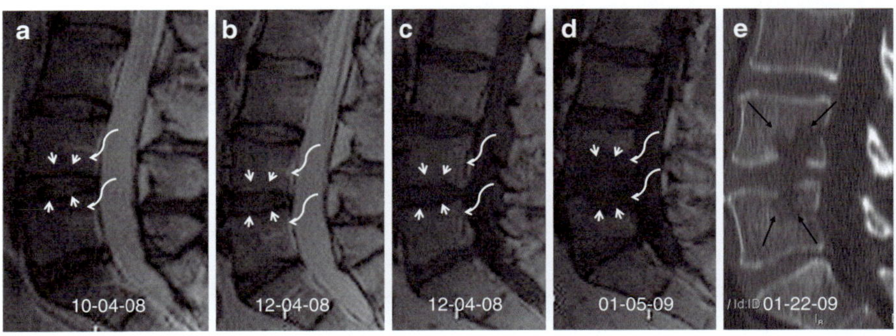


**Fig. 13.23** (**a–e**) Sagittal T2-weighted (**a**) taken before injection of BMP-7 and sagittal T2-weighted (**b**) sagittal T1-weighted (**c** and **d**) MR images and sagittal CT reconstruction (**e**) images taken from a 44 year old male after injection of BMP-7 at the L4-5 level done on 10-22-08. The dates are displayed at the bottom of each image. Signal and endplate alterations are seen progressing from the normal pre-procedure and early post-injection appearance of the endplates (white arrowheads in **a**, **b** and **c**) and the marrow (curved white arrows in **a**, **b** and **c**) to erosions of the endplates best seen on the T1-weighted images (white arrowheads in **d**) and prominent endplate edema best seen as decreased signal on the T1-weighted MR images (curved white arrows in **d**). The CT images taken 3 months after the injection of BMP-7 show prominent endplate erosions at the L4–5 level (black arrows in **e**). The edema was first noted when the patient initially presented with pain at 10 weeks after injection (curved white arrows in **d**). Disc biopsy done 3 months after the injection showed no bacteria and the culture of this specimen was negative. The patient's sed rate and C-reactive protein levels were normal at 14 and 0.9 respectively and the patient improved with supportive treatment resulting in a provisional diagnosis of non-infectious reactive changes rather than discitis primarily due to the time course of appearance of symptoms and the negative inflammatory markers

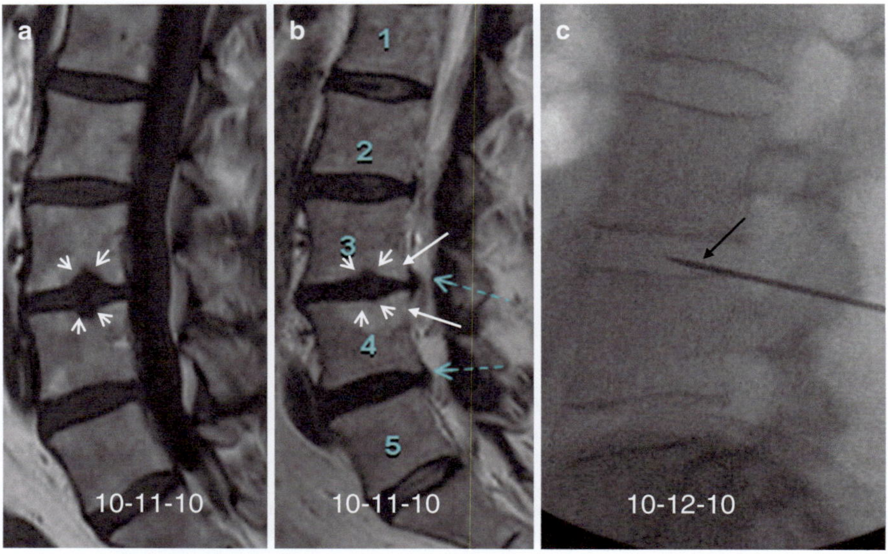


**Fig. 13.24** (**a–c**) Sagittal T1-weighted (**a**), sagittal T2-weighted (**b**) and lateral fluoroscopic image from a 56 year old female after injection of a fibrin sealant (Tisseel) done on 08-30-10. The dates are displayed at the bottom of each image. Endplate erosions are seen on both the T1 and T2-weighted MR images (white arrowheads in **a** and **b**) and marrow edema is seen adjacent to these erosions on the sagittal T2 weighted image (white arrows in **b**). Disc bulging at both the L3–4 and L4–5 levels was also present and best seen on the sagittal T2-weighted images (blue dashed arrows in **b**). The edema was first noted when the patient initially presented with pain less than 6 weeks after injection (white arrows in **b**). Disc biopsy (black arrow in **c**) done 6 weeks after the injection showed numerous gram positive cocci. The diagnosis of discitis was made and the patient was treated with intravenous antibiotics

biopsy and aspiration should be considered. The most effective method of acquiring a sample of the nucleus is by using a mechanical biopsy device such as a core biopsy needle or an auger type device such as the Dekompressor (Stryker Corporation, Kalamazoo, MI). These techniques typically produce a large enough sample for gram stain and culture. During a biopsy, the disc can be flushed with antibiotics and, depending on the results of the biopsy, intravenous antibiotics can be started.

Noninfectious discitis has been documented after numerous types of biologic injections into the intervertebral disc. These changes are usually seen between 8 and 16 weeks after the disc injection procedure which is a longer time interval than changes due to infection that usually occurs within 4 weeks post-procedure (Table 13.6). The incidence of noninfectious discitis after biologic intradiscal injection cannot be accurately defined at this time due to the uncommon occurrence of this entity and the inconsistency of the various biologic products. Each of the products tested have potentially different mechanisms of actions within the intervertebral disc but the biologic reactive response may appear similar on the follow-up imaging evaluations. The exact etiology of these types of inflammatory reactions is

**Table 13.6** Potential complications associated with injection of biologics into the intervertebral disc and the post-injection timeframe in which these complications usually occur

| Timeline of potential complications with intradiscal biologics | |
|---|---|
| Timeline, weeks | Complication |
| 0–2 | Pain with injection<br>– Under 2 cc causes minimal irritation and pressure<br>– Over 2 cc can begin to cause mechanical expansion of disc<br>– Spasm (consider lumbar corset, muscle relaxant) |
| 2–4 | Infection |
| 8–16 | Biologic flare |

still a point of debate but are probably different from product to product. Bone morphogenetic protein-7 (BMP-7), for example, is a protein that stimulates bone and cartilage growth. In a long bone fracture model, this protein initially causes osteolysis followed by osteogenesis. It has also been shown to promote cartilage growth, and the intradiscal study was based on an animal model that showed improvement of disc hydration. The inflammatory changes seen with BMP-7 (Fig. 13.23) was one of the first well-documented examples of noninfectious discitis with a biologic agent.

Early treatment of reactive and/or inflammatory changes in and around the intervertebral disc was initially very aggressive and consisted of a biopsy, intradiscal antibiotics, and subsequent intravenous antibiotics for at least 4–6 weeks or more. As we have seen the noninfectious inflammatory response more frequently, we have learned that the changes do not necessarily indicate and infect and our treatment has evolved. The current recommended treatment, once infection has been excluded, is palliative. Pain control and other supportive measures are applied with a watch-and-wait approach.

## 13.6 Intradiscal Exosomes

As previously discussed, cellular MSC-based regenerative treatments offer great potential in treating discogenic back pain. The cellular therapies are known to supplement the existing cell population by injecting cells either with or without a carrier. These treatments have been shown to promote nucleus pulposis cell proliferation, decrease inflammation, lessen apoptosis, and contribute to multipotent cell differentiation [54]. It has been shown that MSCs cocultured with nucleus pulposis cells can differentiate along the nucleus pulposis lineage either by direct or indirect contact methods and can cause the degenerated nucleus pulposis cells to regain a normal phenotype [55].

The cell-to-cell communication has been known to occur by secreted molecules and by cell surface molecules that contact other cells by specialized molecules in connected channels [56, 57]. The secretion occurs via extracellular microvesicles known as exosomes that are released by cells and are an essential component of the intercellular environment [58–60]. Exosomes are microvesicles that are produced in the endosomal compartment of most cells and, when they fuse with the cell surface, these microvesicles are released as exosomes.

The presence of microvesicles was originally reported by Chargaff and West in the 1940s and for many years were considered inert debris until De Broe et al. suggested these microvesicles may result from a specific process [61, 62]. It is now accepted that most cells release exosomes and recent studies indicate they have important roles in the function of stem cells [63].

Recently, attention has been turned to the function of exosomes which have been found in nearly all biological fluids including blood, urine, semen, and milk [64–66]. Exosomes are nanosized and range in diameter from 30 to 120 nm [67]. They contain multiple components including proteins, mRNAs, miRNAs, lipids, cytokines, noncoding RNAs (ncRNA), and ribosomal RNAs (Fig. 13.25) [67]. They also contain proteins involved in membrane fusion and transport including annexins, flotillin, and GTPases [67]. The two-layer membrane of the exosomes protects the integrity of their contents so that they are stable over long distances and during the interaction with target cells [64].

The exosomes can play unique roles in cell-to-cell communication based upon their cellular origin, and MSC-derived exosomes may provide an acellular alternative to traditional MSC treatment of the intervertebral discs [68]. This possibility has been investigated previously, and it has been shown that exosomes taken from nucleus pulposis cells can stimulate MSCs to differentiate into a nucleus pulposis cell phenotype and can stimulate the existing degenerated cells to regain a nondegenerate phenotype that produces and enhances matrix production [69]. This study suggests that exosomes can potentially stimulate repair of degenerated intervertebral discs and may play a role in the treatment of discogenic back pain. The variety of different functions of exosomes along with the potential to deliver a very concentrated dose of subcellular material taken from specific cell types offers great

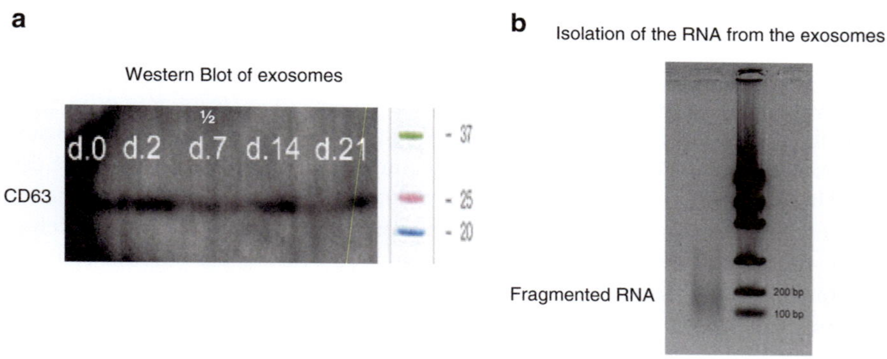


**Fig. 13.25** (**a**) Western blot of fluid taken from a preparation of MSCs show the presence of a protein with a CD63 antigen. This antigen is mainly associated with membranes of intracellular vesicles or exosomes. (**b**) Agrarose gel electrophoresis using 1% agarose gel stained with ethidium bromide on an acellular fluid taken from a preparation of MSCs shows fragmented RNA observed around the 100 and 200 bp DNA standards

potential to regenerate the existing nucleus pulposis cells of degenerated intervertebral discs and could be used alone or in combination with MSCs. Additional investigation of the use of exosomes for this purpose will be essential to determine both the effectiveness of this therapy and the optimal use of these nano-biologics.

## 13.7 Conclusions

Back pain from DDD and IDD is exceedingly common, costly, and a very debilitating disorder. If this disorder can be accurately diagnosed and characterized, treatment may be accomplished with a combination of simple medications or biologically active treatments that are largely needle-based and can be delivered percutaneously. Stable discogenic back pain is not entirely adequately treated with conventional surgery or nonsurgical management but recently developed intradiscal needle-based therapies including the intradiscal biologic treatments are showing great promise.

While some biologic materials such as fibrin sealant and other isolated growth factors such as BMP-7 and GDF-5 have not been shown to be efficacious in treating discogenic back pain, other biologics such as platelet-rich plasma, alpha-2-macroglobulin, and MSCs have. Possibly the greatest promise for the treatment associated with the greatest safety and efficacy are the treatments that involve cellular augmentation of the intervertebral disc. The traditional lack of substantial data and large clinical trials is being remedied by recent RCTs that are producing high quality data and by the continued development of new technologies such as carriers for the cellular therapy.

Techniques for delivery of the intradiscal biologics will need to be reasonably standardized with good clinical practices followed to keep the treatment success high and the peri-procedural complications low. This is mostly refinement of existing techniques combined with a recognition of the nuances of the technical delivery of the new biologic materials.

The increase in the use of biologics will likely to continue to produce some unknown effects including the reactive changes to most of these biologics that have the characteristic of noninfectious immunogenic inflammatory changes. It is important to identify this as different from an infectious inflammatory condition as the treatments for these two conditions are entirely different.

Newer materials such as exosomes have great potential and promise as a biologic nanotechnology but its use in the intervertebral disc has not been studied to any significant degree. Further investigation will be necessary to determine the dose, method of delivery, and the optimal degenerative stage for optimally effective exosome treatment.

Overall intradiscal biological and cellular treatment of patients with discogenic low back pain holds great promise and potential. In patients who have not adequately been benefitted from conventional therapies, these treatments may be the therapeutic tool that produces the most optimal result.

## References


1. DePalma MJ, Ketchum JM, Saullo T. What is the source of chronic low back pain and does age play a role? Pain Med. 2011;12:224–33.
2. Zhang YG, Guo TM, Guo X, Wu SX. Clinical diagnosis for discogenic low back pain [published correction appears in Int J biol Sci. 2010;6(6):613]. Int J Biol Sci. 2009;5(7):647–58.
3. Frymoyer JW. Back pain and sciatica. N Engl J Med. 1988;318(5):291–300.
4. Mooney V. Presidential address. International Society for the Study of the Lumbar Spine. Dallas, 1986. Where is the pain coming from? Spine (Phila Pa 1976). 1987;12:754–9.
5. Cypress BK. Characteristics of physician visits for back symptoms: a national perspective. Am J Public Health. 1983;73(4):389–95.
6. Frymoyer JW. Are we performing too much spinal surgery? Iowa Orthop J. 1989;9:32.
7. Dagenais S, Caro J, Haldeman S. A systematic review of low back pain cost of illness studies in the United States and internationally. Spine J. 2008;8:8–20.
8. Crock HV. A reappraisal of intervertebral disc lesions. Med J Aust. 1970;1:983–9.
9. Manchikanti L, Singh V, Pampati V, Damron KS, Barnhill RC, Beyer C, Cash KA. Evaluation of the relative contributions of various structures in chronic low back pain. Pain Physician. 2001;4:308–16.
10. Singh K, Ledet E, Carl A. Intradiscal therapy: a review of current treatment modalities. Spine (Phila Pa 1976). 2005;30:S20–6.
11. Peng BG. Pathophysiology, diagnosis, and treatment of discogenic low back pain. World J Orthop. 2013;4(2):42–52. https://doi.org/10.5312/wjo.v4.i2.42.
12. Peng B, Fu X, Pang X, Li D, Liu W, Gao C, Yang H. Prospective clinical study on natural history of discogenic low back pain at 4 years of follow-up. Pain Physician. 2012;15:525–32.
13. Kuijpers T, van Middelkoop M, Rubinstein SM, Ostelo R, Verhagen A, Koes BW, van Tulder MW. A systematic review on the effectiveness of pharmacological interventions for chronic non-specific low-back pain. Eur Spine J. 2011;20:40–50.
14. Carragee EJ. Clinical practice. Persistent low back pain. N Engl J Med. 2005;352:1891–8.
15. Benyamin RM, Manchikanti L, Parr AT, Diwan S, Singh V, Falco FJ, Datta S, Abdi S, Hirsch JA. The effectiveness of lumbar interlaminar epidural injections in managing chronic low back and lower extremity pain. Pain Physician. 2012;15:E363–404.
16. Helm S, Hayek SM, Benyamin RM, Manchikanti L. Systematic review of the effectiveness of thermal annular procedures in treating discogenic low back pain. Pain Physician. 2009;12:207–32.
17. Fritzell P, Hägg O, Wessberg P, Nordwall A. 2001 Volvo award winner in clinical studies: lumbar fusion versus nonsurgical treatment for chronic low back pain: a multicenter randomized controlled trial from the Swedish lumbar spine study group. Spine (Phila Pa 1976). 2001;26:2521–32; discussion 2521–32.
18. Lee CK, Vessa P, Lee JK. Chronic disabling low back pain syndrome caused by internal disc derangements. The results of disc excision and posterior lumbar interbody fusion. Spine (Phila Pa 1976). 1995;20:356–61.
19. Irmola TM, Hakkinen A, Jarvenpaa S, Marttinen I, Vihtonen K, Neva M. Reoperation rates following instrumented lumbar spine fusion. Spine. 2018;43:295–301.
20. Peng B, Pang X. Regeneration and repair of intervertebral disc degeneration. In: Sanders S, editor. Regenerative medicine in China. Washington, DC: Science/AAAS; 2012. p. 52–3.
21. Orozco L, Soler R, Morera C, Alberca M, Sánchez A, García-Sancho J. Intervertebral disc repair by autologous mesenchymal bone marrow cells: a pilot study. Transplantation. 2011;92:822–8.
22. Wu T, Song HX, Dong Y, Li JH. Cell-based therapies for lumbar discogenic low back pain: systematic review and single-arm meta-analysis. Spine. 2018;43:49–57.
23. Beall DP, Wilson G, Bishop R, Tally W, Temple HT, Ganey T. Viable Allograft as a supplemental therapeutic for disc regeneration. BioSpine: 7th international congress on biotechnologies for spine surgery, 4 Apr 2019.

24. Bae HW, Amirdelfan K, Coric D, et al. A phase II study demonstrating efficacy and safety of mesenchymal precursor cells in low back pain due to disc degeneration. The Spine Journal. 2014;14(11):S31–2.
25. Fraser RD, Osti OL, Vernon-Roberts B. Discitis after discography. J Bone Joint Surg. 1987;69-B:26–35.
26. Osti OL, Fraser RD, Vernon-Roberts B. Discitis after discography. J Bone Joint Surg. 1990;72B:271–4.
27. Buser Z, Liu J, Thorne K, et al. Inflammatory response of intervertebral disc cells is reduced by fibrin sealant scaffold in vitro. J Tissue Eng Regen Med. 2014;891:77–84.
28. Buser Z, Kuelling F, Liu J, et al. Biological and biomechanical effects of fibrin injection into porcine intervertebral discs. Spine. 2011;36(18):E1201–9.
29. Scuderi GJ, et al. Intradiscal injection of an autologous alpha-2-macroglobulin (a2m) concentrate alleviates back pain in FAC-positive patients. Ortho Rheum Open Access J. 2017;4(2):OROAJ.MS.ID.555634.
30. Sanapati J, Manchikanti L, Atluri S, Jordan S, Albers SL, Pappolla MA, Kaye AD, Candido KD, Pampati V, Hirsch JA. Do regenerative medicine therapies provide long-term relief in chronic low back pain: a systematic review and metaanalysis. Pain Physician. 2018;21:515–40.
31. Tuakli-Wosornu YA, Terry A, Boachie-Adjei K, Harrison JR, Gribbin CK, LaSalle EE, Nguyen JT, Solomon JL, Lutz GE. Lumbar intradiscal platelet-rich plasma (PRP) injections: a prospective, double-blind, randomized controlled study. PM R. 2016;8:1–10.
32. Monfett M, Harrison J, Boachie-Adjei K, Lutz G. Intradiscal platelet-rich plasma (PRP) injections for discogenic low back pain: an update. Int Orthop. 2016;40:1321–8.
33. Navani A, Ambach MA, Navani R, Wei J. Biologics and lumbar discogenic pain: 18 month follow-up for safety and efficacy. IPM Rep. 2018;2:111–8.
34. Akeda K, Ohishi K, Masuda K, Bae WC, Takegami N, Yamada J, Nakamura T, Sakakibara T, Kasai Y, Sudo A. Intradiscal injection of autologous platelet-rich plasma releasate to treat discogenic low back pain: a preliminary clinical trial. Asian Spine J. 2017;11:380–9.
35. Levi D, Horn S, Tyszko S, Levin J, HechtLeavitt C, Walko E. Intradiscal platelet rich plasma injection for chronic discogenic low back pain: preliminary results from a prospective trial. Pain Med. 2016;17:1010–22.
36. Kirchner F, Anitua E. Intradiscal and intra-articular facet infiltrations with plasma rich in growth factors reduce pain in patients with chronic low back pain. J Craniovertebr Junct Spine. 2016;7:250–6.
37. Pettine K, Suzuki R, Sand T, Murphy M. Treatment of discogenic back pain with autologous bone marrow concentrate injection with minimum two year follow-up. Int Orthop. 2016;40:135–40.
38. Pang X, Yang H, Peng B. Human umbilical cord mesenchymal stem cell transplantation for the treatment of chronic discogenic low back pain. Pain Physician. 2014;17:E525–30.
39. Orozco L, Soler R, Morera C, et al. Intervertebral-disc repair by autologous mesenchymal bone marrow cells: a pilot study. Transplantation. 2011;92:822–8.
40. Mochida J, Sakai D, Nakamura Y, et al. Intervertebral disc repair with activated nucleus pulposus cell transplantation: a three-year, prospective clinical study of its safety. Eur Cell Mater. 2015;29:202–12.
41. Coric D, Pettine K, Sumich A, Boltes MO. Prospective study of disc repair with allogeneic chondrocytes presented at the 2012 joint: spine section meeting. J Neurosurg Spine. 2013;18:85–95.
42. Meisel HJ, Ganey T, Hutton WC, et al. Clinical experience in cell based therapeutics: intervention and outcome. Eur Spine. 2006;15(Suppl 3):S397–405.
43. Liebscher T, Haefeli M, Wuertz K, et al. Age-related variation in cell density of human lumbar intervertebral disc. Spine Phila Pa 1976. 2011;36:153–9.
44. Allon AA, Schneider RA, Lotz JC. Co-culture of adult mesenchymal stem cells and nucleus pulposus cells in bilaminar pellets for intervertebral disc regeneration. SAS J. 2009;3(2):41–9. https://doi.org/10.1016/SASJ-2009-0005-NT; eCollection 2009.

45. Vadala G, Sowa G, Hubert M, et al. Mesenchymal stem cells injection in degenerated intervertebral disc: cell leakage may induce osteophyte formation. J Tissue Eng Regen Med. 2012;6:348–55.
46. Yoshikawa T, Ueda Y, Miyazaki K, et al. Disc regeneration therapy using marrow mesenchymal cell transplantation: a report of two case studies. Spine (Phila Pa 1976). 2010;35:E475–80.
47. Vadala G, Russo F, Di Martino A, Denaro V. Intervertebral disc regeneration: from the degenerative cascade to molecular therapy and tissue engineering. Tissue Eng Regen Med. 2015;9:679–90.
48. Beall DP, Gainey T. Stem cell augmentation for the intervertebral disc: current evidence and future directions. St Petersburg, FL: Calusa Ambulatory Spine Conference; 2017.
49. Beall DP, Wilson G, Bishop R, Tally W, Temple HT, Ganey T. Viable allograft as a supplemental therapeutic for disc regeneration. 46th annual meeting of the international society for study of the lumbar spine, Kyoto, Japan, 6 Jun 2019.
50. Griffith JF, Wang YX, Antonio GE, Choi KC, Yu A, Ahuja AT, Leung PC. Modified Pfirrmann grading system for lumbar intervertebral disc degeneration. Spine (Phila Pa 1976). 2007;32:E708–12.
51. Pobiel RS, Schellhas KP, Pollei SR, Johnson BA, Golden MJ, Eklund JA. Diskography: infectious complications from a series of 12,634 cases. Am J Neuroradiol. 2006;27(9):1930–2.
52. Hong SH, Choi JY, Lee JW, Kim NR, Choi JA, Kang HS. MR imaging assessment of the spine: infection or an imitation? Radiographics. 2009;29:599–612. https://doi.org/10.1148/rg.292085137.
53. Yeom JA, Lee IS, Suh HB, Song YS, Song JW. Magnetic resonance imaging findings of early spondylodiscitis: interpretive challenges and atypical findings. Korean J Radiol. 2016;17(5):565–80. https://doi.org/10.3348/kjr.2016.17.5.565.
54. Ma CJ, Liu X, Che L, Liu ZH, Samartzis D, Wang HQ. Stem cell therapies for intervertebral disc degeneration: immune privilege reinforcement by Fas/FasL regulating machinery. Curr Stem Cell Res Ther. 2015;10(4):285–95.
55. Yang SH, Wu CC, Shih TT, Sun YH, Lin FH. In vitro study on interaction between human nucleus pulposus cells and mesenchymal stem cells through paracrine stimulation. Spine (Phila Pa 1976). 2008;33(18):1951–7.
56. Martin PE, Evans WH. Incorporation of connexins into plasma membranes and gap junctions. Cardiovasc Res. 2004;62:378–87.
57. Hynes RO. Integrins: bidirectional, allosteric signalling machines. Cell. 2002;110:673–87.
58. Cocucci E, Racchetti G, Meldolesi J. Shedding microvesicles: artefacts no more. Trends Cell Biol. 2009;19:43–51.
59. Majka M, Janowska-Wieczorek A, Ratajczak J, Ehrenman K, Pietrzkowski Z, Kowalska MA, Gewirtz AM, Emerson SG, Ratajczak MZ. Numerous growth factors, cytokines, and chemokines are secreted by human CD34 (_) cells, myeloblasts, erythroblasts, and megakaryoblasts and regulate normal haematopoiesis in an autocrine/paracrine manner. Blood. 2001;97:3075–85.
60. Ratajczak J, Wysoczynski M, Hayek F, Janowska-Wieczorek A, Ratajczak MZ. Membrane-derived microvesicles: important and underappreciated mediators of cell-to-cell communication. Leukemia. 2006;20:1487–95.
61. Chargaff E, West R. The biological significance of the thromboplastic protein of blood. J Biol Chem. 1946;166:189–97.
62. De Broe ME, Wieme RJ, Logghe GN, Roels F. Spontaneous shedding of plasma membrane fragments by human cells in vivo and in vitro. Clin Chim Acta. 1977;81:237–45.
63. Malda J, Boere J, van de Lest CH, van Weeren PR, Wauben MH. Extracellular vesicles – new tool for joint repair and regeneration. Nat Rev Rheumatol. 2016;12:243–9. https://doi.org/10.1038/nrrheum.2015.170.
64. Cocucci E, Meldolesi J. Ectosomes and exosomes: shedding the confusion between extracellular vesicles. Trends Cell Biol. 2015;25(6):364–72.
65. Simons M, Raposo G. Exosomes—vesicular carriers for intercellular communication. Curr Opin Cell Biol. 2009;21(4):575–81. https://doi.org/10.1016/j.ceb.2009.03.007.

66. EL Andaloussi S, Mäger I, Breakefield XO, Wood MJ. Extracellular vesicles: biology and emerging therapeutic opportunities. Nat Rev Drug Discov. 2013;12(5):347–57. https://doi.org/10.1038/nrd3978.
67. Kourembanas S. Exosomes: vehicles of intercellular signaling, biomarkers, and vectors of cell therapy. Annu Rev Physiol. 2015;77:13–27.
68. Rani S, Ryan AE, Griffin MD, Ritter T. Mesenchymal stem cell-derived extracellular vesicles: toward cell-free therapeutic applications. Mol Ther. 2015;23(5):812–23.
69. Lu K, Li HY, Yang K, et al. Exosomes as potential alternatives to stem cell therapy for intervertebral disc degeneration: in-vitro study on exosomes in interaction of nucleus pulposus cells and bone marrow mesenchymal stem cells. Stem Cell Res Ther. 2017;8(1):108. https://doi.org/10.1186/s13287-017-0563-9.

# Surgical Disc Replacement and Fusion Techniques

# 14

Youssry Elhawary and Mohamed Fawzy Khattab

Chronic low back pain may be anticipated due to facet joints, ligaments, muscles, and intervertebral disc pathologies. Proper history taking, clinical examination, radiological investigations, and diagnostic injection techniques can help to identify the exact cause.

Over the past decades, many surgical options were described as treatment for disabling discogenic low back pain (LBP). Fusion was considered as gold standard with different techniques. Each has its advantages, tips, and tricks. Lumbar interbody fusion can be done through anterior or posterior approaches. Anterior approach can offer better removal of the disc, bigger lordotic cage can be applied, and better correction of sagittal balance. Approach-related complications are limiting cause for wide spread of this technique. Posterior approach is much common technique; most of the surgeons are familiar with such techniques. Currently different minimally invasive posterior or anterior approaches are used to treat LBP after failure of conservative treatment.

Motion preserving technology was the idea behind introduction of lumbar total disc replacement (TDR) aiming to surgically treat LBP with non-inferior results when compared to fusion.

This chapter will present different case scenarios; all have disabling LBP and managed surgically with different techniques. Each case will be managed according

---

Medical knowledge and professional surgical practice in the spine field are continuously changing. Spine surgeons need to rely on their own surgical experience and knowledge in evaluating different surgical techniques. Patient selection and safe spine surgeon are the keys of success in spine procedures.

---

Y. Elhawary (✉)
Faculty of Medicine, Cairo University, Cairo, Egypt

M. F. Khattab
Faculty of medicine, Ain Shams University, Cairo, Egypt





L. Manfrè, J. Van Goethem (eds.), *The Disc and Degenerative Disc Disease*, New Procedures in Spinal Interventional Neuroradiology,
https://doi.org/10.1007/978-3-030-03715-4_14

to the authors preferred method, tips, and tricks and best available evidence will be formulated in the discussion.

## 14.1 Case 1

Female patient 80 years old, presented with long-lasting disabling low back pain, not responsive to conservative treatment including medications, physical therapy, and local spinal injections. Her back pain visual analog scale (VAS) rating was eight out of ten and constant. The Oswestry Disability Index (ODI) score was 58%, with moderate lower extremity intermittent claudicating pain. Past medical and surgical histories are unremarkable.

Clinically, the patient has back muscle spasm, low back tenderness, negative straight leg raising test, and limited lumbar spine range of motion.

Radiological investigations: Plain radiographs (Fig. 14.1a) showed collapsed L4–L5–S1 disc spaces narrowing with double-level degenerative spondylolisthesis Grade one at the L4–5 and L5–S1 levels. Dynamic lateral flexion-extension lumbosacral x-ray shows fixed spondylolisthesis. Patient global sagittal profile is aligned and accepted. MRI scans show narrow spinal canal at these two levels with severe spondylosis and degeneration at the L4–5 and L5–S1 levels (Fig 14.1b).

Posterior L4–L5–S1 decompression and instrumented posterolateral fusion was done (Fig 14.1c).

### 14.1.1 Technical Notes

Under spinal anesthesia, a urinary Foley catheter is placed and a preoperative prophylactic antibiotic (usually third-generation cephalosporin) is given. The patient is positioned prone over a four-bolster frame, and all pressure points of the face, torso, and extremities are carefully padded. The patient belly hangs free to limit pressure on the inferior vena cava, which aids in minimizing intraoperative blood loss. Tranexamic acid 10 mg/kg bolus is given and 1 mg/kg infusion till the wound closure. Patient hips kept extended to help in lumbar lordosis restoration. Elastic stocking is applied to both the legs. L4–L5–S1 image-guided transpedicular trajectory identification is used to mark incision site. The skin is sterilized and draped in hospital standard sterile fashion. Posterior midline skin incision is made. Bovie electrocautery is used to subperiosteally dissect the paraspinal muscles so that the facet capsules and transverse processes are exposed bilaterally at each level. Care is taken not to injure the facet capsules that do not need to be fused. Using mammilary process as a clinical intraoperative landmark, for the L4–L5–S1 pedicles identification. This can be confirmed radiologically by image intensifier in two views. Bilateral laminotomies (fenestration) from L4 through S1 were performed with flavectomy and partial facetectomies. Decompressions were done centrally and along the lateral recesses to improve patient intermittent claudication. While decompression, the neural structures with undercutting medial facetectomy, the surgeon should ensure

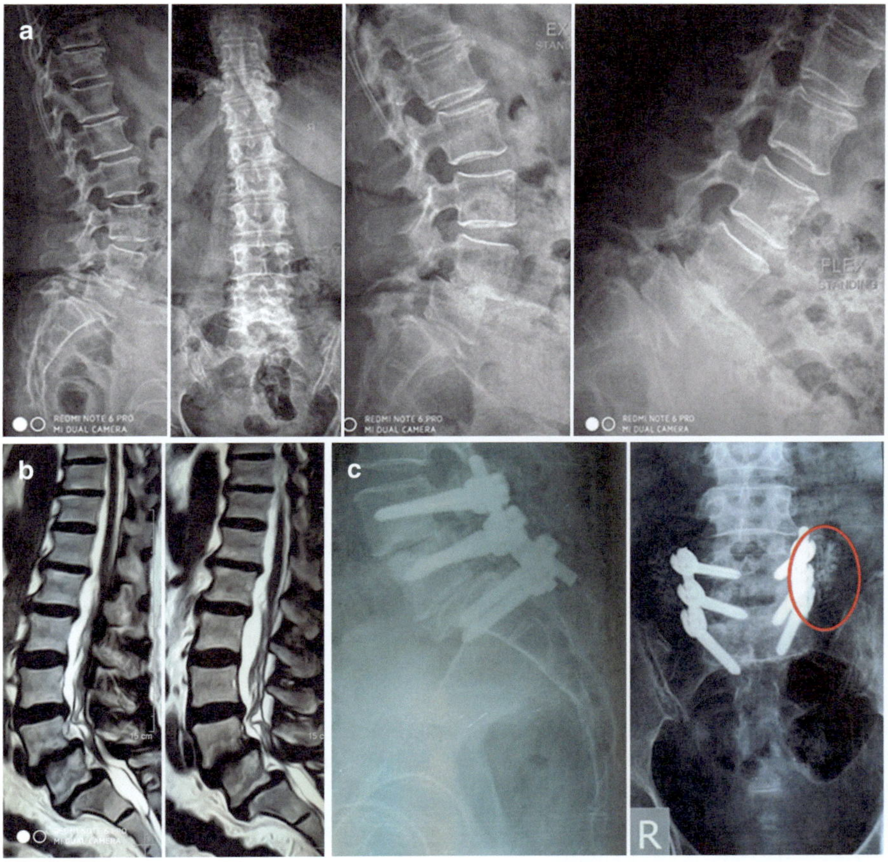


**Fig. 14.1** (**a**) Eighty-year-old female patient, her plain X ray lateral, Ap, flexion and extension show grade 1 degenerative spondylolithesis at L4–5–S1 levels. (**b**) MRI Lumbosacral spine sagittal cuts show modic changes at the disc and spinal canal stenosis at L4–5–S1 with fixed spondylolithesis. (**c**) Postoperative lateral and A-p plain X ray show the screws in good position and the posterolateral bone graft

that at least 50% of a functional facet joint complex remains, inclusive of a functioning superior facet and inferior facet. A nerve hook is used to palpate the pedicle and assess nerve root canal after decompression to ensure that adequate bilateral foraminotomies have been performed. Decortications of the transverse processes bilaterally and the facet complexes are done. Locally harvested bone autograft from the lamina and facets is morselized and placed in the lateral gutters to achieve posterolateral fusion (Fig 14.1c). The low back pain experienced by the patient described in the case presentation was related to the mechanical instability at L4 through S1, and posterior instrumentation with a pedicle screw and rod construct provides immediate fixation and symptomatic improvement.

## 14.2 Case 2

Male patient, 62 years old presented with long-lasting disabling low back pain, mechanical, increase with motion and standing, not responsive to conservative treatment including medications, physical therapy, and local spinal injections. His pain scale rating was nine out of ten. The Oswestry Disability Index (ODI) score was 60%, with lower extremity intermittent claudication pain. The patient is diabetic, hypertensive but controlled past surgical history is unremarkable.

Clinically, the patient has back muscle spasm, low back tenderness, negative straight leg raising test, and limited lumbar spine range of motion.

Radiological investigations: Plain radiographs was done, lumbosacral MRI (Fig. 14.2a) showed collapsed degenerated L4–L5 disc spaces with degenerative spondylolisthesis at the L4–L5. Patient sagittal profile showed kyphotic L4–L5 level with lost lumbar lordosis.

Posterior L4–L5 decompression and instrumented, transforaminal lumbar interbody fusion (TLIF) was the decision. The authors prefer TLIF as there is less traction to the neural structure, no need to do midline generous laminectomy, and more possible to apply the cage anteriorly and correcting the sagittal alignment (Fig. 14.2b).

TLIF is the technique recommended by the authors in revision cases as you can approach disc posterolaterally through the foramen away from the tethered or adherent neural midline structures.

Interbody fusion help to remove the degenerated disc and apply interbody cage with bone graft. Bone fusion is better in interbody fusion because bone graft under compression loads with big surface of cancellous bone anteriorly.

### 14.2.1 Surgical Technique

Under general or spinal anesthesia, the surgery can be done; we used spinal anesthesia for most of our patients, a urinary Foley catheter is placed and a preoperative prophylactic antibiotic (usually third-generation cephalosporin) is given. The patient is positioned prone over a four-bolster frame, and all pressure points are carefully padded. The patient belly hangs free. Tranexamic acid 10 mg/kg bolus is given and 1 mg/kg infusion till the wound closure. Patient hips kept extended to help in restoring the lumbar lordosis. Elastic stocking is applied to both the legs to decrease the incidence of deep venous thrombosis. To locate the incision over L4–L5 level, image intensifier is used to mark L4–L5 transpedicular line. The skin is sterilized and draped in hospital standard sterile fashion. Posterior midline skin incision is made. Bovie electrocautery is used to subperiosteally dissect the paraspinal muscles so that the facet capsules and transverse processes are exposed bilaterally at each level. Care is taken not to injure the facet capsules that do not need to be fused. While dissection, it is important to preserve supraspinous and interspinous ligaments to decrease incidence of adjacent level degeneration or failure. Using

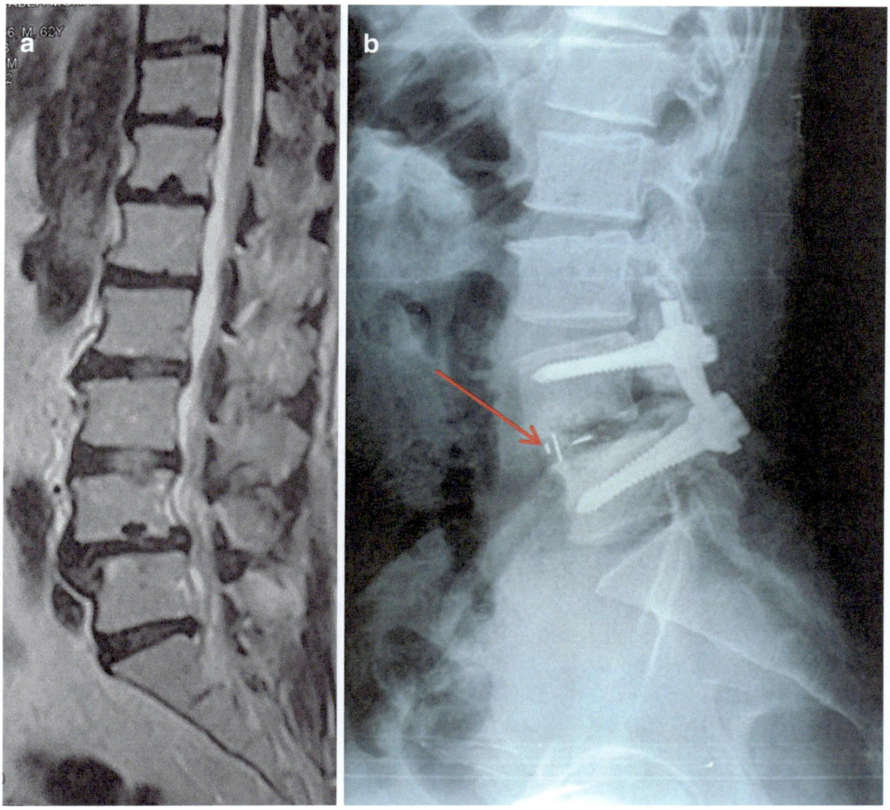


**Fig. 14.2** (**a**) Sixty-two-year old male, his MRI sagittal cut show collapsed disc, degenerated L4–5 disc with spondylolithesis. Lost segmental lordosis. (**b**) Anteriorly located cage red arrow with restoration of segmental lordosis,and disc height

mammilary process as a clinical intraoperative landmarks, for the L4 and 5 pedicles identification. This can be confirmed radiologically using anteroposterior and lateral images by C-arm. We usually do facetectomy and decompression starting from the site of patient complaint. We may decompress (flavectomy and partial facetectomy) the contralateral side if stenotic or symptomatic.

In degenerative scoliosis, we prefer to apply the cage from the concave side. In lost lumbar lordosis, we may do bilateral facetectomies and putting higher cage anteriorly in the intersomatic space then compression at the end of the procedure posteriorly (deformity TLIF), aiming to restore the segmental lordosis.

After facetectomy and decompression, we remove the intervertebral disc and the cartilaginous endplate. Care should be taken while disc preparation for fusion; do not over distract between the screws, to decrease incidence of screw loosening. It is better to use intervertebral distracters gradual increase in reamers and shavers heights to remove disc material.

We used to apply locally harvested bone graft anterior to the cage and inside the cage for fusion.

The highest cage possible to be applied in the anterior part of the disc space is chosen. Care should be taken in revision cases to avoid over distraction and over stretch of tethered neural elements by previous scar tissue and fibrosis.

A nerve and disc hook are used to palpate the pedicle and assess nerve root canal after decompression to ensure that adequate bilateral foraminotomies have been performed. It is important to check there is no any bone fragments around the neural structures. Decortications of the transverse processes bilaterally and the contralateral facet complex if preserved are done. Locally harvested bone autograft from the lamina and facets is morselized and placed in the lateral gutters to achieve posterolateral fusion.

Proper hemostasis and irrigation of the wound by saline. We do not use suction drain. We close the wound in sequential manner.

Patient is allowed to move out of the bed after fully recovering from anesthesia. And usually discharged two days after surgery.

The low back pain experienced by the patient described in the case presentation was related to the mechanical instability and disc degeneration at L4–L5 disc level. Posterior instrumentation with a pedicle screw and rod construct with interbody cage provides immediate fixation and symptomatic improvement. Interbody cage provides maximum translational stability and provides tool to correct sagittal and coronal alignment.

## 14.3 Case 3

Male patient, 50 years old presented with long-standing disabling low back pain, mild bilateral leg pain, his back pain increase with motion and standing, not responsive to conservative treatment including medications and physical therapy. Local spinal injections give him pain relief for short time then his back pain recurred. His back pain scale rating was eight out of ten. The (ODI) score was 60%, with mild lower extremity intermittent claudication pain. The patient has no medical comorbidities and past surgical history is unremarkable.

Clinically, the patient has back muscle spasm, low back tenderness, negative straight leg raising test, and limited lumbar spine range of motion.

Radiological investigations: Plain radiographs show gas sign in L3–4–5 disc and abnormal upper endplate at L3–4–5 disc (Fig. 14.3a); Lumbosacral MRI (Fig. 14.3b) showed collapsed degenerated L3–L4–L5 disc spaces with degenerative disc disease (DDD). L3–4–5 posterior lumbar interbody fusion (PLIF) was done with mild improvement in the patient back pain, and the patient mild leg pain did not improve. Figure 14.3c with follow-up patient complaint was constant and no improvement with conservative medical and physiotherapy treatment. Local injection selective root block at L5–S1 was given with improvement of patient complaint.

New MRI was done, and narrow L5–S1 foramen in the sagittal cut was diagnosed. Figure 14.3d Extension of fusion to L5–S1 was decided. Intraoperative conjoint nerve root was diagnosed and to do interbody fusion from posterior approach was impossible. L5–S1 extension of fusion with posterolateral fusion using local autograft was done (Fig. 14.3e).

Postoperatively patient improve clinically but one month later he got surgical site infection with significant back pain and leg pain; so, debridement and change implant was the decision, S1 screws was loose so we removed it and the fixation was extended distally to S2-alar-iliac screw as distal anchorage point (Fig. 14.3f).

The patient improved but still has back pain, he scheduled for anterior lumbar interbody fusion (ALIF) L5–S1 with improvement of his back and leg pain (Fig. 14.3g).

ALIF at L5–S1 was the decision taken by the authors. The authors prefer ALIF as there is less traction to the neural structure, bigger diameter, and higher anterior cages can be applied under better physiological condition for fusion. Indirect decompression of the neural foramen can be achieved by restoring disc height and indirectly increasing the foraminal height. Better removal of the entire disc can be achieved from anterior approach. Higher cage in the disc can better restore segmental lumbar lordosis.

Absolute contraindications for ALIF approach are significantly calcified aorta or prior reconstructive vascular surgery. Relative contraindications are morbid obesity, previous intraabdominal surgery, history of severe pelvic inflammatory disease (PID), and previous anterior spinal surgery.

### 14.3.1 Surgical Technique

PLIF is a posterior procedure for interbody fusion, while patient in prone positioning, after general or spinal anesthesia, paravertebral muscle dissection with exposure of the spinous processes and lamina over the appropriate levels midline laminotomy (medial to the facet) were done, and the dural sleeve was retracted to approach disc. After disc space preparation, we apply bullet-like cage in the disc space, unlike TLIF more retraction to the neural midline structure is needed.

In this case scenario, we will discuss the anterior L5–S1 lumbar interbody fusion (ALIF), which allows better disc space clearance. Under general anesthesia, a urinary Foley silicone catheter was placed under complete aseptic condition, and a preoperative prophylactic antibiotic was delayed till harvesting culture from L5–S1 disc space. (Usually third-generation cephalosporin is given.) The patient is positioned supine, and all pressure points are carefully padded. Elastic stocking to the patient legs was applied. Tranexamic acid 10 mg/kg bolus is given and 1 mg/kg infusion till the wound closure. Sterilization and draping according to the hospital standards. The L5/S1disc space is reached through a Pfannenstiel surgical incision. An 8-cm transverse skin incision is performed after localization of the corridor by image intensifier in A-P and lateral view (Fig. 14.3h). A right retroperitoneal route to L5/S1 was performed through the linea alba of the rectus sheath. The incidence of retrograde ejaculation is much lower when a retroperitoneal approach is used compared to when a transperitoneal approach is used. Beside we keep the

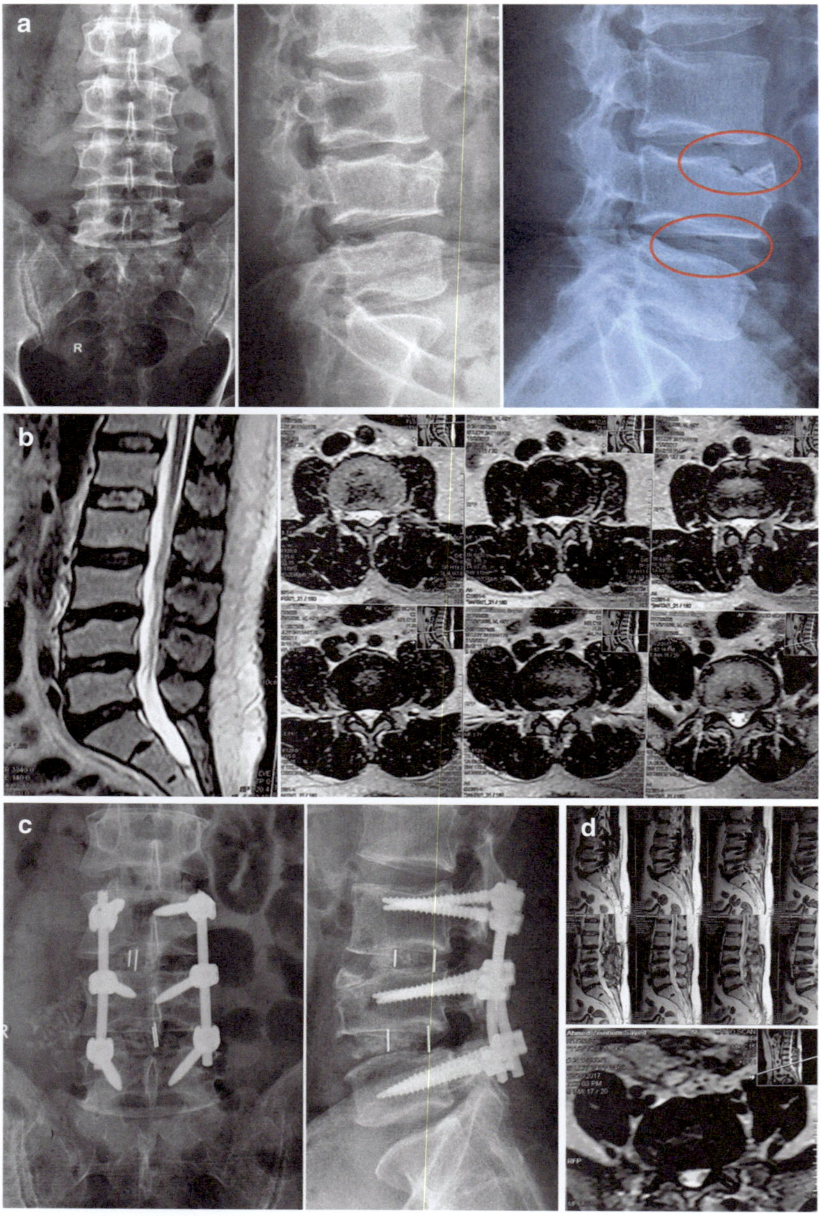


**Fig. 14.3** (**a**) Male patient 50 years old with LBP, Plain X ray Lumbosacral spine show degenerated disc with gas sign at L3–4–5 with abnormal upper endplate. (**b**) MRI sagittal and axial T2 weighted images showed degenerated disc with no stenosis. (**c**) Postoperative lumbosacral plain x ray Ap-Lateral show pedicular screws and PLIF cages in place at L3–4–5 with restoration of segmental lordosis and good amount of bone graft in the disc space and posterolateral. (**d**) Postoperative lumbosacral MRI sagittal and axial T2 cuts show degenerated disc at L5–S1 with stenotic foramen with signs of screw at L3–4–5. (**e**) immediate postoperative lumbosacral plain X ray Ap-Lateral

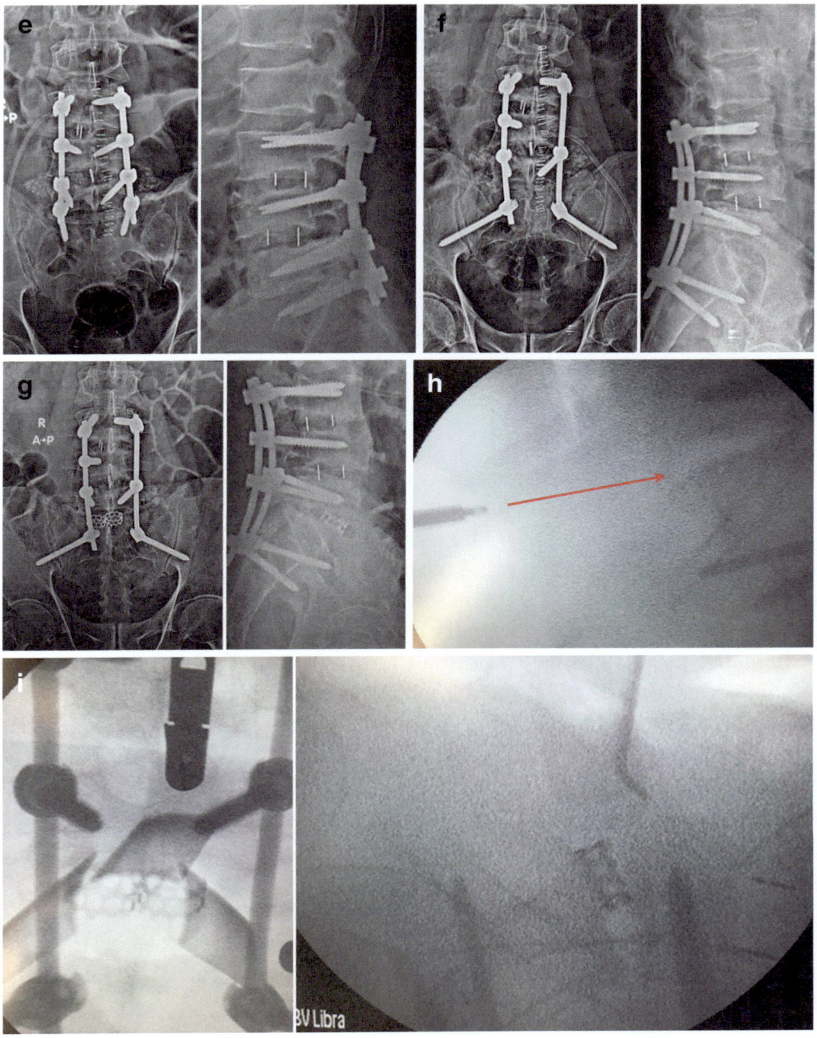


**Fig. 14.3** (continued)

show L3–S1 pedicular screws and PLIF cages in place at L3–4–5 with posterolateral instrumented fusion at L5–S1. Skin stables and portovac can be seen in the X ray. (**f**) Immediate postoperative (debridement and change of implant) lumbosacral plain X ray Ap-Lateral show removal of the infected loose s1 screws and left L4 screw. L3–S2 alariliac fixation and PLIF cages in place at L3–4–5 with posterolateral instrumented fusion at L5–S1. Skin stables and portovac can be seen in the X ray. (**g**) Last lumbosacral plain X ray Ap-Lateral show big anterior L5-S1 cages after ALIF. With posterolateral instrumented fusion at L5–S1. (**h**) Prior to skin incision, intraoperative image intensifier photo to lumbosacral region lateral projection show trajectory of L5–S1 disc at patient skin. (**i**) intraoperative image intensifier photo to lumbosacral region AP and lateral projection to confirm proper cage position at L5–S1 disc prior to skin closure transperitoneal approach for revision anterior surgery. The arcuate line is identified and released. The peritoneum and ureter are retracted from lateral to medial with a special soft-tissue retractor. The psoas muscle is identified and great vessels. L5–S1 approached in between the bifurcation. The median sacral vessels are ligated and dissected, and it is important to use only the bipolar cautery at the anterior surface of L5–S1 disc and by soft gauze dissect the superior hypogastric plexus to avoid retrograde ejaculation. Once the anterior circumference of L5/S1 intervertebral disc is exposed, interbody fusion using titanium mesh cage filed with autologous iliac crest bone graft is performed after debridement of the disc material. Assessment of cage location was done clincally and by the use of image intensifier (Fig. 14.3i). Hemostasis then closure of wound in layers.

## 14.4 Case 4

Female patient, 46 years old presented with long-lasting disabling low back pain, not responsive to conservative treatment including medications, physical therapy, and local spinal injections. But she showed improvement on disc analgesia test. Visual analog pain scale rating was 8 out of 10 and constant. The Oswestry Disability Index (ODI) score was 60%, with no lower extremity radicular or intermittent claudication pain. The patient is medically free.

Clinically, the patient has back muscle spasm, low back tenderness, negative straight leg raising test, and limited lumbar spine range of motion.

Radiological investigations: Plain radiographs showed narrow L4–5, L5–S1 disc space. Lumbosacral MRI showed collapsed degenerated L4–L5 disc spaces with degenerative hyperintenisty zone sign and degenerated L5–S1 disc space with Modic changes. Patient sagittal profile showed lost lower lumbar lordosis. Axial MRI show good facet state and can help to assess vascular topography of the patient (Fig. 14.4a, b).

L4–5, L5–S1 lumbar disc arthroplasty was the decision taken by the author to remove the degenerated disc and restore the mobility at the index levels (Fig. 14.4c). The authors prefer this method of surgical treatment for her disabling LBP because the patient is young with stable spine and the posterior facets are not degenerated.

The surgery was uneventful done through an open retroperitoneal approach. At 6 years of follow-up, the patient was free of back pain and visual analog scale and Oswestry Disability Index score are improved significantly. She required no pain medication and was able to return to her household activity.

### 14.4.1 Surgical Technique

Under general anesthesia, the patient is positioned supine, urinary catheter was applied. It is important to allow hyperextension of the lumbar region using the bed controls. Also, the plane of the anterior superior iliac spines must be horizontally kept parallel to the floor; the patient must be centralized properly and this is checked

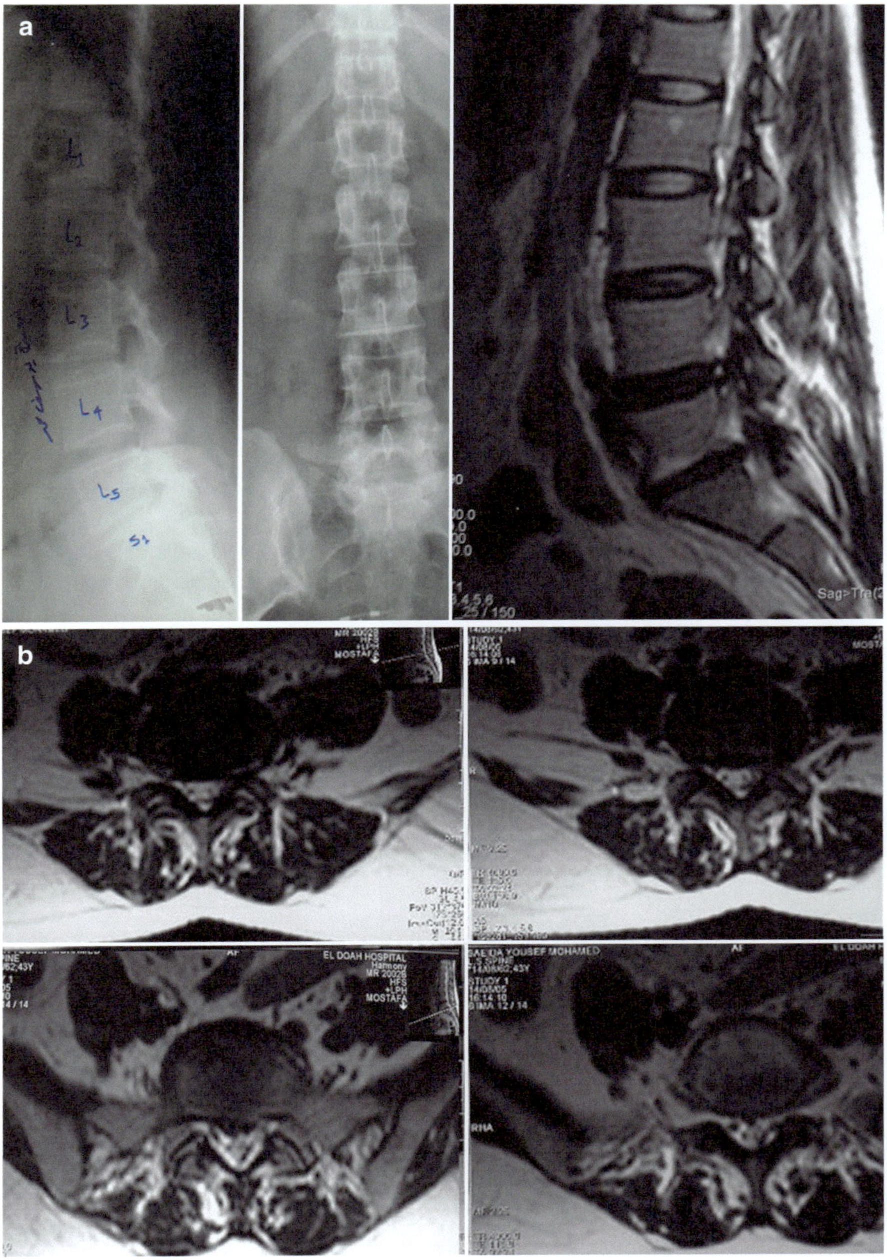


**Fig. 14.4** (**a**) 46 years old female with LBP plain X ray Ap/Lateral show degenarative narrow disc at L4–5–S1 MRI show degenerated disc with modic changes at L5–S1 and Hyperintenisty zone at L4–5. (**b**) Axial cut at L4–5–S1 disc level show good facet state, show vascular topography at L4–5–S1. (**c**) Postoperative plain X ray showing double level SB Charetє III Lumbar disc prosthesis in place and mobile in dynamic view. (**d**) Intraoperative image intensifier to assess proper centralization of the disc prosthesis in AP view and as posterior as possible in lateral view

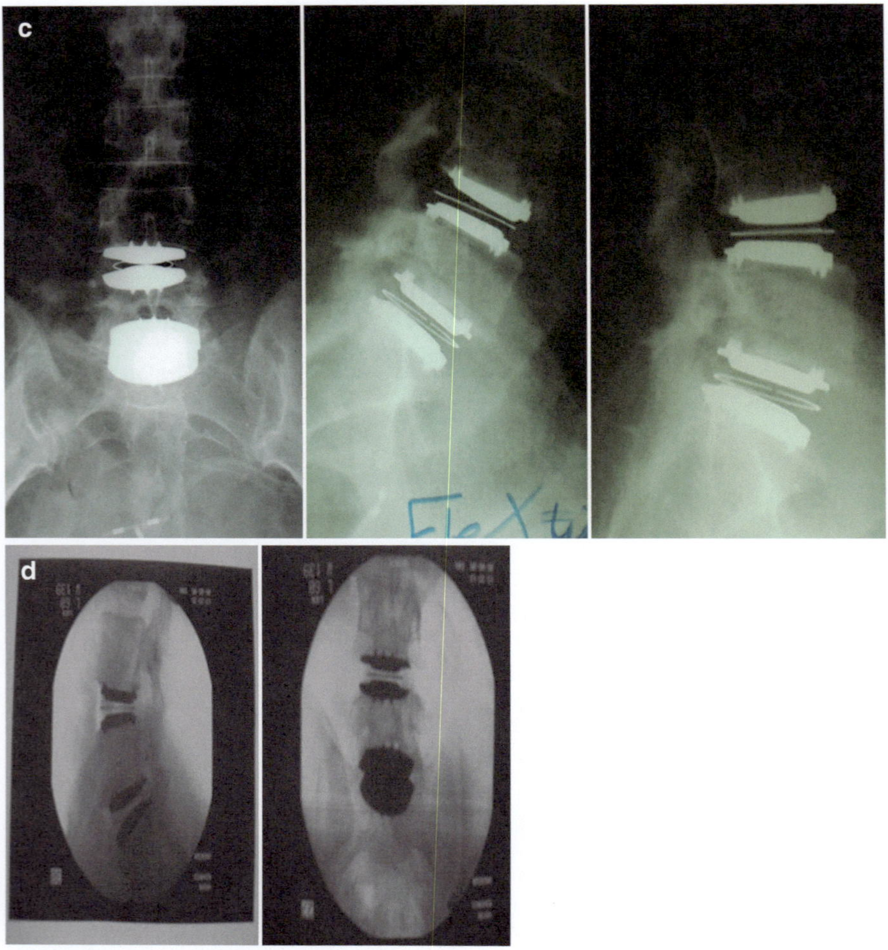


**Fig. 14.4** (continued)

by image intensifier prior to sterilization and draping. The pressure points should be properly protected. Both lower limbs should be kept in neutral position, with mild knee flexion. We used to have the help of access surgeon to help us while manipulating great vessels; a paramedial, left-sided retroperitoneal approach is preferred.

At lower abdomen 12-cm left-sided paramedical vertical incision is made. After the skin incision, subcutaneous tissue is dissected by electrocautery to expose the anterior rectus sheath. Identification of the midline fascial raphe of the rectus, and the left rectus is mobilized to the left side with careful attention to avoid injury to the inferior epigastric vessels. Blunt finger dissection is then used to develop the retroperitoneal plane and release of the arcuate ligament. The peritoneum is bluntly dissected and retracted off the abdominal wall. The ureter should be identified and retracted with the peritoneum. The genitofemoral nerve can usually be identified on the surface of the psoas muscle. It is mandatory to identify and ligate the iliolumbar vein, to allow mobilization of the great vessels to the right side, when operating L4–5 level. We usually start by operating L5–S1 level, it is approached between the bifurcation of the great vessels. Care should be taken while dissecting the anterior surface of L5–S1 to avoid injury of the superior hypogastric plexus injury. It is recommended to use blunt dissection at that level and no use of monopolar electrocautery to avoid hypogastric plexus injury. Identification and transection after ligation of median sacral artery is necessary. Median sacral artery helps to identify midline. Table-held retractors can be used on each side of the spine to create a safe corridor to approach L5–S1 disc. L5–S1 disc midline is confirmed by image intensifier.

An anterior annulotomy is completed using a knife, centered on the midline mark. Symmetrical complete discectomy and cartilaginous endplate removal are carried out. For lumbar spinal arthroplasty, it is mandatory to fully restore the disc height to recreate segmental mobility.

Special intervertebral distractor used to aid in remobilization of the degenerated segment, and release of the posterior longitudinal ligament may be needed in collapsed segments.

Trial implants can be inserted into the disc space. The trial implants should be centered on the previously marked midline. The operating table break at the level of the operated disc space can aid in placing the trial implant by putting the patient torso into extension and thereby opening the anterior disk space. Once a trial implant of the appropriate size is placed, an AP image is taken to verify the central midline position and neutral rotation of the implant in the midline. The SB Charité III device was applied at L5–S1 then at L4–5 disc. It has spikes on the endplate surface for initial stabilization. Anteroposterior and Lateral fluoroscopic images should be made frequently to verify the trajectory angle and the proper location of the prosthesis (Fig. 14.4d). The device should be inserted exactly in the midline in AP view, and as far posterior as possible in lateral view.

## 14.5 Discussion

The degenerative process in the functional spine unit usually starts from the intervertebral discs leading to pathological changes in the surrounding ligaments, vertebral bodies, and posterior bulging of posterior disc surface, narrowing of the central spinal canal, decrease disc height, buckling of the ligamentum flavum, osteophyte formation, and sliding of vertebral bodies [1].

This degenerative cascade leads to different clinical symptoms like lower back pain (LBP), radicular pain, and neurogenic intermittent claudication. There are many conservative treatment options, including physiotherapy and steroid local injections. Where conservative management fails, surgery may be indicated. Currently, surgical management involves decompression only, which may potentially destabilize the spine, or decompression followed by fusion to prevent further destabilization [2].

Spinal functional unit fusion is the mainstay to treat degenerative disc conditions, many spinal fusion techniques were described in the literatures. Posterolateral intertransverse fusion (PLF) is a useful procedure with good fusion rates for most degenerative disc conditions. Interbody fusion techniques involve placement of an implant (cage, spacer, or structural graft) within the intervertebral space after complete discectomy and endplate preparation; interbody fusion can be done either anterior lumbar interbody fusion (ALIF) or posterior lumbar interbody fusion, (PLIF) approaches were described to restore the structural integrity of degenerated functional spine unit or degenerated unstable discs. There is no solid evidence showing that the functional outcome scores are better after anterior column support than other posterior fusion techniques [3, 4].

In 1982, Harms from Germany introduced transforaminal lumbar interbody fusion (TLIF) to avoid neural structures, dural manipulation, and subsequent epidural fibrosis [3].

To have 360-degree solid fusion, PLF can be combined with posterior interbody fusion techniques to circumferentially stabilize the relevant unstable segment, but it is unclear whether this improves the fusion rates [4, 5].

Different techniques are described in the literature: posterior lumbar interbody fusion (PLIF), transforaminal lumbar interbody fusion (TLIF), minimally invasive TLIF (MI-TLIF), oblique lumbar interbody fusion/anterior to psoas (OLIF/ATP), anterior lumbar interbody fusion (ALIF), lateral lumbar interbody fusion (LLIF), and extreme lateral interbody fusion (X-LIF). There is no clear definitive evidence for one approach being superior to another in terms of fusion or clinical outcomes. Minimally invasive surgical techniques (MIS) mean to achieve the target with less collateral damage. MIS has the advantage of less hospital stay, less blood loss, and early reintegration in the daily life activity [6].

The aims for all types of lumbar fusion are the same: reduction of the back pain with or without radicular symptoms by neural decompression, restabilizing the degenerated segment, and the restoring intervertebral disc height (in interbody fusion techniques) [7].

Postoperative we examine patient radiologically for spinal fusion criteria were based on presence of bonebridge between the endplates of both adjacent vertebral bodies inside and/or outside the cage, no osteolysis around the implant or loosening, no angular motion in lateral flexion-extension radiographs more than 3°, and no cage migration [8, 9].

In recently published meta-analysis to compare posterolateral fusion versus interbody fusion for degenerative spondylolisthesis, they concluded that, according to the available literature there was no statistically significant difference in functional and operative outcomes following fusion alone versus with interbody [10].

There is a large volume of literature detailing clinical and radiological outcomes following specific interbody fusion techniques; however, little are class 1 data comparing the various available techniques. Surgeons who have been trained in one specific fusion technique will favor that technique; most of the literature uniformly supports the concept of interbody fusion techniques over on-lay posterior spinal fusion for sagittal and coronal plane deformities corrections [11].

When comparing clinical outcomes, of anterior and posterior surgeries, most studies showed that clinical outcomes in ALIF were similar to TLIF [12].

Available data in the literature suggests that anterior fusion techniques are superior to posterior in terms of disc space height restoration, lumbar lordosis, and spinal deformity correction, and that clinical, functional outcome, and fusion rates were similar to those in posterior fusion techniques [13].

The advent of total disc replacement (TDR) offered a new alternative that aims to restore and maintain mobility and stability at the diseased functional spine unit. The history of lumbar disc arthroplasty began in the 1950s with insertion of stainless steel metal spheres into the disc space after discectomy by Fernström [14].

The lumbar disc replacement prosthesis continued to evolve during the 1970s as a partial replacement by nuclear implant, going from a metal sphere to a silicone rubber prosthesis to a polyurethane injectant. It was in 1984 that the modern lumbar disc prosthesis began to be developed. In Charité hospital in Berlin, Dr. Büttner-Janz and Dr. Schellnack designed a modular three-piece TDR device known as the SB Charité, and it was implanted in September 1984. The prosthesis was evolved and finally SB Charité III (DePuy Spine, Raynham, MA) came to use worldwide in 1987. Many prosthesis are now available in the market with different designs.

TDR is done through anterior approach, it is contraindicated in active systemic infection or infection localized to the site of implantation, osteopenia or osteoporosis, bony lumbar spinal stenosis, allergy or sensitivity to implant materials, isolated radicular compression syndromes, especially due to disc herniation, pars defect, and spondylolisthesis.

There is reported long-term follow-up data for lumbar spine arthroplasty with greater than an 80% excellent or good long-term (more than 10 years) clinical outcomes. TDR was done using the SB Charité lumbar disc prosthesis. This study concluded that 90% of prostheses were still mobile at a mean of 13.2 years of follow-up. The reoperation rate was 7.5%, and the rate of adjacent-level degenerative pathology was found to be 2.8%. Almost 90% of the patients returned to their work after the procedure. As for complications, David reported a 4.6% rate of posterior facet joint arthrosis, a 2.8% rate of implant subsidence, and less than a 2% rate of core subluxation [15].

According to the FDA IDE prospective randomized studies for TDR, comparing lumbar spine arthroplasty to fusion, TDR-produced clinical and functional outcomes are at least similar or non-inferior to those of fusion and superior to fusion results on some measures [16, 17].

## 14.6 Conclusion

Different treatment modalities are available to manage patients with disabling low back pain due to degenerative disc disease. It should be stressed that appropriate patient selection and meticulous surgical technique are paramount in obtaining successful clinical outcomes.

Surgeon experience and following good level of evidence help to improve patient's health-related quality of life.

## References


1. Leone A, Guglielmi G, Cassar-Pullicino VN, Bonomo L. Lumbar intervertebral instability: a review. Radiology. 2007;245:62–77.
2. Koreckij TD, Fischgrund JS. Degenerative spondylolisthesis. J Spinal Disord Tech. 2015;28:236–41. https://doi.org/10.1097/BSD.0000000000000298.
3. Humphreys SC, Hodges SD, Patwardhan AG, Eck JC, Murphy RB, Covington LA. Comparison of posterior and transforaminal approaches to lumbar interbody fusion. Spine (Phila Pa 1976). 2001;26(5):567–71.
4. Christensen FB, Hansen ES, Eiskjaer SP, et al. Circumferential lumbar spinal fusion with Brantigan cage versus posterolateral fusion with titanium Cotrel-Dubousset instrumentation: a prospective, randomized clinical study of 146 patients. Spine (Phila Pa 1976). 2002;27(23):2674–83.
5. Fritzell P, Hagg O, Wessberg P, Nordwall A, Swedish Lumbar Spine Study Group. Chronic low back pain and fusion: a comparison of three surgical techniques: a prospective multicenter randomized study from the Swedish lumbar spine study group. Spine (Phila Pa 1976). 2002;27(11):1131–41.
6. Mobbs RJ, Sivabalan P, Li J. Minimally invasive surgery compared to open spinal fusion for the treatment of degenerative lumbar spine pathologies. J Clin Neurosci. 2012;19:829–35.
7. Harms JG, Jeszenszky D. Die posteriore, lumbale, interkorporelle fusion in unilateraler transforaminaler technik. Oper Orthop Traumatol. 1998;10:90–102.
8. Abbushi A, Cabraja M, Thomale UW, Woiciechowsky C, Kroppenstedt SN. The influence of cage positioning and cage type on cage migration and fusion rates in patients with monosegmental posterior lumbar interbody fusion and posterior fixation. Eur Spine J. 2009;18:1621–8.
9. McAfee PC, DeVine JG, Chaput CD, Prybis BG, Fedder IL, et al. The indications for interbody fusion cages in the treatment of spondylolisthesis: analysis of 120 cases. Spine (Phila Pa 1976). 2005;30:S60–5.
10. Cambpell RC, Mobbs RJ, Lu VM, Xu J, Rao PJ, Phan K. Posterolateral fusion versus interbody fusion for degenerative spondylolisthesis systematic review and metaanalysis. Global Spine J. 2017;7(5):482–90.
11. Kowalski RJ, Ferrara LA, Benzel EC. Biomechanics of bone fusion. Neurosurg Focus. 2001;10:E2.
12. Kim JS, Kang BU, Lee SH, et al. Mini-transforaminal lumbar interbody fusion versus anterior lumbar interbody fusion augmented by percutaneous pedicle screw fixation: a comparison of surgical outcomes in adult low-grade isthmic spondylolisthesis. J Spinal Disord Tech. 2009;22:114–21.
13. Faundez AA, Schwender JD, Safriel Y, et al. Clinical and radiological outcome of anterior-posterior fusion versus transforaminal lumbar interbody fusion for symptomatic disc degeneration: a retrospective comparative study of 133 patients. Eur Spine J. 2009;18:203–11.
14. Fernström U. Arthroplasty with intercorporal endoprosthesis in herniated disc and in painful disc. Acta Chir Scand Suppl. 1966;357:154–9.
15. David T. Long-term results of one-level lumbar arthroplasty: minimum 10-year follow-up of the Charité artificial disc in 106 patients. Spine. 2007;32:661–6.
16. Blumenthal S, McAfee PC, Guyer RD, et al. A prospective, randomized, multicenter Food and Drug Administration investigational device exemptions study of lumbar total disc replacement with the CHARITE artificial disc versus lumbar fusion. Part I: evaluation of clinical outcomes. Spine. 2005;30:1565–75.
17. Zigler J, Delamarter R, Spivak JM, et al. Results of the prospective, randomized, multicenter Food and Drug Administration investigational device exemption study of the ProDisc-L total disc replacement versus circumferential fusion for the treatment of 1-level degenerative disc disease. Spine. 2007;32:1155–62.

MIX
Papier aus verantwortungsvollen Quellen
Paper from responsible sources
FSC® C105338

If you have any concerns about our products,
you can contact us on
**ProductSafety@springernature.com**

In case Publisher is established outside the EU,
the EU authorized representative is:
**Springer Nature Customer Service Center GmbH**
**Europaplatz 3, 69115 Heidelberg, Germany**

Printed by Libri Plureos GmbH
in Hamburg, Germany